Aromatherapist Danièle Ryman offers a new approach to nutrition and healing—that lets you enjoy the benefits of aromatherapy through simple changes in your diet. This technique—grounded in wisdom that reaches back to ancient times—is both natural and effective and can make a difference in the way you feel today!

Aromatherapy in Your Diet

AROMATHERAPY IN YOUR DIET

How to Enjoy the Health Benefits
of Aromatherapy
Without Using Essential Oils

Danièle Ryman

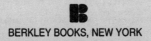

BERKLEY BOOKS, NEW YORK

This Berkley Book contains the complete text of the previous edition. It has been completely reset in a typeface designed for easy reading and was printed from new film.

AROMATHERAPY IN YOUR DIET

A Berkley Book / published by arrangement with Piatkus Books

PRINTING HISTORY
Piatkus Books edition published 1996
Berkley edition / September 1997

The Putnam Berkley World Wide Web site address is http://www.berkley.com

ISBN: 0-425-15978-7

BERKLEY®
Berkley Books are published by The Berkley Publishing Group, a member of Penguin Putnam Inc., 200 Madison Avenue, New York, New York 10016.
BERKLEY and the "B" design are trademarks belonging to Berkley Publishing Corporation.

PRINTED IN THE UNITED STATES OF AMERICA

10 9 8 7 6 5 4 3 2 1

To my mother, Jacqueline

CONTENTS

ACKNOWLEDGMENT

I WOULD particularly like to thank Susan Fleming for the enormous contributions she has made to this book. It owes much to her meticulous research and thoughtful organisation of my work. I have really appreciated her help over the last two years, and, as always, she encouraged me at every stage. Susan and I share an understanding of so many things. She is a pleasure to work with.

HOW TO USE THIS BOOK

THIS BOOK is, as the title states, about aromatherapy in your diet. It does not, therefore, cover external uses of aroma-therapeutic products, such as skin and hair treatments or ointments for wounds and injuries, which are dealt with in my other books on the subject (see Bibliography).

Part One consists of an alphabetical list of common foods, including herbs and spices. It explains their major therapeutic uses, and suggests how you can incorporate these foods in everyday cooking and eating so as to obtain the best value from them; the principal nutrients are given for all foods other than herbs and spices. Some entries in Part One appear under type of food rather than individual food (for instance, Dairy Products, Grains and Pulses): if you do not immediately find the food you are looking for, consult the index.

Part Two outlines the workings of the human body, de-scribes the common ailments that affect it, and tells you which foods are appropriate for which complaint: at-a-glance tables are included for speedy reference. You can then look up these foods in Part One for more detailed in-formation.

INTRODUCTION

FOR NEARLY 30 years now I have been practising aromatherapy, a natural therapy which promotes health and well-being through the use of aromas and the essential oils of plants. But a consciousness of the importance of aroma has been with me for very much longer. For instance, I still feel a sense of love and security every time I smell a rose perfume, one my mother used to wear. I had always been conscious of the importance of aromas in the kitchen, too—but then I do happen to be French! My mother and grandmother were both talented, natural and resourceful cooks, and I "digested" an amazing amount of culinary—as well as health—knowledge in their kitchens. It was my father who was to teach me about the subtleties of smell and taste in wine, an introduction I shall never forget. And in the last few years, I have come to the conclusion that one of the most significant ways in which I, and indeed all of us, can practise aromatherapy is through the food that we smell, taste and eat. Aromatherapy starts in the kitchen.

We all need food, and we couldn't survive for long without it. Every system of the body relies on the nourishment that food provides, and when deprived of food, or the right sort of food, each of those systems can degenerate or fail in any number of ways. So our bodies rely on food—but what else encourages us to eat? I believe it is the aroma and taste of foods that are the principal conscious stimuli in the process of eating. It is also aroma and taste that contribute to the enjoyment and pleasure we get from eating. The part of the brain associated with the sense of smell—the primitive limbic region—

controls feelings of contentment as well, and the association probably arose because the body had to make the processes necessary for survival (collecting and eating foods) emotionally rewarding—a form of aromatic blackmail! Think of how you react to the smell of coffee being ground and made. The volatile substances in the beans immediately dynamise you, acting like an electric shock on the system. It is the *smell* that gives me such pleasure, and I often don't need to drink it all—just a sip can be enough for me to enjoy it to its full.

If we experience pleasure in a food, then we will eat it again, and it is the aroma and taste that will bring us back to that food. It is a characteristic that has been explored and exploited by the present-day food industry, knowing, for instance, that once a child has tasted a chocolate bar, he or she will usually clamour for the same thing again. It is the stimulant essential oils of the cocoa bean which form and flavour chocolate that create "chocoholics," those who crave ever more and more of the substance: if chocolate didn't taste or smell of anything, nobody would want to buy or eat it!

These essential oils in foods are often the same oils that are extracted for use in aromatherapy. The latter come from very many aromatic plants, and from very many parts of plants—from leaves, flowers, roots, seeds, buds, bark, rhizomes, resins and rinds. These oils, being present in the foods themselves, can therefore have much the same effect on the body as the extracted essential oils used in the therapy. Most food plants are aromatic to some degree or other, and even though oils may not actually be extracted from them, they still exist, and create aroma, flavour and satisfaction as well as benefits to health.

If foods did not contain these aromas and flavours I think we would eat to live but we would not enjoy it, and we would become depressed. Too many people are depressed these days—the obese who experience no satisfaction except in overeating; the anorexics and bulimics who learn to hate food in order to stay fashionably and depressingly thin. The reason for this is because we are all suffering from a form of malnutrition. We have lost sight of the vital necessity of aroma and flavour in food—of the "vitality" of food, perhaps—and as a result we are undernourished. This is primarily the fault of the food industry, who for so long have done our cooking for us, who deprive us of our requirement to see, touch, smell and taste. Supermarkets may pull us in with that homely smell of baking bread at the entrance (the best way to sell your house, estate agents tell us!), but then they lock the foods away from us behind glass partitions, or hermetically seal them in clingfilm in chill cabinets. No longer do we judge readiness or ripeness by aroma, and very seldom can we do so by touch. Instead meats are reddened by colourings, chickens are plumped up with water and phosphates, and melons and other fruit, in the interests of commerce, are plucked from the plant before they are properly ready, ripe, sweet and juicy.

The food industry is feeding us illusions, rather than real food, and it is this malnourishment of the body, as well as of the spirit, that has inspired me to write this book.

A History of Aromatherapeutic Eating

It was with the Ancient Egyptians that the use of edible plants as medicine truly began. Certain extant papyri record how they grew, ate and cooked aromatics for both pleasure and health. They cultivated fields of cucumbers, leeks, radishes and garlic—all extremely active and therapeutic plants—and highly valued other herbs and spices. They were aware of the specific dietary merits of many foods, as well as of their demerits: knowing, for instance, that their bread, made from millet or rye, was a little hard to digest, they included in the dough aromatic and digestive seeds such as coriander, aniseed and caraway. They cooked beans with thyme to preempt flatulence, and before cooking fish would rub it with aromatics to cleanse and purify it. The slaves building the Great Pyramid at Giza were given a clove of garlic per day to lend them strength and keep infections at bay, and indeed garlic is still valued highly today for its antibacterial and antiviral properties.

The Ancient Greeks also utilised aromatics in cooking and medicine, and may have been influenced by the Egyptians. Hippocrates, the "Father of Medicine," prescribed onions for water retention, chervil for those depressed because of a liver or stomach malady, rosemary for liver disorders and mustard for sciatica. Epicurus, the renowned gourmet philosopher, would insist on the use of at least five aromatic herbs if he were to enjoy a meal. Theophrastus, the "Father of Botany," was distinguished by his use of digestive plants in cooking—caraway and pepper with oysters, oregano and fennel with fish, parsley and oregano with meat.

The Romans had originally eaten very plain foods, but as they conquered further afield they brought back many new plants, herbs and spices, and ways of using them in cooking. They would protect themselves from plague by burning aromatic herbs and by using them in their dishes; among them were rosemary, juniper berries, hyssop and basil. Like the Greeks, the Romans became great eaters, sitting down to enormous banquets which must only have been made possible by the inclusion of aromatic and digestive herbs, spices and other foods.

In Asia, too, foods and their cooking were regarded as medicinal. The *Ayurveda*, an ancient collection of Hindu knowledge of food and health, was the main dietary and medicinal influence on the majority of Indians. Basically, Ayurvedic principles require the body to be treated by food first, and only then by medicine, and food treatments are based on the six tastes—sweet, sour, salty, pungent, bitter and astringent. The sour taste, for instance, would be provided by something like lime, for the purpose of stimulating digestion and benefiting the heart (citrus fruit are rich in vitamin C, which does indeed benefit the heart). In another ancient civilization, that of the Chinese, the same types of eating principles were being formulated: that for health, aroma and flavour, five tastes should be combined—salty, sweet, sour, bitter and pepper hot. The principles of yin and yang (cooling and heating properties respectively) were and still are very important in Chinese cooking; the Chinese believe that there is a direct correlation between the properties of the food you eat and the yin-yang, or healthy balance in your body.

The culinary spices used in India and China were probably spread throughout the West by the Arabs, who still incorporate many Asian rather than African aromatics in their cooking. They civilised Europe in a number of ways, introducing architecture, science, medicine and foods—oranges, lemons, rice, almonds and many spices were introduced to Spain during the seven-hundred-year Moorish occupation, and an Arab co-founded the famous School of Salerno, near Naples, which used food in medicine.

Odd as it may seem, the chilli which now provides the heat of curries was not introduced to India until after the great explorations of the fifteenth century, when Christopher Columbus discovered the Americas. (Before then, to counter bacterial infections in meats, the Indians had used ginger, pepper, mustard and other hot spices.) As a result of these explorations many new plants were introduced: tomatoes, maize, tobacco and potatoes to Europe, among other foods, and broad beans, melons and cucumbers to the Americas. Some of these new foods were viewed with distrust in Europe: the potato, for instance, because it was a member of the same family as deadly nightshade, was suspected of causing leprosy. It was first mentioned in print in 1597 by Gerard, one of the great English herbal writers of the sixteenth and seventeenth centuries, at a time when foods, spices and herbs and their place in health and medicine were particularly valued.

It is from these centuries of cooking certain foods and combining them with other aromatics—for both pleasure and therapy—that our modern modes of cooking have developed. The Chinese and Indians still cook in the traditional ways, making in every meal a happy union of the diverse tastes considered essential for health. We can learn from their approach, as we can from the Arabs, and ideas such as their marriage of sweet things such as dried fruit, and the antibacterial lemon and oranges, with meat. But we have our own traditional combinations which are just as valuable and therapeutic. The British roast beef and horseradish or mustard was not simply a fortuitous taste combination; both the spices are preservative in action, with very strong essential oils, so they were primarily used to make the meat wholesome. The mint served with lamb in Britain is again acting as an antiputrefactive. However, at the same time as they make the meats safer to eat, the spice and herb accompaniments boost the flavour and aroma of the meats, making them more palatable and satisfying to the sense of smell and taste. (It is interesting that meat is very rarely eaten by itself: it is almost invariably accompanied by some sort of plant flavouring because the meat by itself is not very interesting in taste. See also page 102.)

The same applies in the French tradition. A French cook would not dream of simmering a pot of haricot beans without adding sprigs of thyme and parsley to enhance the aroma and taste and, echoing the wisdom of the Ancient Egyptians, to aid digestion. Thyme is used a lot in country cooking, possibly because yet another of its properties is that it makes the iron in meats and other foods easier to assimilate. The French cook a lot with wine, and this too is protective; at the same time the wine adds incomparable flavour plus a range of nutrients of its own. As well as flavouring, marjoram makes mushrooms succulent and easy to digest; lemon juice dissolves fat and cleanses fish or meat. Garlic, *the* characteristic of French cooking to many people, is the ultimate flavouring, but it is its potency as an antibiotic that makes it so valuable (although it is also a good source of iodine). The humble orange is almost a medicine chest in itself, and every part of it is used in cooking in France and in herbal therapy. Duck and orange, a classic French partnership, combines the antiputrefactive properties of the orange juice and essential oils in the rind with the fatty and potentially rather toxic flesh of the duck, rendering it safer to eat and easier to digest.

These food combinations are not accidental, but came about through the culinary wisdom, garnered through centuries, of our forefathers. We are aware that they exist, but we do not know why they should exist, nor why plants are so beneficial to health in general. Now, towards the end of the twentieth century, when our general health is under stress from lifestyle, pollution and chemical solutions to illness, we should turn again to the old traditions, to the natural remedies, to the healing powers of the essential oils contained in simple plant foods.

Preparing and Eating Aromatherapeutic Foods

Essential oils are primarily antibacterial or disinfectant and digestive, stimulating all the glands and organs involved in the process of digestion, arguably the most important process in the whole body. They also cleanse, dynamise, remineralise, reconstitute, sedate and encourage appetite, amongst many other properties. Like the essential oils used in aromatherapy, they can penetrate skin externally, and body tissue internally, and can also directly benefit individual parts of the body. Many plants, for instance, contain good quantities of natural hormones, so something like sage, which is highly oestrogenic, has a very beneficial effect on the female reproduction system, stimulating the ovaries and regulating the menstrual cycle. Plants are actually very high in hormones as they are "sexually" much more active than humans, reproducing seasonally. Pulses and beans, ovary-shaped themselves, are particularly beneficial to women, as they are too when sprouted and rich with the nutrients necessary for the next generation.

The fresher the plant food is, and the less it has been tampered with, the more therapeutic it will be. It will then have its full complement of vitamins, minerals and other nutrients, which can largely be lost in processes such as canning, freezing and refining. Raw foods are "alive," and when subjected to high temperatures, or when their structural integrity is destroyed, they lose their energy as well as their essential oils. Another consideration concerning freshness is the natural "season" of foods. Foods that are local and in season—English asparagus in May and June, for instance—will be much fresher and therefore much more valuable to eat. Apples and carrots out of season may have been stored for some time, and nutrients inexorably decrease the longer any plant food is away from the soil or its parent plant.

It is best, therefore, to eat most plant foods raw, although a few, such as pulses, rice or potatoes, have to be cooked before they are edible, let alone palatable. Many people find raw foods difficult to digest, but the addition of complementary herbs and spices will make digestion easier. Chewing foods efficiently can help the digestion of raw (and other) foods as well, and it always surprises me that, although we teach our children how to brush their teeth, we do not teach them how to chew—which is just as important for the health of the teeth and gums and for the rest of the body too.

Chopping foods small, or grating them, is another way of making them easier to assimilate: you can grate carrots, turnips, swedes, celeriac, radishes, beetroot and so on; slice mushrooms, tomatoes, onions, peppers, cauliflower, fennel and celery; and shred cabbage and other greens. Wash them well first, perhaps adding some lemon juice or cider vinegar to the water to cleanse them thoroughly. If possible, try to buy organically grown plants, as many can store in their flesh the chemicals used in insecticides and fertilisers.

Steaming or lightly grilling are other ways of preparing plant foods; both are fast, and ensure that most of the nutrients remain locked within the foods. If foods have to be boiled, water-soluble nutrients can be lost in the water, so try to keep your vegetable-cooking water for a soup or sauce, or make it the basis of a healthy tisane.

Eating seasonally is also important. When the weather is coldest we tend to eat heavier and fattier foods, but aromatic foods can be just as satisfying: herbs hydrate us and keep us warm, and nuts and dried fruits, which are richly concentrated sources of nutrients, can be cooked in compotes or nibbled. Lighter foods such as salads and new vegetables are appropriate in the summer months and usually our bodies dictate to us what they require. The trouble is that most people do not listen to what their bodies tell them, and this is when obesity and other health problems can make an appearance.

It surprises people when I tell them that everything they smell and put into their mouths has significance for their health. They have to understand that every fruit, vegetable, pulse, nut, herb or spice can help to balance our nervous system or our digestive system, can help growth and cell regeneration, and can help us heal both mentally and physically. All of nature's wonders are there for us to take and benefit from, and they can all be kept in the kitchen. In the fridge and cupboards you can have a pharmacopeia of foods that will keep you alive, alert, active, satisfied and healthy. To be a good and imaginative cook, combining these nutrients, is to be a do-it-yourself doctor, and indeed many top chefs, very often without knowing it, hit the jackpot by composing something sublime for the nose and palate in a dish which brings energy, pleasure, flavour and health into harmony, creating a culinary symphony.

Look upon the kitchen as the brain of your house, where everything can be found to keep you and your family as well as possible.

IMPORTANT NOTE

Never use bought essential oils in cooking, whether to add flavour or therapeutic benefit. Oils are extremely strong, and unfortunately many oils commonly used these days are chemically based, so they could do untold harm. Manufacturers use essential oils in certain foods, which is bad enough, but they work to very carefully estimated proportions. On your very much smaller scale you could get the proportions extremely wrong, turning what is essentially a benefit into a virtual poison. Essential oils should *never* be taken internally.

USING AROMATHERAPEUTIC FOODS

The aromatic foods that will benefit you when you eat them can also be used in other ways—in herbal teas and tisanes, in inhalations, as compresses and poultices, as well as in juices, wines and spirits, oils and vinegars. This book, however, is concerned principally with aromatherapy in your daily diet.

Herbal Teas and Tisanes

These will contain all the essential properties of the aromatics—normally herbs and spices, although some fruits and vegetables can be utilised—and should replace the stimulants tea and coffee when you change to a healthy aromatherapeutic diet. You can buy herbs in teabag form in health food shops (or grow your own, of course), and you should use whole spices, not ready ground.

Follow the instructions in each aromatic section. In general, though, use a dessertspoon of chopped fresh herbs or half that quantity of dried per teapot full of boiling water. Infuse for seven minutes, then drink, sweetened to taste with honey if needed. (You can even make an aromatic honey, by infusing your chosen herb or sweet spice in runny honey.) Spices and other aromatics may need a slightly longer infusing time.

Juices

Many vegetables and fruit can be juiced, and as they are uncooked they are extremely nutritious, containing all the properties of the food. The Swiss pioneer of raw food eating, Dr. Bircher-Benner—who was to introduce the world to muesli—made raw juices the basis of many of his treatments. They must be drunk fresh, though, immediately after making.

Electric juicers are vital for this, but they are not too expensive, and the benefits to your family's health will more than outweigh the cost. Blenders and liquidisers can be used for some fruit and vegetables.

Wines and Spirits

As you will see throughout the book and in the Appendix on the benefits of wine, I am not advocating teetotalism. Wines can in themselves benefit the body in a number of ways, as can spirits. The key is moderation.

Some wines and spirits can actually be made more aromatic by the addition of fruits, herbs or spices and other plants such as ginseng. In general, macerate the chosen aromatic in a wine or spirit for a week or so, stoppering tightly and shaking every now and again. Aromatics include angelica, apricots, blackberries, cinnamon, ginseng, quince, sloes and vanilla. And remember one important point: do not use your best wines for making aromatic wine—save them to accompany a special dinner!

Herb Oils and Vinegars

Making these at home is much more effective—and much more fun—than buying them. Both oils and vinegars are best used in cooking, in marinades and in salad dressings, but they can also form the basis of more strictly aromatherapeutic practised—in massage, and in skin cleansing and toning.

Roughly speaking, you need 225 g (8 oz) fresh herbs (half that quantity if dried) per 600 ml (1 pint) olive, grapeseed, soya or other chosen oil (it's best to use bland oils). Follow your own taste if using spices, garlic, ginger and so on. About 50 g (2 oz) crushed garlic cloves would be pungent in the above amount of oil, as would 1–2 tablespoons crushed spice seeds.

Macerate together (see below), tightly sealed, for 2–3 weeks in a sunny place. Adding aromatics to something like a cold-pressed olive oil can actually add to its kitchen life, as well as enhance its therapeutic properties.

Use the same amounts of herb or other aromatic per 600 ml (1 pint) cider vinegar. Keep in the dark for at least 10 days, shaking every so often.

Infusions

These are generally used as a compress for the eyes or facial skin. The basic method is the same as for herbal teas and ti-sanes above, using fresh or dried herbs, whole spices or other aromatics as appropriate. Soak pieces of lint or real cotton wool in the warm strained infusion, then apply, or soak when cold.

Decoctions and Macerations

Use this method for harder stems, roots and seeds. Bruise with a mortar and pestle, then bring to the boil in water for 1–2 minutes. Cover and leave to infuse. For a decoction, strain after 15 minutes. For a very much stronger macera-tion, strain after several hours.

PART ONE

A–Z OF
AROMATHERAPEUTIC
FOODS AND FLAVOURINGS

Agar Agar, *see* Seaweeds

Allspice
Pimenta officinalis/dioica
Myrtaceae family

ALLSPICE BERRIES—known variously as pimento, myrtle pepper and Jamaica pepper—are the fruit of a small ever-green tree native to the tropical forests of South America. It is now cultivated extensively in Jamaica. Named *pimienta* or pepper by the early Spanish explorers because of the slightly peppery overtones, it is known as allspice because it seems to combine the flavours and aromas of cinnamon, nutmeg and cloves.

Therapeutic Uses
The spice, allspice, has been used for years in therapy, pri-marily as a digestive. The berries should be added, crushed or ground, to any foods which are difficult to digest.

The essential oil—pimento—is distilled from the berries, and is used in the treatment of arthritis and rheumatism. Be-cause of the phenol content (60–80 per cent eugenol) the oil is highly antibacterial, so the berries could be used in cook-ing for much the same effect.

In the Kitchen
A versatile spice, it can be used in sweet and savoury dishes. As with any whole spice, the flavour and aroma are best when newly ground. Put allspice berries in a pepper grinder for instant use, or grind in a mortar and pestle.

- Allspice was used in South America as a flavouring for chocolate; it is very good, whole or ground, as a warming ingredient in mulled wines and hot punches.
- Add whole berries to meat and poultry stews or curries, to bean soups and pulse dishes (for digestive benefit), and to marinades for seafood, meat, poultry and game.
- Add ground to pâtés, ham, sweet cakes and biscuits.
- Add whole to pickles, preserves and chutneys.

ALMOND, *see* Nuts

ANGELICA
Angelica archangelical/officinalis
Umbelliferae family

THIS TALL PLANT is native to the northern hemisphere, and all parts—leaves, stems, roots and seeds—are aromatic. The name derives from a tenth-century French story that the Archangel Raphael revealed its virtues to a monk so that he might use it against the plague. The stems were chewed in the Middle Ages in England to keep plague at bay, and the seeds and roots burned to purify the air.

Angelica is cultivated in many countries in Europe, as well as in China, for its medicinal properties.

Therapeutic Uses
The leaves and seeds have long been used as a general tonic and as a remedy against infections, particularly of the respiratory system. If you eat angelica regularly—say, slices of dried root twice a day for 6 months—you càn build up resistance to many infections.

Angelica stimulates the brain, so can help nervous depression and other nerve-related disorders. It also enhances the appetite and stimulates the digestion: Dr. Leclerc, a distinguished doctor, and head of the Phytotherapy School in France earlier this century, prescribed it for anorexia. Chew angelica stems after meals to prevent flatulence and indigestion, or make tisanes of the leaves, stems and seeds.

Take angelica in infusion—5-10 g (a scant 1/4-1/2 oz) of root per cup of boiling water—or, for a good general tonic, especially effective for PMT and the menopause, in wine. Add 60 g (a good 2 oz) sliced or grated angelica root to about 1 litre (1 3/4 pints) of a fortified wine (Malaga, sherry or port) or a sweet wine and leave for 6 weeks. This is as effective in the West as ginseng in the East. In China ginseng is prescribed as an aphrodisiac for men, angelica for women. You can add a small ginseng root as well if you would like to enhance the effects of the tonic.

Separate essential oils are distilled from the seeds and roots of angelica.

In the Kitchen

Try to get hold of fresh plants rather than rely on the crystallised angelica available in grocers. The plants are easy to grow but do so at the back of beds, as they can reach a height of 2 metres (6 ft 6 in).

- Crystallise the hollow stems and use in confectionery and cakes. These can also add flavour to jam and other preserves, and sweetness to tart fruit such as plums and rhubarb.
- Use raw stems and leaves in fish-poaching liquids.
- Use stems or leaves in milky desserts such as rice puddings and custards. They will sweeten, give flavour and keep infections at bay.

ANISE

Pimpinella anisum
Umbelliferae family

ALSO KNOWN as aniseed, this is an annual related to dill, caraway and fennel. Native to the Middle East, it is now cultivated around the Mediterranean and elsewhere, but does not set seed in colder climates. It was introduced to Europe by the Romans, who, like the Ancient Egyptians, ate the seeds as an aid to digestion.

Therapeutic Uses

Tisanes made from the seeds will help nervous indigestion and nervous palpitations as well as flatulence and hiccups. A tisane made from 2 teaspoons bruised seeds boiled in 600 ml (1 pint) water for 3 minutes is also good for PMT and menopausal symptoms, particularly fluid retention.

The essential oil of aniseed, which is extremely toxic, is distilled from the seed fruits.

In the Kitchen

Buy the seeds whole and grind them in a mortar and pestle. If you grow the plant in your garden, use the young leaves in salads, sweet or savoury, or cook briefly in vegetable dishes and soups.

- Use the seeds, which are similar in flavour to fennel seeds, in fish and vegetable dishes, soups and curries.
- Also use the seeds in fresh and dried fruit dishes: they go particularly well with figs.
- Anise (or star anise) is the principal flavouring of many alcohols in Europe and around the Mediterranean: the pastis of France—Ricard, Pernod, anisette—and ouzo, raki and arrack. Use these in cooking for their outstanding anise flavour and some therapeutic effect.

APPLE
Malus sylvestris
Rosaceae family

PRINCIPAL NUTRIENTS
Vitamins: A, B, C
Minerals: calcium, magnesium, phosphorus, potassium

Eating and cooking apples have been cultivated from the native European crab apple for over three thousand years. By Roman times there were some 36 varieties in existence according to Pliny the Elder, and today there are tens of thousands (over six thousand in Britain alone), although few of these are grown anymore because of the demands of commerce.

Therapeutic Uses
The apple is a treasure chest of therapeutic properties with its natural sugars, its pectin, amino acids, vitamins and minerals. Throughout the centuries it has been prescribed for virtually every ailment. It particularly benefits the digestive system, helping constipation as well as diarrhoea, and all intestinal problems, especially intestinal bacteria. The pectin in the fruit is an antidiarrhoeal used in many over-the-counter remedies. For home treatment, grate an apple, sprinkle with a little lemon juice to prevent it browning, and eat 1 tablespoon every hour. Drink the following tea too, which

is also useful when you have a cold or flu, when you have lost your voice, and to prevent infection. Keep the skins of any apples you eat or use in remedies, and mix them and a whole apple, cut into chunks, with 1 litre (1 3/4 pints) water and a few pieces of liquorice. Boil for 20 minutes, then strain and drink, without sugar, at room temperature. A chopped Bramley apple by itself, cooked similarly, would make a wonderful pick-me-up drink.

Apples are good for rheumatic conditions such as gout, for the mouth (slow chewing allows the aromatic oils to massage inflamed gums), for general fatigue (both physical and mental), for stress, anaemia, demineralisation (as in those recovering from illness), and weaknesses of the liver. In France an apple a day is prescribed to prevent heart attack, and two apples to patients who have had heart surgery. Dr. Leclerc in fact recommended a kilo or over 2 lb of apples (about six) per day, because of the content of vitamins and minerals, to those who tend to suffer from heart problems in general. The pectin in the fruit is believed to "soak up" fats and cholesterol, preventing them from being absorbed by the body.

In the Kitchen
As with many foods containing vitamin C, apples are best eaten raw and with their skin, so try to buy organic, untreated fruit. Apples are also best eaten in the morning, when they can give you the energy required to face a stressful day. You could eat them cooked at night, when they will help you sleep due to their bromine, a soother of the nervous system.

- Eat them whole, or sliced or chopped into fruit salads. Always cut them at the last minute or acidulate with lemon juice, because enzyme activity turns the flesh brown.
- At breakfast, eat them grated or chopped into cereal or porridge. The therapeutic properties will be greatest if the cereal is freshly milled. (Do this in a food processor, coffee grinder or spice mill.)
- My favourite breakfast recipe is one I learned from my great mentor, Marguerite Maury, who in turn learned it from a doctor in Switzerland, the home of muesli. Soak 1

large tablespoon of your chosen milled cereal—rye, wheat, oat, buckwheat—in 5 tablespoons cold water for 12 hours. Mix in some freshly squeezed lemon juice, 3 large tablespoons live yogurt, and 1 coffeespoon honey. Grate in an apple (with its skin) and add a few almonds, hazelnuts or walnuts. This is very simple but very delicious. It must be prepared just before eating, otherwise it will lose most of its nutritive values and active properties.

- Eat apples with cheese for a snack lunch or after dinner.
- Use apple and cheese diced as an omelette filling, or apple alone, raw or cooked, as a pancake filling.
- Use chopped apples in savoury salads, with celery, avocado, ham or other meats, nuts, lettuce etc.
- Make apples, tart or sweet, into apple sauces, flavouring them as appropriate—with horseradish, mixed spice, cloves, lemon juice, wine vinegar and so on. The acidity of the apple (from malic acid) balances the fattiness of meats such as pork, duck and goose, and helps you to digest them.
- Serve briefly fried apple slices or small whole baked apples as a garnish for the meats above and for game birds.
- Bake large cored apples—tart or sweet—stuffed with sugar, nuts and dried fruits. Baste with a citrus juice, syrup or liqueur, and serve with a sweet sauce or cream.
- Slice firm apples and use in pies and flans. If you want the apple pieces to keep their shape, avoid varieties such as Bramleys, which cook to a mush. The English, French and American culinary traditions are rich in apple desserts.
- Juice apples, and drink or use in cooking.
- Use cider and Calvados (apple brandy) in your cooking, as well as cider vinegar. Perhaps it is the digestive properties of the apple that gave rise to the traditional *"trou Normand,"* the "hole" in the middle of a large meal allotted to a glass of Calvados which allows the remainder of the meal to be eaten and enjoyed.
- Slice apples into rings and dry them as you would any herb or fruit. In this way the vitamins, minerals and other nutrients are concentrated.

APRICOT
Prunus armeniaca
Rosaceae family

PRINCIPAL NUTRIENTS
Vitamins: A, B, C, K
Minerals: calcium, iron, magnesium, phosphorus, potassium

PROBABLY a native of eastern Asia, apricots have been cultivated in China for at least four thousand years. They thrive in warm, subtropical climates. They flower early (the name comes from the Latin *praecox*, meaning "precocious") and are therefore vulnerable to frosts. The Romans knew apricots and thought they came from Armenia—hence their botanical name; later the Moors grew them in Spain. The fruit was known in France in the fifteenth century, but was only introduced to England in 1542, when one of Henry VIII's gardeners, a French priest and plant expert, brought some apricots from Italy.

Apricots do not travel very well, but can be dried very successfully. The most therapeutic are those grown in the Hunza Valley of Kashmir. If you pay a little more you can buy apricots which do not need the customary soaking before cooking.

Therapeutic Uses
Fresh apricots are very high in betacarotene, the vitamin A derived from vegetable sources, which concentrates when the fruit is dried. The potassium and niacin content concentrate too. Ounce for ounce, dried apricots contain up to ten times the iron and ten times the fiber of the fresh fruit.

Apricots, both fresh and dried, are powerhouses of nutrition. Because of the antioxidant vitamin A (see page 278), apricots are believed to be significant in the fight against ageing and cancer. The people of the Hunza Valley, for instance, eat a simple diet, including lots of the local apricots. Many live to well over a hundred and do not fall victim to the ageing diseases common in the West. The vitamin A content is also good for growth of both bones and skin. The vitamin B in the fruit helps the nervous system, alleviating nervous depression as well as menopausal and menstrual problems. The iron is good for anaemia. Apricots are also helpful when you lose your voice, as with laryngitis.

In the Kitchen

Neither cooking nor drying reduces the nutritive levels of apricots much, apart from the vitamin C which is water soluble and therefore lost in cooking water.

- Eat fresh apricots whole, or lightly poached in a syrup along with complementary spices such as cardamom.
- Stuff halved fresh apricots with an almond or a little marzipan—a popular Arab sweetmeat. (It makes natural taste sense too, for almond is the flavour of the kernel in the apricot stone.)
- Use halved fresh or dried apricots in open tarts and flans and puddings such as crumbles.
- Cook fresh or dried, and use in cakes, soufflés, fools, ice creams, sorbets etc.
- Use fresh or dried soaked apricots in cereals, with muesli or yogurt for breakfast.
- Eat unsoaked dried apricots as a snack, perhaps with almonds (the perfect remedy for PMT).
- Make a hearty salad with lettuce and chicory leaves, banana chunks, sliced onion and apple, dried apricots, raisins, sunflower seeds, walnuts, firm tofu and cubes of cheese (Emmenthal, Mozzarella, Gouda, Gruyère, mature Cheddar). Dress with a sauce of natural yogurt, olive oil and lime juice.
- Cook dried apricots in stuffings for duck and goose to counterbalance the fattiness of the birds, or in a lamb stew (a favourite combination in the Middle East, where apricots are used often with meat).
- Make dried or fresh apricots into jam, with or without split almonds.
- Cook with apricot liqueurs, or make one for yourself, using vodka or brandy as a base.

ARTICHOKE, GLOBE
Cynara scolymus
Compositae family

PRINCIPAL NUTRIENTS
Vitamins: A, B, C
Minerals: calcium, potassium

THE GLOBE ARTICHOKE (no relation to the potato-like Jerusalem artichoke) is a type of thistle native to the Mediterranean and has been cultivated for centuries. It was known to the Greeks and Romans; early Arab civilizations called it *kharchiof*, echoed in the present-day Italian *carciofo* and Spanish *alcachofa*. Catherine de' Medici is said to have imported it to France in the sixteenth century, from where it spread to the rest of Europe.

The vegetable is actually the unopened flower bud of the plant. The scale-like leaves are too tough to eat except at the base, and they and the prickly central choke (which would become the flower) must be pulled away to get at the delicious heart.

Therapeutic Uses
Rich in carbohydrate, globe artichokes are energising, stimulant and tonic, particularly for the liver and kidneys. Cynarine, a sweet-tasting chemical present in all parts of the plant, is thought to improve liver function and increase bile production, and thus assist in fat metabolism in general. The endocrine glands benefit as well. Globe artichokes also purify the blood, fortify the heart and benefit the nervous system. For intestinal illness and/or diarrhoea, eat the vegetable or use its leaves in a tisane. Boil a handful of leaves in 600 ml (1 pint) water for 10 minutes. Drink cool, first thing in the morning, to help liver, kidney and digestive problems.

Make a tea from artichoke leaves. Boil 50 g (2 oz) leaves in 600 ml (1 pint) water for 10 minutes, leave to stand for about 10 minutes, then drink, with honey if you like.

Some essential oils contained in globe artichokes may cause contact dermatitis.

In the Kitchen

Globe artichokes are usually quite large in Britain and have to be cooked before eating. In Mediterranean areas, particularly Italy, many varieties can be found. Some are picked when so small and tender that they can be eaten whole and raw, or very lightly cooked.

The cynarine makes anything in your mouth taste sweet, so never try to drink good wines with artichokes.

- Boil whole in salted acidulated water until a leaf pulls off easily, then eat cold with a vinaigrette or mayonnaise, or hot with melted butter or hollandaise. Pull off the leaves one at a time, and scrape the fleshy base off with your bottom teeth. After removing most of the leaves you can take out the hairy choke and eat the tender heart with a knife and fork rather than your fingers. This makes a delicious hors d'oeuvre or light lunch.

- Cook whole and remove the leaves (keep the tender base flesh for a soup or purée) to get at the heart. Use this sliced or whole in or with salads, or fry lightly and serve with a sauce made of lemon juice, walnut oil, chopped parsley and sesame seeds.

- Whole artichoke hearts can accompany many meat, fish and pasta dishes. The vitamin A and B content makes protein fats easier to digest.

- If you can get hold of baby artichokes, use them whole or slice them and coat in a light batter before deep-frying (see pages 168–169). Alternatively, fry with some of the following typically Mediterranean ingredients and serve as a cold hors d'oeuvre: olive oil, anchovies, ripe plum tomatoes, capers, lemon juice and grated lemon peel.

ASPARAGUS

Asparagus officinalis
Liliaceae family

PRINCIPAL NUTRIENTS

Vitamins: A, B, C
Minerals: manganese, potassium, sulphur

THIS LUXURIOUS member of the lily family was eaten by the Ancient Egyptians, Greeks and Romans. It was reintroduced to England by the French in Tudor times. There are different varieties: plump white stalks are prized on the Continent; slender green or purple stalks are more popular in the USA and Britain; and the cheaper thin stalks known as sprue (good for soup) are unappreciated except in Britain.

Therapeutic Uses

Asparagus is a strong diuretic, which is very useful for those suffering from oedema, toxaemia, high blood pressure, water retention, kidney problems, gout and some rheumatic conditions. (In fact, after we eat asparagus we excrete a smelly waste product in our urine, caused by a sulphur compound in the vegetable.) It is good for people who suffer from diabetes or hypoglycaemia, and can decongest the liver. It is a natural blood cleanser due to its vitamin A, manganese and nitre content and therefore has an effect on the skin, particularly on eczema. The vitamin B content is also good for nervous disorders and asthma.

In the Kitchen

The fresher the plant, the more nutrients it contains. In the northern hemisphere the season for asparagus is extremely short—from about late May to the end of June in the UK—so asparagus should be eaten as often as possible during that time.

Trim minimally, and use the trimmings in soup or stock. Never drink wine and eat asparagus at the same time: that sulphur content makes the wine taste metallic.

- Asparagus is usually cooked, but it is much better nutritionally when raw. Grate it into salad. If you freeze it for a while the flesh softens a little, and so can more easily be eaten raw.
- One of my favourite salads is a combination of raw grated asparagus, carrot, sweet potato and parsnip. Dress with olive oil and citrus juice.
- Cook lightly in as little boiling salted water as possible, head in the steam, feet in the water, until still crisp (use

the water in stock). Serve hot or lukewarm with melted butter, plain or flavoured with a citrus juice (particularly lime) and herbs, or with hollandaise. Serve lukewarm or cold with vinaigrette, mayonnaise (plain, green herb or orange) or a béarnaise. This makes a good dinner starter or a main course for lunch.

- Make the stems into a soup, saving the tips for a garnish.
- Cook in a soufflé, use in a risotto or bake in a quiche.
- Juice asparagus and have a glass a day for a week. The benefits will far outweigh the cost!

AUBERGINE
Solanum melongena
Solanaceae family

PRINCIPAL NUTRIENTS

Vitamins: B
Minerals: manganese, phosphorus, potassium

THE AUBERGINE is a low bushy plant, often prickly along the stems and leafstalks, with a fruit which can be round, ovoid or cucumber-shaped, and in colours from white to purple. It is native to Asia and has been grown in India for over four thousand years. Aubergines were thought to have been introduced to Europe by the Moors, and at first were viewed with great suspicion, being associated with epilepsy.

Therapeutic Uses
Aubergines are not rich in any particular nutrient, but are low in calories, sodium, fat and cholesterol. They are diuretic, and stimulate the kidneys, intestines, liver and pancreas. They also calm the nerves.

In the Kitchen
Aubergines should always be smooth and unwrinkled—a wrinkled skin indicates age. Large ones may need to have their bitter juices removed: slice, sprinkle with salt and leave for about 30 minutes. Discard the liquid that comes out of the vegetable, and rinse the slices. If you don't do this only

cut the aubergine at the last minute, or it will turn brown through enzymic reactions.

Aubergines are usually eaten cooked. Their prime culinary virtue lies in their adaptability and their ability to take up spices and other flavourings. Aubergine cells are full of air which escapes when the vegetable is heated. If this is done in oil the aubergine soaks it up, which is why some aubergine dishes can be very greasy. For the healthiest result choose recipes that use little oil.

- Braise, with onions, peppers, tomatoes and courgettes, to make a Provençal ratatouille.
- Grill or barbecue thick slices, lightly brushed with oil, until brown. Serve with other grilled vegetables as an hors d'oeuvre or vegetable accompaniment. Spread with pesto and sprinkle with Parmesan, as advocated by the famous Swiss chef Anton Mosimann, to make a wonderful starter.
- Bake an aubergine gently in the oven at 180°C/350°F/Gas 4 for 30 minutes, then cut in half and spread the cut sides with olive oil, chopped parsley and garlic. Put the two halves together again and bake for another 30 minutes. Serve as a main course with whole rice, millet or couscous, or as a starter or accompaniment to grilled poultry, lamb, beef or fish.
- Cut an aubergine in half, pour some olive oil and 1 teaspoon miso (fermented soy sauce) on to each cut side, and bake in the oven at 180°C/350°F/Gas 4 for 45 minutes or more.
- Cook in Indian or Middle Eastern dishes, choosing recipes that require braising, grilling and baking rather than frying.

Aubergine Pâté

This can be used as a dip, but I like it best spread on toasted country or wholemeal bread and served with a watercress or rocket salad.

SERVES 2

1 aubergine, baked plainly (see previous page)
1 large mild white onion, peeled and minced
1/2 fresh chilli, seeded and very finely chopped
1/2 coffeespoon salt
1–2 garlic cloves, peeled and crushed
2 tablespoons chopped parsley
2–3 tablespoons olive oil

Remove the softened aubergine flesh from the shells, and when cool mix with the onion, chilli, salt, garlic and parsley. Add as much oil as you need to make the mixture paste-like. Let it rest for about 10 minutes for the flavours to mingle.

AVOCADO
Persea americana/gratissima
Lauraceae family

PRINCIPAL NUTRIENTS
Vitamins: A, B, C
Minerals: potassium

THE AVOCADO is the fruit of a tropical and subtropical evergreen tree. There are hundreds of varieties differing in shape, size, colour and skin texture. It was eaten by the Aztecs, and by the Spanish in the early sixteenth century, but was not universally known until the early twentieth century when its commercial cultivation in the USA began.

Therapeutic Uses
The avocado has the highest fat content of any fruit—over 20 per cent of its weight—but over 80 per cent of this is composed of the healthier monounsaturated and polyunsaturated fatty acids. It has a high vitamin C content and is also easy to digest, so it is recommended for stomach and intestinal trouble and for stimulating the liver. Avocados help to reduce the proliferation of bacteria in the intestines and those which cause problems in the bladder, such as cystitis. The vitamin A and B content are good for the nervous system.

In the Kitchen

Because of its firm, buttery texture, avocado can easily replace meat. It is also perfect for a quick and nutritious meal.

- Halve, stone and eat from the skin, with salt and pepper or some citrus juice (because enzyme activity turns the flesh brown after contact with the air) or a simple vinaigrette. Fill the hole with a savoury dip such as taramasalata or with shrimps.
- Chop the flesh and add to lettuce or spinach salads: sprinkle with a few toasted pine kernels.
- Serve sliced with slices of ripe tomato and Mozzarella cheese for an Italian *tricoloure* salad.
- Mash and spread on toasted wholemeal or rye bread.
- Add slices to sandwich fillings.

Guacamole

Some people find avocados boring in taste and texture, but this Mexican dish—to be used as a spread or dip, with biscuits, crudités, potato crisps, miniature tortilla chips or pitta bread—sings with both flavour and health.

SERVES 4

2 large avacados
2–3 tablespoons lime or lemon juice
3 medium tomatoes, skinned, seeded and diced
1 large garlic clove, peeled and crushed
2 tablespoons chopped fresh coriander
salt and freshly ground black pepper
chilli sauce to taste, or a little very finely chopped
    fresh seeded chilli pepper

Halve the avocados, stone them and scoop the flesh carefully out of the skins. Mash with the lime juice, then mix in the remaining ingredients. Eat straightaway, or brush with lemon juice and cover with clingfilm to prevent the avocado turning brown.

BANANA

Musa sapientum
Scitamineae family

PRINCIPAL NUTRIENTS

Vitamins: A, B, C
Minerals: calcium, iron, magnesium, phosphorus, potassium

Bananas grow in bunches on a plant which can be up to 10 metres (32 ft) high. Originating in India and southern Asia, the plants are now cultivated all over the world in frost-free climates. They were established in the Canaries in 1402; taken to the West Indies in 1516; and must have been introduced at some point to Hawaii, because Captain Cook found them there when he arrived in 1778.

Bananas consist mainly of starch, which turns to sugar as they ripen. When a banana is fully ripe and the skin is bright yellow, the flesh consists of over 90 per cent natural sugars.

Plantains (*Musa paradisiaca*) grow in the same way, but are not sweet like bananas: the starch does not convert into sugar and so they need to be cooked before eating and for their nutrients to be released.

Therapeutic Uses

Bananas are very easily digested which makes them a good food for children, invalids and old people. They help growth in the young and counter calcium deficiency and brittle bones in the elderly. They restore the equilibrium of the nervous system—due to the potassium—and are also recommended as a cure for diarrhoea.

British research in the 1980s suggested that powdered plantain helped prevent the formation of gastric ulcers caused by aspirin consumption, and healed existing ulcers.

In the Kitchen

Due to enzyme activity banana flesh browns in contact with air, so if peeled or cut and not eaten straightaway it should be immersed in lemon juice or the juice used in a fruit salad.

- Eat a raw one daily, perhaps at breakfast mixed with muesli or on porridge.
- Mash ripe bananas for a sandwich filling for children.
- Bake bananas in their skins in the oven, or wrap in foil and grill on the barbecue. Bananas become even sweeter and more intense in flavour when cooked.
- Bananas can also be fried briefly in a little butter with a complementary spirit or liqueur such as rum.
- Deep-fry bananas, whole or in chunks, in an egg white fritter batter (see pages 168–169). Sprinkle with sesame seeds and serve with maple syrup, or serve as a savoury fritter with chicken as they do in the Southern United States.
- Bake mashed bananas in a soufflé, cake or teabread.
- Slice plantains thinly and deep-fry until brown and crisp. These are served as an appetiser with drinks in the Caribbean.
- Add chunks of ripe plantain to stews and casseroles, or bake in their skins in foil instead of potatoes.

BARLEY, *see* Cereal Grains

BASIL
Ocimum basilicum
Labiatae family

THE BASIL PLANT originated in India and is thought to have reached Europe in the sixteenth century. It has long been considered an aphrodisiac.

Therapeutic Uses
Basil is a good diuretic, and fortifies the digestive and nervous systems. It helps those suffering from menstrual problems, insomnia and migraine. Eat the leaves in some of the ways outlined on the next page, or drink basil tisanes.

The essential oil is distilled from the flower tops and young shoots and leaves.

In the Kitchen
In Britain, grow basil plants outside in a warm summer, otherwise inside on a sunny windowsill. Avoid dried basil,

which is minty and curry-like in flavour. Tear rather than cut the leaves, and do so at the very last moment.

- Use fresh basil leaves as a garnish for a tomato salad (basil and tomatoes have a unique affinity), or a vegetable soup. This adds flavour as well as helping with digestion. Use the flower heads as well when available.
- Add the torn leaves at the last moment to egg, mushroom and rice dishes, spaghetti sauces and vegetable stews (basil is delicious in ratatouille).
- Put fresh leaves in a food processor with garlic, pine kernels, grated Parmesan and olive oil to make pesto, a wonderful sauce for pasta that can be used in lots of other dishes as well.
- Preserve the summer fragrance of basil by macerating leaves in olive oil: they will turn black, but the flavour of the oil is magically transformed.

Bay Leaf
Laurus nobilis
Lauraceae family

THE SWEET BAY or bay laurel is an evergreen shrub or tree which originated in Asia, but is now well established in Europe. It arrived in England around the sixteenth century, but was well known to the Greeks and Romans long before; it was the bay laurel leaf that was made into the crowns worn by victors in battle and sport. (Beware: do not confuse bay leaves with the related but poisonous laurel.)

Therapeutic Uses
Bay leaves have long been considered curative in many ways. Dr. Leclerc considered them beneficial for virus infections, influenza, coughs, bronchitis and digestive problems such as flatulence. Boil 5 g (1/4 oz) leaves with the same weight of organic orange peel and 300 ml (10 fl oz) boiling water, and infuse for 10 minutes. Strain and drink for its ability to promote sweating, especially valuable if you are feverish.

For rheumatism, lie in a hot bath in which some fresh bay leaves have been infused.

In the Kitchen
Bay leaves may be used fresh, but are less bitter if dried. Avoid ground bay leaves. The warm spicy flavour is useful— and therapeutic—in a variety of dishes, sweet and savoury.

- Use bay leaves in meat marinades: the phenol content is an aromatic bacterial and tenderiser. (These antiseptic properties can be used in other protective ways: keep bay in bags of grain or flour to keep insects away—the reason for the bay leaf found in packets of dried figs.)
- Use bay leaves in stocks, sauces and bouquet garnis, and in or on pâté mixtures.
- Boil bay leaves in the milk for rice and other milk puddings.

BEANS, BROAD, *see* Pulses

BEANS, GREEN
Phaseolus spp
Leguminosae family

PRINCIPAL NUTRIENTS
Vitamins: A, B, C
Minerals: calcium, iron, magnesium, phosphorus, potassium, zinc

BY GREEN BEANS, I mean beans that are eaten pod and all. These include the numerous varieties of haricots verts or French beans (string or snap beans in the USA) and runner beans. These beans are native to Central and South America, and were eaten by the Aztecs; they were not introduced to Europe and Asia until after the discovery of the New World by Columbus.

If French beans *(Phaseolus vulgaris)* and other legumes are left to mature, they produce beans which are dried for the protein-rich pulses of winter (see page 152). In Continental Europe the freshly matured beans, out of their pods and before they are dried, are a prized vegetable.

Therapeutic Uses

Green beans provide a lot of energy due to their mineral salts, hydrocarbon, chlorophyll and vitamin content. Dr. Leclerc believed that the inositol they contain is a bonus for weak hearts and kidneys. They are diuretic and can therefore treat fluid retention, gout and rheumatic conditions. French doctors prescribe a daily half glass of juice for kidney stones.

In the Kitchen

French beans come in a variety of sizes, and only need to be topped and tailed before use. Runner beans need to be stringed as well; when topping and tailing, pull off the strings running down the sides, or shave them off with a sharp knife. Cut into diagonal lengths or push through a bean cutter.

- Eat raw, sliced thinly and added to salads of lettuce, cucumber, beetroot, tomatoes, raw courgettes and so on. Flavour with garlic and good olive oil dressings, and sprinkle with toasted almonds, pine kernels or sunflower seeds.
- Add raw or lightly cooked cold beans to protein salads of tuna, eggs, anchovies or cheese (such as Emmenthal, mature Cheddar, Cantal, Mozzarella or Parmesan).
- Steam beans (French, whole, runners, cut) for just a few minutes to keep them crisp, and to retain as much of their nutritive value as possible. Serve plain or with a little butter, or add garlic, parsley and butter. Cold and dressed with a good dressing, they make a delicious starter.
- If boiling (when vitamins can be quickly lost), use plenty of water, adding the beans when it is at a full boil, and boil only for a few minutes. This retains the colour well, for enzymes which attack chlorophyll (responsible for the green colour and many therapeutic properties) are rapidly inactivated by the high temperature. Do not cover the pan, as acids released by the beans could leach back into the

pan after condensing on the lid and discolour the vegetables.
- Sprinkle cooked beans with sesame seeds, raw or toasted, for delicious flavour and texture, and extra nutrients.
- Use beans, whole or in pieces, in stir-fries.

Terrine of Green Vegetables

You could substitute any green vegetable such as spinach, peas, mange-tout, courgettes and so on. Use a 150 ml (5 fl oz) cup as a measure.

SERVES 4

2 cups minced green beans
2 cups cubed, slightly stale bread
1 cup soya milk
4 shallots, peeled and minced
2 onions, peeled and minced
3 teaspoons sesame oil
freshly grated nutmeg
2 eggs, beaten
1 garlic clove, peeled and halved

Preheat the oven to 180°C/350°F/Gas 4. Mince the beans immediately before use. Soak the bread in the milk to soften it. Fry the shallot and onion in most of the oil, then add to the milk along with nutmeg to taste, the eggs and beans. Mix well.

Grease the inside of an ovenproof dish with the remaining oil, then rub thoroughly with the cut garlic. Pour in the mixture, and bake for 30 minutes. Serve hot, with a tomato sauce if you like, some whole rice or a salad, or as an accompaniment to meat.

BEANS, KIDNEY, *see* Pulses

BEANS, SOYA, *see* Pulses

BEETROOT
Beta vulgaris
Chenopodiaceae family

PRINCIPAL NUTRIENTS
Vitamins: B, C
Minerals: iron, magnesium, phosphorus, potassium

THERE ARE four types of beet—table beet, spinach beet or chard, sugar beet and mangel wurzel. All varieties are rich in the sugars for which they are grown commercially on a massive scale in Europe.

Therapeutic Uses
Because of its high sugar content, beetroot is highly energising; it also dynamises the digestive system. The magnesium helps bone growth, while phosphorus and vitamin B have a sedative effect. Vitamins B and C together are extremely effective in the treatment of neuritis, an inflammation or deterioration of the nerves. Beetroot is highly recommended for anaemia and general disability, and is very useful for old people.

In the Kitchen
Cooked beetroot loses a lot of its properties, particularly vitamin C, so it is best eaten raw. Scrub and peel first, but beware of the juice which stains very easily.

- Use raw and grated in salads with other herbs and flavourings such as apples, chives, garlic and parsley. Cider vinegar, orange, lemon and lime juice and zest, and walnut oil are also good. Beetroot's earthy taste can even mingle well with strong flavours such as anchovies, capers, mustard and horseradish.
- A combination of grated raw beetroot and carrot is wonderful for convalescents, giving them back their appetite.
- Stir-fry grated raw beetroot with some of the above flavourings.

- Scrub and trim carefully and boil whole for up to 1 1/2 hours, depending on size. Skin, and slice or dice.
- Make into a soup, using potato or apple as a partner.
- Make into Russian bortsch, which can be a deep pink consommé or a thick red vegetable soup.
- Pickle cooked beetroot in vinegar.
- Serve cooked or pickled beetroot with strong-tasting fish such as herring or complement with soured cream.
- Cook the leaves lightly as you would spinach—they contain vitamin C and other nutrients.
- Juice beetroot and drink every day for 3 weeks during the season. This forms part of a cure for cancer at clinics in Switzerland.

BILBERRY
Vaccinium myrtillus
Ericaceae family

PRINCIPAL NUTRIENTS
Vitamins: A, C
Minerals: potassium

THE VACCINIUM genus includes the European bilberry (also known as blaeberry, whinberry and whortleberry), the American cranberry, blueberry and huckleberry, and the Scandinavian lingonberry. They all grow wild in northern hemisphere moorland or on mountainsides and some are cultivated. All have long been known as food and medicine.

Therapeutic Uses
These berries contain vitamin A and C and fruit acids. The bilberry has often been recommended for heavy periods, dysentery and diarrhoea because of its astringent properties, which are so gentle that bilberries can be used for weaned babies with loose bowels. Quarter fill a container with bilberries and fill it up with water, then cook slowly for about an hour. Add the juice to their yogurt or fruit salads.

Bilberries, like other berries in the genus, are highly antiseptic and antibacterial. Laboratory tests have shown that bilberries can kill bacteria such as *Escherichia coli* and *Bacillus enteridis* in the space of 24 hours. Berries are therefore often used for throat infections such as laryngitis or tonsillitis. Juice the berries, or make an infusion and drink slowly.

You can dry the berries and turn them into a tisane: use 1 dessertspoon per 600 ml (1 pint) and boil gently for 10–15 minutes. Strain, and drink with honey. Add some water for children.

If you have loose teeth and receding gums, chew the berries slowly to give the gums a good massage.

In the Kitchen

Blueberries are slightly larger than bilberries and both are sweet and fragrant, best eaten soon after picking. Cranberries are much sourer, so are not eaten raw, and are interesting in a culinary sense because they contain benzoic acid, a preservative: cranberries can survive for up to eight months in the refrigerator.

* Eat bilberries and blueberries raw and whole, with cream, fromage frais or yogurt. Crush them slightly and mix with thick cream or yogurt for an easy and delicious pudding.
* Use raw in fruit and savoury salads.
* Cook bilberries and blueberries in pies, American-type muffins, teabreads and Summer Pudding, and for a pancake filling and cheesecake topping.
* Make ice creams with bilberries and blueberries.
* Cook cranberries for the famous sauce to accompany turkey, or add them to sauces for rich meats like duck, game or lamb. Their acidity also goes well in sauces for certain fish.
* Cook cranberries with sweet fruit in pies and crumbles, or instead of raisins or sultanas in teabreads.
* Make any of the berries into jams and jellies—cranberries have a particularly high pectin content and therefore gell easily.
* Make a syrup (see Blackberry).

BLACKBERRY
Rubus fruitcosus
Rosaceae family

PRINCIPAL NUTRIENTS

Vitamins: A, B, C, E
Minerals: calcium, potassium

THE RUBUS genus, which includes the raspberry and dewberry, originated in Asia, but blackberries grow wild and are cultivated all over the world. The loganberry is a cross between the blackberry and raspberry, producing a fruit that is larger than either and excellent for cooking.

Therapeutic Uses
Blackberries can be used in the same ways, and for the same purposes, as other berries and currants (see Bilberry, Currants and Raspberry). Blackberry leaves are described by Dr. Leclerc as a good remedy for diabetes.

Make a wonderful syrup for sore throats by mixing and heating fruit and sugar in equal proportions, then adding 40 percent of alcohol (gin or vodka). Leave to macerate in a cool place for a few weeks. Strain and use. Blackcurrants, redcurrants, cranberries, bilberries or blueberries could replace the blackberries.

Blackberries can be implicated in allergic reactions such as hives and facial swelling.

In the Kitchen
Blackberries are not difficult to grow—in fact, it's sometimes difficult to stop them taking root everywhere. Or go blackberrying in the country—but avoid fruit growing beside main roads.

- Use and cook much as you would raspberries (see page 162).
- Bake in the classic blackberry and apple pie.
- Make into sauces to accompany meat and game, or desserts.

BLUEBERRY, *see* Bilberry

BORAGE
Borago officinalis
Boraginaceae family

This hairy, bristly green herb with star-shaped, blue-purple flowers originated in the middle East, and was spread throughout Europe by the Romans.

Therapeutic Uses
The leaves contain a natural gum, which is useful for digestive problems, constipation in particular, for respiratory problems such as coughs and bronchitis, and for liver deficiencies. It is a natural blood cleanser as well, which make it good for skin problems such as acne and herpes.

Borage is a natural kind of "pep pill", and a drug derived from borage is used by French homeopathic doctors to treat depression, fevers and nervous disorders. Some experts also assert that borage can help cure a hangover.

In the Kitchen
One of borage's most familiar uses is in the English summer drink, Pimms. Both flowers and leaves have a mild cucumber flavour.

- Add the leaves and flowers to salads. The leaves go particularly well with watercress, in equal proportions.
- Cook the leaves with spinach for 2–3 minutes to make a highly nutritious accompaniment to chicken or meat.
- For a vegetarian dish, cover borage and spinach leaves with a white sauce enriched with ground oats and rye, and flavoured with mature Cheddar or Emmenthal cheese.
- The leaves can be chopped in stuffings, or fried in batter as fritters (see pages 168–169); shredded in cold sauces such as mayonnaise, or added to hot sauces at the last minute.
- Use the leaves and flowers in summery drinks and claret cups etc, or freeze flowers in ice cubes and use to cool and decorate drinks.
- Make borage leaves into a refreshing tisane (see page xxii).

- Make a borage vinegar (page xxiii).
- Crystallise the flowers to use as cake and pudding decorations.

BRAZIL NUT, *see* Nuts

BROCCOLI AND CAULIFLOWER
Brassica oleracea botrytis
Cruciferae family

PRINCIPAL NUTRIENTS
Vitamins: A, B, C, E, K
Minerals: calcium, iron, potassium

THESE ARE both members of the cabbage family. Cauliflower is thought to have come from the Orient, and has been cultivated in Europe since about the sixteenth century. Broccoli is a later arrival, a type of "flowering cabbage" developed in Calabria in Italy—hence its alternative name calabrese.

Therapeutic Uses
Cauliflower contains vitamins A, B and C, and iron, potassium, calcium, copper and zinc, although less than its green relative, broccoli. Both also contain good quantities of folic acid, a B vitamin which is rare in vegetables, and the blood-clotting agent vitamin K, a lack of which can cause haemorrhages. Antibiotics and some other drugs interfere with the functioning of the latter, so these vegetables are useful if you have been prescribed such medication.

Both vegetables are recommended for arthritic and rheumatic conditions, and for those who retain fluid (PMT sufferers, menopausal and ageing women).

In the Kitchen
Buy fresh, use fresh, and for preference eat raw, to obtain the full benefit from the vitamins.

- Eat both, chopped into tiny florets, raw in salads. Dressed with ground walnuts, chopped parsley and a flavourful dressing, this makes a good starter.
- Use raw in florets as crudités, with a dip.

- Lightly cook florets of both and serve warm, dressed as above if you like. Try sprinkling ground caraway seeds over the top.
- Eat the leaves and stalks as well, as they are full of nutrients. If your recipe only requires the florets, cut the rest small and eat raw, or use in stir-fries or cook in a soup. Broccoli stalks in particular are really tender and tasty.
- Both vegetables are delicious in stir-fries, with minimal meat and lots of flavourings, to be served with rice or another grain.
- Both can be served in a white or cheese sauce (with hard-boiled eggs and freshly grated nutmeg as well, if you like), and are particularly nutritious when served with another vegetable such as spinach.
- Florets of either can be deep-fried in a light batter as fritters (see pages 168–169).
- Never throw away the cooking water, which contains many of the nutrients. Use in gravy, sauces or soups: onion soup made with cauliflower water is delicious.

BRUSSELS SPROUTS, *see* Cabbage

BUCKWHEAT, *see* Cereal Grains

BUTTERMILK, *see* Dairy Products

CABBAGE
Brassica oleracea spp
Cruciferae family

PRINCIPAL NUTRIENTS
Vitamins: A, B, C
Minerals: calcium, iodine, iron, magnesium, phosphorus, potassium, sulphur

CABBAGES of all varieties have been cultivated for thousands of years, by the Ancient Greeks and Romans, and by the Chinese, who served pickled cabbage to the builders of the Great Wall (although Chinese cabbages are of a different genus). The Celts and Saxons also ate cabbage and valued it medicinally, which is probably why it still plays such a major part in the cuisines of northern Europe.

Red cabbage *(Brassica oleracea capitata rubra)* and Brussels sprouts *(Brassica oleracea gemmifera)* are also varieties of cabbage.

Therapeutic Uses

Cabbage and Brussels sprouts are most useful for respiratory ailments—asthma, coughs, colds and flu—and I make the following cabbage syrup, although eating them will also help. Liquidise a large red cabbage and add to the juice the same proportions of sugar; then cook until it becomes a thick syrup. When cool, bottle and use one dessertspoon per day in winter to keep colds and flu at bay; one dessertspoon two to three times per day to help a cough; and one teaspoon when an asthma attack is on the way. The syrup is also good for anaemia (although the iron content of cabbage is not very high) and glandular problems such as tonsillitis. The iodine content is good for the thyroid.

People who sweat a lot should eat raw cabbage every day, according to Dr. Leclerc, because of its magnesium, potassium and calcium content. The only people who should perhaps not eat cabbage are those who suffer from flatulence. Indigestible fibre in the cabbage is degraded in the gut by benign bacteria which produce a noxious gas in the process.

In the Kitchen

To obtain maximum nutritional benefit cabbage and Brussels sprouts should be eaten raw, for the vitamin C is lost in cooking. Also, do not cut cabbage or other vitamin C-rich vegetables until just before eating, as cutting releases the enzymes responsible for oxidation and thus vitamin loss. Cooking releases the mustard oils in cabbages; these break down into sulphur compounds and cause the familiar smell which gets worse the longer the cabbage is cooked.

- Shred or grate cabbage or Brussels sprouts and use in salads, alone or with grated carrot. Dress as for coleslaw or with a lemon juice and olive oil vinaigrette. Add raisins, sliced onions, chopped apples and walnuts. This is good with courgettes stuffed with rice, or with grilled chicken or meat.

- Buy sauerkraut—shredded green cabbage pickled in a salt solution. The salt kills off harmful bacteria and breaks down proteins in the cabbage, producing a characteristic lactic acid flavour.
- Cook cabbage in soups with beetroot, as they do in Russia. Both are very good at countering cold-weather respiratory problems because of the sulphur.
- Cook shredded cabbage very briefly in lots of boiling salted water, to keep it crisp and sweet. Alternatively cook it in cider, beer, orange juice or gin. Add crushed garlic, juniper berries or caraway seeds (the latter will help digestion). Do the same with Brussels sprouts, or steam them; flavour with shreds of crispy bacon, toasted almonds, pine kernels or a nut oil. Chestnuts and Brussels sprouts are a traditional and delicious combination.
- Blanch cabbage leaves and use as a crisp wrapping for other ingredients (meats, rice, etc.).
- Stir-fry shredded cabbage and Brussels sprouts with other flavourings like onion and garlic.
- Cook shreds of either vegetable in soups thick or thin. For the best texture and flavour, add at the last moment.
- Cook and purée Brussels sprouts as a vegetable accompaniment to meat or fish, or use as the basis of a creamy vegetable soup.

CARAWAY
Carum carvi
Umbelliferae family

NATIVE to south-eastern Europe, the caraway plant is a member of the same family as cumin and coriander. The Ancient Egyptians used the seeds in religious rituals and to make food more digestible. The latter use was echoed by the Greeks and Romans, and by medical practitioners throughout the ages.

Therapeutic Uses

Chew the seeds slowly before or after a meal—they are often included in *paan,* the digestive seeds cum breath fresheners offered in Indian restaurants. Or drink an infusion of 1/2 teaspoon seeds per 300 ml (10 fl oz) boiling water. This will relieve dyspepsia, colic and colitis, and can also help dysmenorrhoea.

An essential oil is distilled from the seeds.

In the Kitchen

If you grow the plant in your garden, you can use both the fresh leaves (in salads or as a garnish) and the tap roots (cook and eat like parsnips).

- Use as a seasoning for flavour and digestion in meat mixtures such as sausages and pâté, in cabbage, potato and beetroot dishes, and in heavy or rich meat dishes, particularly of duck, goose or pork.
- Add seeds to cake or bread doughs, as they do in parts of Europe.
- Add seeds (or a mixture of caraway, anise and fennel seeds) to soft cheeses.

Herring with Caraway

Herrings are very fatty (although the oils are nutritious), so cook them with a digestive spice and serve with a salad of lettuce, apple and cucumber dressed with oil and cider vinegar. (Herrings are also delicious with mustard or horseradish, which serve the same purpose as caraway.)

PER PERSON

1 medium herring
salt
1 tablespoon wholewheat, plain, soya or corn flour
1 tablespoon caraway seeds, crushed to a powder
2 tablespoons soya oil

TOPPING

1–2 tablespoons natural yogurt
1/2 teaspoon caraway seeds, crushed
1/2 tablespoon chopped parsley

Cut each herring open along the stomach. Remove any roe (which can be fried separately if liked). Clean the fish thoroughly, and bone if you like. Wash and dry, then sprinkle with a little salt. Mix the flour and crushed seeds together, and coat the herrings.

Heat the oil in a frying pan and fry the herrings on a medium heat for 6 minutes per side until crisp and golden. Drain well.

Serve topped with a mixture of the yogurt, seeds and parsley, seasoned with a little salt and pepper, along with the salad.

CARDAMOM
Elettaria cardamomum
Zingiberaceae family

THE PODS AND SEEDS which form the spice cardamom come from a tall herbaceous plant belonging to the ginger and turmeric family. Native to India and Sri Lanka, it was known to the Greeks and Romans.

Therapeutic Uses
The seeds are a good digestive stimulant often included in the Indian *paan* offered after a meal. You could boil a teaspoon of seeds in 600 ml (1 pint) water for 2 minutes and drink after meals, adding a little honey if desired. Or infuse whole crushed pods in the boiling water to be used for conventional tea, or add ground seeds to black coffee as the Bedouins do.

Use the spice in cooking for its diuretic properties—it is particularly good for premenstrual and menopausal fluid retention.

An essential oil is distilled from the seeds.

In the Kitchen
Buy whole green or bleached white pods rather than black, and avoid loose seeds or ground cardamom.

- Use whole pods—lightly crushed so that the flavour of the seeds can filter out—in rice dishes like *pullaos*, in curries, pâtés, sausages and meat stews.
- Bake cardamom seeds in cakes, bread and pastries as they do in Scandinavia.
- Add freshly ground cardamom seeds to fruit salad for a stupendous flavour.
- Infuse hot milk or cream for a custard, rice pudding or ice cream with several bruised cardamom pods.

CARRAGHEEN, *see* Seaweeds

CARROT
Daucus carota
Umbelliferae family

PRINCIPAL NUTRIENTS
Vitamins: A, B, C, D, E, K
Minerals: copper, iron, magnesium, manganese, phosphorus, potassium, sulphur

CARROTS have been eaten for at least two thousand years. They are thought to have originated in Asia, and were known to the Greeks and Romans. It was not until the seventeenth century, though, that the familiar fat, long, orange carrot was developed by the Dutch; up to then they had resembled the thin white wild carrot still found throughout Europe and North America.

Therapeutic Uses
Many digestive problems such as colitis and diarrhoea can be treated with carrots. French doctors recommend them for duodenal ulcers, and two in particular, Leclerc and Dexment, claim that carrots can save people with intestinal bleeding when all other medication has failed.

Carrots are revered also for their ability to stimulate the

liver and fluidify the bile. Betacarotene (responsible for the colour of carrots) converts in the intestine to vitamin A, which is stored in the liver. (Liver eaten as food is rich in vitamin A.)

The carotene in carrots also reinforces the body's immune system, making it more resistant to disease. Many experts believe that cancer may be prevented by a diet rich in vitamin A. The anti-epidemic and antiseptic properties can benefit the respiratory system particularly (eat carrots if you suffer from hay fever, for instance).

Eating carrots is good for the blood and the skin and enables wounds, ulcers and burns to heal more quickly.

The essential oil in raw carrots helps stop tooth decay, and chewing them maintains healthy gums. Give a teething baby a raw carrot stick to "chew" on. One of the most famous properties attributed to the carrot is an ability to improve eyesight: an early symptom of vitamin A deficiency is night blindness, and this vitamin is very important for eye health in general.

In the Kitchen

As carrots are so valuable they should be eaten often—every day if possible. They are best crisp and raw, although cooking does not actually destroy their vitamin A content. It is normally better to scrub rather than peel them, because most of the nutrients are just under the skin. However, in light of recent alarms about chemical residues, peeling is perhaps wise. Or buy organic carrots, which have the best flavour anyway.

- Cut into thin circles or julienne sticks or grate, and add to salads of lettuce, tomatoes, fennel, radishes and so on.
- Cut into long chunks and eat as a crudité, with dips.
- Grate as a salad, and dress with lemon, lime or orange juice. Mixed with grated raw beetroot it is particularly good for loss of appetite.
- Cut into small pieces and steam or boil until still crisp, or glaze with citrus juice, a little butter and seasoning.
- Boil or steam until tender, and then purée. Enrich with a little cream or crème fraîche if you like.

- Herbs and spices that go well with carrot are caraway seeds, chervil, coriander (fresh or seeds), dill, ginger, horseradish, hyssop, marjoram, parsley and thyme. Walnut or hazelnut oils go well, too, as do pieces of shelled nuts—walnuts, hazelnuts or pine kernels.
- Sprinkle carrot salads or cooked carrot dishes with seeds for texture—caraway, celery, dill, fennel, poppy, sesame or sunflower.
- Mix carrots with a flavouring or another fruit or vegetable (such as apple or spinach) and cook either as a creamed soup, or cut in small chunks in a thick vegetable and/or meat soup.
- Use as an ingredient in stews and casseroles.
- Bake grated carrot in a carrot cake—they are very sweet indeed—or as the filling for a quiche with onions, sourced cream and egg, some grated Gruyère or Emmenthal cheese, and lots of grated nutmeg.
- Turn carrots into the most nutritious juice of all. (Dilute with mineral water for children.)

CASSIA, *see* Cinnamon and Cassia

CAULIFLOWER, *see* Broccoli and Cauliflower

CELERIAC
Apium graveolens var. *rapaceum*
Umbelliferae family

PRINCIPAL NUTRIENTS
Vitamins: B, C
Minerals: calcium, phosphorus, potassium

THE BULBOUS stem-base of a type of celery, celeriac has been popular for centuries in Continental Europe but has only recently become familiar in Britain. It is celery-like in aroma and flavour, but more like a root vegetable in appearance and texture.

Therapeutic Uses

Celeriac has more fibre and more potassium than celery, and about the same content of vitamin C. Due to its mineral content it is a builder and cleanser of the blood. It helps the drainage of the liver and kidneys because of its essential oils, which are very similar to those of celery. It also helps in the absorption of calcium, which is useful for arthritis sufferers.

In the Kitchen

Celeriac must be peeled fairly thickly to get rid of all the knobbly bits. Do so after cutting the bulb into pieces, so that you can see what you are doing. Put the pieces immediately into acidulated water or they will turn brown.

- Grate celeriac and combine with a mustardy French dressing or mayonnaise to make the classic French rémoulade, an excellent hors d'oeuvre.
- Stir-fry grated celeriac briefly in a good oil.
- Steam small pieces above salted water for a few minutes, then add chopped chives and celery leaves.
- Steam chunks or boil them (use the water for soup or stock), and then purée to accompany meat dishes.
- Juice celeriac with some lemon, lime, grapefruit or carrot juice to make a wonderful cocktail for a tired nervous system.
- Cut into chunks, peel, then put in an ovenproof dish. Sprinkle with coarse salt and olive oil and bake in the oven at 180°C/350°F/Gas 4 for 30 minutes. Serve with meat, fish, or with whole rice or salad.

CELERY

Apium graveolens var. *dulce*
Umbelliferae family

PRINCIPAL NUTRIENTS
Vitamins: B, C
Minerals: iron, phosphorus, potassium

OUR FAMILIAR modern celery was developed by the Italians in the seventeenth century from the wild plant still found in damp areas of Europe and Asia. Although very strong-smelling and bitter it was much appreciated by the Romans, who used it as both vegetable and seasoning.

Therapeutic Uses

Celery is not particularly rich in nutrients, but is still useful for a number of complaints due to its high content of aromatic substances. It fortifies the stomach, kidneys and liver, is a nerve tonic and stimulates glandular action. It also helps to remineralise your body after illness, due to its sodium and potassium content. It is very gentle on the digestive system, helping other foods to be more easily assimilated. Celery is one of the best remedies for gout, rheumatism, nephritic colic and jaundice. For the liver and for rheumatism, or when recovering from a cold or flu, juice celery stalks and drink half a glass every day for 2–3 weeks.

In the Kitchen

Celery should always be crisp, so do not buy limp or bruised stalks. The seeds have the same flavour as the stalks, but are rather bitter.

- Eat celery raw, sliced in salads, in chunks as a crudité with a dip, or with cheese (often Stilton) after dinner. This seems to be a uniquely British habit, but it is sensible, for the aromatics in the celery help the digestion of the cheese.
- Celery is a "foundation" vegetable, rather like onions and carrots, and is a useful flavouring in stocks, soups and stews.
- As a vegetable, use the chopped stalks in stir-fries, or braise the hearts to accompany roast game, beef or ham.
- Never throw away the leaves, which can be used as a herb. They contain much of the flavour and can be used fresh or dried. They are very useful for those on low-salt or reduced-salt diets, as they add so much spicy flavour.
- To make your own celery salt, grind the dried leaves with coarse sea salt in a mortar and keep in an airtight jar. Use as a condiment on top of rice, pasta, meat and fish dishes.

CEREAL GRAINS

The word "cereal" comes from Ceres, the Roman goddess of corn. The term is used to describe any grain from a domesticated grass, and includes the Old World grains barley, millet, oats, rice, rye and wheat, and the New World maize and quinoa.

Cereal grains are packed with energy and nutrients for the next generation of plants, and therefore form the chief source of energy (carbohydrate) for the majority of the world's population. Cereal intake decreases in direct proportion to a country's wealth: in China rice, eked out by a few vegetables, forms about 80 per cent of the total energy intake; in richer Britain we eat a lot more animal proteins, and flour and bread provide only about 20 per cent of our daily energy intake.

Cereals also supply protein, although it is incomplete since most lack the essential amino acid lysine. The protein in wheat and rye is gluten, which is stretchable and this enables these grains to be made into a risen bread. Most cereals contain good amounts of B vitamins, potassium, magnesium and phosphorus, with some calcium and iron. Many, however, contain phytic acid which make these minerals unavailable to the body.

Several grains can be sprouted (see Seeds), when their nutrients are increased: these include barley, buckwheat, oats and wheat.

BARLEY
Hordium distichon
Gramineae family

PRINCIPAL NUTRIENTS

Vitamins: B
Minerals: calcium, iron, magnesium, phosphorus, potassium

ALTHOUGH BARLEY grows in many countries and climates, its importance as food has diminished; it is, however, still used in beer and whiskey-making.

Try to buy whole or pot barley; if the husk is removed from the whole grain, as for pearl barley and barley flour, most of the nutrients go as well.

Barley contains a little of the protein gluten, so people who suffer from coeliac disease should avoid it.

- Cook whole barley in a soup.
- Alternatively, cook whole barley in a pilaff (retain the water for soup or stock). Serve with meat or pulse dishes to make the most of the proteins.

BUCKWHEAT
Fagopyrum esculentum
Polygonaceae family

PRINCIPAL NUTRIENTS
Vitamins: B, P
Minerals: copper, magnesium, phosphorus, potassium

Not a true cereal or grain, buckwheat used to be a staple in Brittany and eastern Europe (Russian *blini* are made from buckwheat flour, as are Breton *crêpes*). The flavour is strong and more intense than that of other grains.

Buckwheat is very energising due to its carbohydrate content, while its vitamin P (rutin) fortifies the veins and capillaries and is effective in treating atherosclerosis and high blood pressure. Buckwheat is rich in magnesium as well, so it benefits the intestines and the digestive system in general. Because of this and other minerals and the B vitamins, buckwheat is good for the nervous system, uplifting your spirits. It is also of benefit during pregnancy and the menopause, and helps avoid osteoporosis.

- Cook buckwheat as a pilaff, toasting it first briefly in a frying pan with a little olive oil to bring out the flavour. Add salt, some savoury or thyme and boiling water, and cook slowly for at least 15–20 minutes. Serve with grilled tomatoes, aubergines or courgettes, or with a meat or fish dish. I often add raisins, just as it is finishing cooking, to add more flavour and nutrition.

MAIZE
Zea mays
Gramineae family

PRINCIPAL NUTRIENTS
Vitamins: A, B, C
Minerals: calcium, iron, potassium, zinc

A QUICK-GROWING grass native to South America, maize was introduced into the Old World after Columbus. It is now second only to wheat in its production throughout the world. There are two types of maize (or corn, as it is often called): sweetcorn—corn on the cob, popcorn, baby corn and so on—and field corn, which is tougher and starchier, and is processed into cornflour (cornstarch) and corn oils.

Maize that is yellow contains a little vitamin A; it also provides calcium, iron, potassium, zinc and some vitamins B and C. The protein of maize lacks lysine and tryptophan, which are essential amino acids. Corn on the cob and sweetcorn are rich in fibre and so can help constipation.

Corn kernels start to convert their sugar to starch as soon as the cob is picked, so try to buy cobs as fresh as possible, and refrigerate them to retain their sweetness and vitamin C. Maize kernels can be sprouted, when they increase their content of lysine and tryptophan. The protein value of the sprouts is greater than that of the kernels.

• Boil briefly, to lose as little vitamin C as possible, and serve with meats or other foods rich in vitamin C to make the iron in the sweetcorn more available and useful.

MILLET
Sorghum vulgare
Gramineae family

PRINCIPAL NUTRIENTS
Vitamins: B
Minerals: calcium, iron

A MAIZE-LIKE, quick-growing grass, millet is cultivated all over Africa and South America. Unlike most other grains, it does not absorb water and expand when cooked; its slight crunch makes up for its basic lack of flavour. It is nutritious, though, containing calcium, iron and B vitamins, and is the only grain that contains all eight amino acids.

Millet can be sprouted; the sprouts contain natural oestrogens, so are particularly useful during menopause.

OATS

Avena sativa
Gramineae family

PRINCIPAL NUTRIENTS
Vitamins: B
Minerals: iron, phosphorus, potassium

OATMEAL is higher in both protein and fat than other cereals, so goes rancid quite quickly. Rolled oats (grain that has been crushed and partially cooked) are easier and quicker to cook than oatmeal; the partial cooking also destroys the enzymes which cause rancidity.

Oats are rich in fibre, B vitamins, iron, phosphorus and potassium. They also contain a little of the gluten protein which can cause an allergic reaction, so should be avoided by people who have coeliac disease.

Eat oats with milk, as porridge, which will provide the essential amino acid lysine. Oat bran is said to reduce the levels of cholesterol in the blood, and to act as a protection against some forms of cancer.

Oats can be sprouted, when the B vitamin content increases many times.

QUINOA
Chenopodium quinoa

THIS plant, native to the Andes, is not a true grain. The seeds have an acrid outer layer, removed by a basic processing. Quinoa contains more protein than other grains—around 14–15 per cent, compared to 7.5 per cent for rice. It is easily digested and has a good flavour, if perhaps a little grassy, and can be used instead of rice.

RICE
Oryza sativa
Gramineae family

PRINCIPAL NUTRIENTS
Vitamins: B
Minerals: iron, silicon, calcium, potassium

THE STAPLE FOOD of most of Asia, rice is second only to wheat in world nutritive importance. It has been cultivated since time immemorial in the East, and has been introduced to southern Europe and the Americas.

It is a highly valued carbohydrate food, especially when left whole and brown and therefore containing more dietary fibre. The vitamin B in rice is also at risk from processes such as milling and polishing, and the lack of thiamin (vitamin B1) is responsible for beri-beri, a disease of predominantly rice-eating countries. Although it contains less protein than other cereals, the protein is of a higher quality; it is still incomplete, though, lacking in particular the amino acid lysine (brown rice has 20–25 per cent more lysine than white). Rice is rich in silicon, which plays an important part in the fixing of calcium and magnesium. Rice also contains useful amounts of iron.

People with weak hearts and muscles, and those suffering from general fatigue, should eat whole rice. It is easily digested, and can gently detoxify the body. It also helps to combat the degeneration of arteries—useful in heart disease and for other circulatory problems such as haemorrhoids. Eating rice is important during pregnancy as it helps produce a good flow of milk; it is also a useful ally during the menopause.

- Cook rice with aromatics such as onions and thyme to reinforce the uptake of calcium.
- Serve it with pulses and/or vegetables to maximise the protein uptake, and sprinkle when cooked with grated (Parmesan), and/or ground hazelnuts or walnuts.
- Serve with foods that are rich in vitamin C to maximise the uptake of the iron in the rice.

Rice and Chestnut Pilaff

This is an unusual and interesting combination. Serve as an accompaniment to a meat or vegetarian main dish.

SERVES 4

1 cup dried chestnuts
3 cups whole (brown) rice
salt and freshly ground black pepper

Wash the dried chestnuts thoroughly, then soak them in cold water for 1 hour. Drain well. Cover the chestnuts and rice with fresh cold water in a saucepan and cook gently for an hour. Drain if necessary. Season to taste.

RYE
Secale cereale
Gramineae family

PRINCIPAL NUTRIENTS
Vitamins: B
Minerals: calcium, iron

THIS IS a cold climate cereal: rye breads are characteristic of Scandinavia, northern Germany and Russia. It is also grown and eaten in central France, where people are said to suffer much less from arteriosclerosis and bad circulation because they eat rye bread at every meal. Rye is more difficult for weak stomachs to digest than other cereals, but in bread-making it can be mixed half and half with whole wheat, and digestive seeds or herbs like thyme could also be added.

Rye is a nutritious cereal containing calcium, iron and many B vitamins. An energising drink can be made by gently boiling 30 g (1 oz) rye grains per litre (1 3/4 pints) of water for 10 minutes. When cool, strain, and add some lemon juice and honey. This is good as a gentle laxative, and, according to Dr. Leclerc, for those suffering from internal bleeding.

People with coeliac disease should avoid rye because of gluten content, and go instead for rice or maize.

Rye can be sprouted.

- Eat rye bread or pumpernickel with smoked salmon, caviar, beetroot and a good mixed salad. It goes well with herrings and dill, and an accompanying glass of schnapps or vodka would be good in cold weather!

WHEAT
Triticum ssp
Gramineae family

PRINCIPAL NUTRIENTS
Vitamins: B, E
Minerals: calcium, iron, phosphorus, potassium

MORE WHEAT is grown in the world than any other grain. It is available in many forms, all of which are nutritious to some extent. Flours with more of the original grain or berry (up to 100 per cent) are more nutritious, as they contain the proteins of all three parts of the grain—bran, germ and endosperm. They also contain the vitamins B and E of the germ. The protein of wheat is gluten, which sufferers from coeliac disease should avoid.

Wheat bran is best known for its use as fibre in the treatment of constipation. Wheatgerm is most useful nutritionally for its E content: scatter it on other cereals, or on fruit or yogurt.

Wheat can be sprouted, when the B vitamin content increase many times.

CHAMOMILE
Chaemaemelum nobile/Matricaria chamomilla
Compositae family

THE FLOWERS of chamomile were sacred in Ancient Egypt, and later it was grown in medieval monastery gardens as a medicinal herb. There are two major types grown for therapeutic use: the Roman, sweet or common chamomile *(Chaemaemelum nobile)* and the German variety *(Matricaria chamomilla)*. Both yield essential oils distilled from the freshly dried flowers: that from the German variety is stronger and less acrid.

Therapeutic Uses
The plant is a good tonic, digestive, sedative and antiseptic. Chamomile tisanes relieve headaches, migraines, flu, coughs, facial neuralgia and sinusitis. They are particularly effective before going to bed: chamomile is a digestive and, because of its traces of calcium, relaxing and sleep-inducing.

In the Kitchen
Small sprigs of fresh chamomile can be added to salads, sauces, omelettes or bread doughs. Dry the flowers in the kitchen, hanging them from hooks or a clothes pulley, and they will be ready for medicinal use as needed.

CHEESE

PRINCIPAL NUTRIENTS
Vitamins: A, B, D
Minerals: calcium, phosphorus

THERE ARE THOUSANDS of cheeses made throughout the world, all different in look, taste, texture and smell. It is the smell of a cheese which most interests me. However mild its flavour, a cheese should have its own characteristic smell. Cheeses can be classified into three kinds of "aromas":

1. *Fresh, mild taste and smell* These are mostly fresh, full-fat and soft. They include cream, curd and cottage

cheeses. Some pressed cheeses like Mozzarella smell and taste mild too.

2. *Pronounced flavour and smell* These are ripened cheeses and are very variable in type. They include Camembert and Brie, Pont l'Evêque, Caerphilly and white Cheshire, Emmenthal, Gouda, some semi-dry goat cheeses, Parmesan and Cheddar.

3. *Strong flavour and smell* These too are ripened cheeses, and include Munster, Livarot and some goat cheeses.

Blue cheeses can be either pronounced or strong in aroma and flavour.

In many countries people often buy, store and eat cheese wrongly. Try to buy at a proper cheese shop, where cheeses will be on offer at the right temperature and at the right degree of maturity. You cannot judge a cheese wrapped in tight polythene and sitting under lights in a chill cabinet at the supermarket.

If you can smell the cheese before buying, you will know whether it is at the right stage; and if it is at the right stage, it will be digested more easily. I believe that cheese has acquired a reputation for indigestibility because it is sold and eaten before it is ready. People who suffer from rheumatic complaints are told not to eat cheese or other dairy products because these foods produce acidity, and therefore pain in the joints. This acidity, however, could be due to imperfectly matured cheese. People often complain, too, that their breath smells after eating cheese; this could be the result of imperfect digestion of an unripe cheese.

I also think that cheese is often *eaten* in the wrong way. It is traditionally served towards the end of a meal that may already have been rich in protein, making it far too heavy for the digestion. But if cheese is eaten as a first course, or, even more happily, as the main course, the balance is better. You need nothing more than a salad to accompany it.

Therapeutic Uses

Cheese is an excellent source of complete protein, although it is also high in fat and sodium. Cheddar-type cheeses are a rich source of vitamin A (they are coloured with pigments derived from betacarotene), calcium and phosphorus.

The protein of cheese is of great value, particularly since it is easier to digest (if properly ready to eat) than meat. It is also cheaper than meat, so can benefit those on lower incomes, such as the elderly. The calcium is very important too, and again is useful to the elderly, to those in danger of osteoporosis (menopausal women), to pregnant women and to growing children. But do bear in mind that salmonella and listeria are potential dangers associated with cheeses made from unpasteurised milk, and cheeses of this sort should be avoided by those who are particularly vulnerable—the elderly, the very young and pregnant women (those, ironically, who stand to gain most by eating cheese).

The traditional accompaniments to cheese aid in its digestion: the spicy essential oils of radishes help in the assimilation of fats in cheese, as do the oils in celery, apples and grapes. The *penicillium* bloom on some goat cheeses and on Brie and Camembert, as well as the *penicillium* blue of blue cheeses such as Roquefort, are also aids to digestion, and possess natural antibiotic properties which are good for general health.

Whether a cheese is mature or not, it can still be severely indigestible to a proportion of the population who suffer from lactose intolerance—an inability to digest the sugar in milk. The Chinese, for instance, do not eat dairy products and never have; they are said to dislike the smell of Westerners caused by their intake of dairy products. Soya milk and soya products are their alternative. A yogurt or yogurt "cheese" may be the answer.

In the Kitchen

Most cheeses should be eaten ripe, mature and uncooked. I advocate a day of cheese per week, eating it with salad vegetables and fruit. But of course some cheeses add so much flavour to cooked dishes that they are irresistible. Cheeses should only be cooked very lightly, though, and at the last minute: heat coagulates the protein of cheese, separating it from the fat, which is when it forms strings.

- For a delicious lunch or light supper serve a piece of Brie or a Camembert, or some goat's cheese, with a good crisp fresh salad and some fresh crusty bread.
- Experiment with cheese salads: cubes of firm Emmenthal, for instance, could form the protein element of a mixed salad. Or you could crumble blue cheese into a salad dressing.
- Grate Parmesan over risottos and pasta to add a little protein, lots of calcium (Parmesan has more calcium than any other cheese) and masses of flavour. Try flakes or slivers of Parmesan on carpaccio, thinly sliced raw beef which is a Venetian speciality, or on a green salad such as rocket, dressed with a rich olive oil.
- Grate cheeses into and on to fish or vegetable soups for added health and flavour.
- Slice cheeses such as Cheddar or Emmenthal, place over cooked vegetables and bake or grill briefly to melt (see page 55).
- Add grated semi-hard and hard cheeses at the last minute to white sauces to be used in pasta and vegetable dishes.
- Use cheese as a filling for little filo pastry parcels, pasta (ravioli), tarts or quiches.
- Soft cheeses such as Ricotta can be cooked in cheesecakes and cheese tarts.

Aromatic Cheese on Toast

This is a variation on the traditional British cheese on toast.

PER PERSON

15 g (1/2 oz) butter
a good pinch of fresh herb leaves (thyme, rosemary or tarragon)
1 slice wholemeal bread
50 g (2 oz) Cheddar or other firm cheese

Mix the butter and herbs together and leave for at least an hour, or overnight. (You can make this herb butter in much larger quantities of course, and store it in the fridge or freezer for use in other dishes.)

Toast one side of the bread, then spread the herb butter on the untoasted side. Grate the cheese on top, and grill until brown and sizzling. Use any herb you think will help you.

Country Toast

Another good way of eating cheese, especially for vegetarians.

PER PERSON

about 50 g (2 oz) Brie or Camembert
about 40 g (1 1/2 oz) butter, cream or crème fraîche
1 slice wholemeal bread, toasted
a little coarse salt
5–6 almonds, toasted and finely chopped

Pare the skin carefully off the cheese, and then mix the soft insides with the butter or cream (the proportions should be about half and half). Spread on to the toasted bread, then sprinkle with the salt and chopped almonds. Serve with a salad to make a balanced, easy-to-digest light meal.

CHERRY
Prunus avium/Prunus cerasum
Rosaceae family

PRINCIPAL NUTRIENTS
Vitamins: A, C
Minerals: calcium, iron, magnesium, potassium, sulphur

THERE ARE two main types of cherry, the sweet dessert cherry *(Prunus avium)* and the sour cooking cherry *(Prunus cerasum)*. The lighter coloured cherries are usually sweet, the darker red or black ones sour or bitter (though there are exceptions). Sour cherries are used extensively in the making of liqueurs such as Kirsch and Maraschino.

Therapeutic Uses

Because of their high content of mineral salts, cherries have energising and rejuvenating properties. The vitamin A has a rejuvenating effect on the skin as well. When you are tired, mentally and physically, and your body needs to be detoxified, take nothing but cherries for 2 days: drinking their juice (2–3 glasses per day, made without the stones), and eating them can be a wonderful way to regain lost energy. The traces of cobalt, copper and manganese in cherries have a calming effect on the nervous system, making them a refreshing tonic in cases of anxiety, stress and irritability.

Cherries also help with diabetes and other blood sugar problems. Dr. Leclerc recommends them for rheumatic and arthritic conditions, since they act as a natural blood cleanser. They are good too for constipation, stomach and liver disturbances.

Make a tisane of cherry stalks to combat fluid retention and to help cystitis and other bladder problems. Boil a handful of stalks, about 20 g (3/4 oz) for 5 minutes in 2 pints (1.2 litres) water. Let it stand for 10 minutes, then drink throughout the day, adding a little honey if necessary and a few cherries, too, if you like.

In the Kitchen

As the season is so short, eat cherries every day and at every meal if you can—they are best for health if eaten first thing in the morning. To tell fresh cherries, look at their stalks: they should be green, bending easily and snapping back when released.

- Eat sweet dessert cherries raw for the most nutritive value, and to take full advantage of the vitamin C content.
- Eat raw with cheese, or stone and use in fruit salads or on ice cream.
- Cook sour cherries in sauces to accompany duck and game. This cuts the fattiness.
- Cook cherries in tarts, pies, strudels and cakes.

• Make a cherry liqueur using brandy or vodka, sugar and good ripe red cherries.

CHERVIL
Anthriscus cerefolium
Umbelliferae family

A NATIVE of eastern Europe and western Asia, chervil is now cultivated and grows wild in many parts of Europe. There are several varieties, all of which taste fresh, slightly sweet and aniseed-like.

Therapeutic Uses
Chervil is a potent diuretic, so herbal teas should be drunk often to benefit the circulation and associated problems such as cellulite, haemorrhoids, varicose veins, high blood pressure and the fluid retention of PMT and menopause. This property can also benefit bladder disorders such as kidney stones and cystitis, and liver problems: infuse 10 g (a good 1/4 oz) chervil and 20 g (3/4 oz) lettuce in 500 ml (17 fl oz) boiling water, and drink when cool.

Tisanes are good for the puffiness caused by complaints such as hay fever and colds. The skin can benefit hugely from chervil's gentle antibiotic action: drink tisanes often for internal cleanliness.

In the Kitchen
Grow chervil in your garden and use it often. It does not dry very well.

• One of the French *fines herbes*, chervil can be used fresh as a last-minute garnish for soups and stews, in salads, chopped in sauces (béarnaise and mayonnaise particularly), in egg dishes such as omelettes, and in a herb butter.
• If you can get hold of enough, chervil makes a delicious soup or quiche with Emmenthal cheese.
• A soup made from potatoes and chervil is particularly useful for those suffering from kidney stones. If celery is added—to maximise the effects of the chervil—it benefits cystitis sufferers.
• Add seeds to salads.

CHESTNUT, *see* Nuts

CHICKPEA, *see* Pulses

CHICORY AND ENDIVE
Cichorium spp
Compositae family

PRINCIPAL NUTRIENTS
Vitamins: A, B, C
Minerals: calcium, iron, magnesium, phosphorus, potassium

WHAT THE Americans and French call chicory the British call endive, and vice versa. In Britain chicory is a long, silvery white, compact vegetable, while endive is a frondy, lettuce-like, green salad vegetable. They are closely related.

Endive is said to be one of the bitter herbs of the Bible, originating from Asia; chicory was first formally cultivated in Belgium. There are two types of endive, the frizzy one and the broader-leaved type, once known as batavia or escarole, although this name is now given to types of lettuce. Another close relative is the red lettuce, radicchio.

Therapeutic Uses
Chicory contains B vitamins and small quantities of vitamin C and minerals; endive, being green, contains vitamin A as well. Both are stomachic, lubricant and good for the intestines. They are easy to digest and, when cooked, are particularly good for digestive problems.

In the Kitchen
Keep chicory out of the light and, when cut, either brush it with lemon juice or use it straightaway. Wash endive well, but do not soak, and then drain well.

- Eat both vegetables raw to maximise the nutrients. The bitterness and crunchiness of chicory is particularly delicious in a salad of softer, less bitter leaves.
- Use raw chicory leaves as the decoration around a bowl of salad—perhaps even as crudités with a dip or salsa.

- Bake, steam or braise chicory, and serve with a variety of sauces.

Baked Chicory

Preheat the oven to 180°C/350°F/Gas 4. Trim a head of chicory per person and cut in half lengthways. Place in an ovenproof dish and sprinkle with a good olive oil (I occasionally add a teaspoon or two of honey as well). Bake for 30 minutes, then remove from the oven and cover with a soft cheese such as Boursin. Bake for a few minutes more—or place under a hot grill—until the cheese has just started to melt. Serve as a starter or main course.

CHILLIES, *see* Peppers

CHIVES, *see* Onion

CHOCOLATE
Theobroma cacao
Sterculiaceae family

PRINCIPAL NUTRIENTS
Vitamins: B
Minerals: calcium, copper, iron, potassium

COCOA BEANS contain proteins, fibres, B vitamins (1, 2 and nicotinic acid), and various minerals. Cocoa butter is the third most highly saturated fat after coconut and palm kernel oils (bitter chocolate contains the most), but is cholesterol-free. The oxalic acid content is said to inhibit the absorption of calcium but, if cocoa is made into a milky drink or you eat milk chocolate, the calcium content will outweigh that of the oxalic acid.

Chocolate and cocoa are often implicated in allergic reactions such as facial swelling, migraines, and headaches, heartburn and cold sores.

Therapeutic Uses
Cocoa and chocolate contain several central nervous system stimulants, including caffeine and theobromine—the latter is a muscle stimulant as well. There is some truth in the idea that chocolate can give energy, therefore, but don't eat too much because of the fat and sugar content.

CINNAMON AND CASSIA
Cinnamomum zeylanicum/Cinnamomum cassia
Lauraceae family

BOTH THESE SPICES are the bark of evergreen and aromatic trees or bushes. Cassia originated in Myanmar (Burma), cinnamon in Sri Lanka. Both have a long history of medicinal use, cinnamon being revered by the Chinese, Ancient Egyptians, Greeks and Romans. Both are also available as quills or sticks—rolled up tubes. Cassia is redder in colour and more coarsely pungent than cinnamon.

Therapeutic Uses
The major property of both spices is antiseptic because of their very high phenol content, particularly of eugenol in cinnamon. The oils are distilled from the bark and leaves, and are so strong that their use is officially restricted. This property can be utilised by including quills of either in meat cookery, especially in curries (traditional in India to counter any possible putrefaction). Chewing a piece of cinnamon or cassia is antiseptic for the mouth and freshens the breath.

Use either spice in tisanes to help the symptoms of flu and colds, and to stimulate the digestive system. A cup of hot milk scented with either will ease a cough or sore throat. A fortified wine (Malaga, sherry or port) or a sweet wine infused for a few weeks with cinnamon, plus vanilla and ginseng, is a wonderful "cure" for flu, fatigue or depression.

In the Kitchen
Buy in quill form for the most intense flavour or, if ground, in very small quantities as the aroma soon fades.

• Use either spice whole in marinades, meat and game dishes, stuffings, pickles and relishes.

- Use either spice whole in sweet dishes—stew a little with fruits such as rhubarb or apple, or dried apricots or prunes.
- Use whole as a swizzle stick for hot cocoa or chocolate.
- Ground cinnamon or cassia can be added to cakes, biscuits, breads (sprinkle on hot buttered toast for a delicious and therapeutic teatime treat).
- Use either ground spice to flavour the milk for milk or rice puddings or ice creams (or infuse whole spices in milk).

CLOVE
Eugenia caryophyllata
Myrtaceae family

CLOVES originated in south-east Asia, and are now cultivated in many tropical islands, for the evergreen trees grow best near the sea. It is the flower buds that yield the spice, and their medicinal properties—principally antiseptic because of the high eugenol content—have been acknowledged since ancient times.

Therapeutic Uses
For toothache, suck a clove, holding it over the sore tooth both to clean the area and to relieve pain (cloves have sedative and mild anaesthetic properties). Boil a few cloves in water for a few minutes for an antiseptic mouthwash to combat bad breath and general mouth infection such as gum disease. Use as a gargle to relieve an infected and sore throat.

Cloves also stimulate digestion and restore appetite, so foods cooked with them will help those who are convalescing or anorexic. I believe cloves are a tonic for the whole system, and I suck one when I am feeling low or tired.

The sedative, pain-killing properties of cloves can also be helpful for rheumatism, and to relieve the pains of childbirth. Take in infusion form.

The essential oil is one of the strongest antibacterial oils, and is distilled from the leaves and unripe fruit.

In the Kitchen
Buy cloves whole, or if ground, in very small quantities, as the aroma and essential oils soon fade.

- Use a whole clove to flavour a meat stock or stew (embed it in an onion), and stud a ham joint with cloves before baking.
- Use in cabbage, broccoli and cauliflower dishes to help the digestion.
- Use whole cloves in marinades, chutneys, and bread sauce.
- Add one clove to stewed apple or apple pie, and to an apple sauce for pork.
- Use ground cloves in spiced sweet dessert mixtures such as mincemeat, Christmas puddings, cakes and biscuits.

COCONUT, *see* Nuts

CORIANDER
Coriandrum sativum
Umbelliferae family

THIS IS one of those rare plants that supply both a herb and a spice. Indigenous to south-east Europe and Asia, it has been cultivated for thousands of years. The leaves look like flat-leaf parsley and have a faint anise-like flavour, while the seeds are bitter-sweet with overtones of orange zest.

Therapeutic Uses
Coriander is a digestive and can help restore the appetite, so it is good for anorexia. It is mildly antiseptic, and is used as such with meat in Indian curries. It sweetens the breath, and can relieve headaches and depression. It can also help you to sleep.

An essential oil is distilled from the seeds. It is extremely toxic, so its provenance must be certain and its use limited to the most experienced practitioners.

In the Kitchen
Buy coriander seeds whole, and grind just before use. Toast them in a dry pan first to intensify the flavour. Wash the

leaves well—they are usually rather gritty—and use quickly, as they soon wilt and become smelly.

- Use fresh leaves as a wonderfully aromatic garnish for any meat, poultry or vegetable dish that is remotely exotic or Eastern.
- Use fresh leaves in an Indian coriander "chutney", in Mexican salsas, in guacamole (see page 17) or in meatballs.
- Use coriander with pulse dishes (lentils, beans and so on), to help their digestion: add ground seeds during cooking, fresh leaves at the end.
- Use the whole seeds, slightly bruised, in stocks, marinades, chutneys and relishes, or with braised celery or carrot; garnish with fresh leaves.
- Use the leaves and seeds in mushroom dishes to give a wonderful flavour and to help digestion of the mushrooms.
- Grind the seeds and use in meat stews, curries, kebab marinades and soups.
- Mix ground seeds into a bread dough for an unusual flavour.
- Chew coriander seeds after eating garlic to sweeten your breath.

COURGETTE, *see* Marrow and Courgette

CRANBERRY, *see* Bilberry

CUCUMBER
Cucumis sativus
Cucurbitaceae family

PRINCIPAL NUTRIENTS
Vitamins: A, C
Minerals: calcium, iron, magnesium, phosphorus, potassium

CUCUMBERS belong to the same family as squashes, marrows, courgettes and melons, and are perhaps the most mild-tasting and watery of all. There are two types: the familiar hothouse or frame cucumber, and the ridge cucumber which can be grown outside. (Gherkins are a type of ridge cucumber, plucked small for pickling.)

Therapeutic Uses

Cucumbers are some 96 per cent water, so are not rich in any vitamins or minerals. However, the essential oils make that water a good blood purifier, so the vegetable is useful in the treatment of arthritic conditions and gout. A famous Swiss naturopath, Dr. Kousmine, recommends cucumber for people who suffer from intestinal bacteria and bladder irritation. Cucumbers are diuretic, but some people find them indigestible and they can cause wind.

In the Kitchen

Try to eat cucumber as fresh as possible, and unpeeled (preferably, if organic). Do not store it in the fridge. Remove any seeds from older fruit.

- Eat raw, sliced, grated or diced, in salads.
- Use in chunks as a crudité with dips.
- Slice very thinly and use in those most British of sandwiches, with a drop of a pungent vinegar and some salt and pepper.
- Mix cubes of cucumber with yogurt and mint for a delicious and nutritious salad, good to cool down a curry-heated mouth.
- Use scooped-out cucumber as a container for a salsa, a dip, taramasalata, hummus or similar foods.
- Cucumber can be used in cold soups—with tomatoes and peppers in gazpacho, for instance.

CUMIN
Cuminum cyminum
Umbelliferae family

RELATED to dill, fennel and coriander, cumin is native to Egypt but is now grown in many hot countries. The seeds, the only part used, look like caraway but there is no resemblance in flavour. Cumin was cultivated by the Ancient

Egyptians, Greeks and Romans, and was used in biblical times as an antiseptic.

Therapeutic Uses
Cumin makes a good general tonic, digestive, antiseptic and antibacterial. It is also good for cellulite: drink a tisane of the seeds to galvanise the circulation and tissues.

An essential oil is distilled from the seeds.

In the Kitchen
Buy the spice as seeds and ground, as the seeds are difficult to grind smooth at home—but buy ground in small quantities only. Toast the seeds in a dry pan before use to bring out the flavour. Cumin is used extensively in Indian, North African and Middle Eastern cuisines.

- Use the seeds, whole or ground, in curries or spicy meat stews. Sprinkle over lamb to be barbecued, or add to kebab mixtures.
- Use the sweetness of cumin to balance the heat in a dish like chilli con carne (cumin is included in many commercial chilli powders and seasonings).
- Season cooked Eastern-type salads of tomatoes, green peppers, courgettes or aubergines with powdered cumin and other spices such as chilli or coriander.
- Roll small balls of cream cheese or goat's cheese in cumin seeds.
- Use the seeds in pickles and other preserves.

CURRANTS, BLACK, RED AND WHITE
Ribes ssp
Saxifrageae family

PRINCIPAL NUTRIENTS
Vitamins: A, C
Minerals: calcium, phosphorus, potassium

CURRANTS are native to cool, moist parts of the northern hemisphere, red *(Ribes ribrum)* and black *(Ribes nigrum)* growing wild in Europe and Asia. The French turn their blackcurrants into a cordial called cassis or Kir.

Redcurrants (and white, which are a variety of red) are slightly sweeter than black, but blackcurrants are richer nutritionally: they have twice as much vitamin A and five times as much vitamin C (200 mg per 100 g/4 oz).

Currants are often implicated in allergy reactions such as hives and stomach upsets.

Therapeutic Uses: Blackcurrants

These are described by Dr. Leclerc and Dr. Dextrait (another well-known French phytotherapist) as a fortifier of the glandular system and stimulant of the spleen and liver. In large quantities they encourage sweating. A blackcurrant extract recently produced in Sweden is proving effective as an antidote to diarrhoea.

Blackcurrants have long been used to cure sore throats and ailments such as tonsillitis. Suck the fruits slowly when they are in season. I find this particularly useful for the throat irritation caused by hay fever. (See also Blackberry for a useful syrup.)

The leaves can be used in tea for gout, arthritis and rheumatic and kidney conditions, to get rid of uric acid in the system. This tea also benefits women suffering menopausal symptoms as it calms the circulation and palpitations.

Therapeutic Uses: Redcurrants

These have a high sugar content as well as traces of malic, citric and tartaric acids (hence their culinary use as a souring agent). They are alkalinising, diuretic and slightly laxative, and help with rheumatic and digestive problems. To prevent viral infections such as flu or cystitis, juice the fruit and dilute half and half with mineral water. This is also very beneficial for the gums and teeth.

In the Kitchen

Eat currants raw and use in cooking as much as possible during their very short season. If cooked, currants lose a proportion of their vitamin C.

- Eat raw, sugared if you like, with cream, or use in fruit salads, or as garnishes for both savoury and sweet dishes.

- Cook very lightly with other soft fruits to make the classic English Summer Pudding.
- Bake in tarts, pies and puddings.
- Make into jams and jellies: currants are high in pectin and acid, and they also contain lots of juice. They can be sweet enough to use as a conserve or glaze for a fruit tart, but are also tart enough to use in meat and game cookery—redcurrant jelly accompanies game, turkey and lamb, and is an essential ingredient in Cumberland sauce.
- If you have a lot of blackcurrants, make them into a homemade crème de cassis: *Jane Grigson's Fruit Book* has a wonderful recipe. This or bought cassis can be used in cooking for flavour.

CURRANTS, DRIED, *see* Grape

DAIKON, *see* Radish

DAIRY PRODUCTS

PRINCIPAL NUTRIENTS
Vitamins: A, B, D
Minerals: calcium, iodine, manganese, phosphorus, potassium, zinc

THIS ENTRY includes milk and all its products except cheese, which has a separate entry. No dairy products are aromatic, but they are prime sources of the B vitamins, calcium and the elusive vitamin D. They may also contain iodine. Intake must be moderate, though, as these foods are high in saturated fatty acids. They are easy to digest, although many people have a metabolic intolerance (see next page and page 242). Some babies react to cows' milk; if so, use an alternative like goat or soya (useful also for vegans).

Milk skimmed of its fat still contains all its other nutrients, particularly calcium. The fat is made into butter and cream. Their flavour is valuable in cooking, and sometimes there is no real alternative.

Therapeutic Uses: Milk

There is some evidence that milk drunk in infancy and childhood can help prevent osteoporosis. It also has a reputation for calming digestive problems such as ulcers and gastritis (probably because of the calcium content), and a milky drink at night is sedative.

Therapeutic Uses: Cultured Milk Products

Cultured milk products such as yogurt, buttermilk and soured cream are fermented, their lactose or milk sugars having been digested by bacteria; these produce lactic acid which thickens and flavours the milk. In terms of vitamins and minerals these cultured milks are much the same as ordinary milk, but the bacteria appear to be beneficial in a number of ways as yet not properly understood. For instance, research has shown that cholesterol levels are low in people who consume a lot of natural fermented milks; as milk, particularly full-fat, could actually contribute to cholesterol levels, this effect may be due to the bacteria. There is some evidence too that those who cannot consume milk or milk products because of lactose intolerance can actually take yogurts; some of these, through bacterial action, may supply the enzyme needed to digest lactose.

Yogurt eaten with a curry can take away some of its heat; as can lassi, the Indian yogurt drink. Yogurt or buttermilk should be eaten after a course of antibiotics to re-establish the beneficial bacteria.

Home-made Fromage Frais

Bring 2 litres (3 1/2 pints) whole, full-fat milk to the boil, then add the juice of 1 lemon. Stir well and continuously: and the milk should curdle, separating into curds and whey. Suspend a large piece of muslin over a bowl and pour the curds and whey into it: cover with a plate to weight it down, and as the whey drips out the curds will become thicker and cheese-like. Leave to drain for at least 2 hours. Chill.

Either serve as it is, in dollops, or press into little moulds and eat with fruit as a dessert. Alternatively flavour with crushed garlic, chopped parsley and/or chives, or roll balls of it in coarsely crushed black pepper, paprika or chopped herbs. Choose the herb to suit your therapeutic needs as well as your palate.

Serve with toasted rye or pumpernickel. This, with a salad, makes a deliciously healthy, cheap meal. A good salad to accompany it would be chicory, sliced apples and red peppers for colour.

You could add fresh cream to the fromage frais to enrich the flavour (but it pushes up the fat content). You could also make a similar "cheese" with home-made yogurt.

Cultured Milk Products in the Kitchen

- Use yogurt and buttermilk instead of cream in stews and sauces—add at the last moment, though, and off the heat, or they will curdle.
- A cold reduced-fat sauce is excellent for vegetables: make a French dressing in the proportion of 1 teaspoon cider vinegar or lemon juice to 1 tablespoon olive oil, mix in a handful of chopped herbs according to preference and medical need, and just before serving mix in a tablespoon of natural yogurt and seasoning to taste.

DATE
Phoenix dactylifera
Palmae family

PRINCIPAL NUTRIENTS
Vitamins: A, B
Minerals: calcium, iron, magnesium, phosphorus, potassium

THE DATE is one of the world's oldest known fruits, growing in hot, dry, subtropical regions, especially in North Africa and the Middle East where it is an important foodstuff. Palm hearts are often used for distilling the fiery liquor called arrack.

Therapeutic Uses

We need 0.9 mg of iron per day. Since 100 g (4 oz) of dried dates contain 1.6 mg of iron, they are an easy source of iron for vegetarians or those who are anaemic, or lacking in iron.

The high magnesium content is a result of the arid growing conditions. The palm tree's roots take up water from far underground, which includes magnesium salts. Our daily requirement of magnesium is some 100-250 mg: 100 g (4 oz) of dried dates contain a useful 59 mg. Magnesium is one of the heart's three principal nutrients and helps to combat tiredness and fatigue. The high sugar and energy content (some 248 calories per 100 g/4 oz of dried dates) is also a factor here.

Vitamin B1 helps the regeneration of nerve cells, while the phosphorus in dates stimulates the nervous system.

In the Kitchen

Dates are available in Europe in three forms: as fresh fruit (brown, unwrinkled and shiny); as semi-dry fruit (brown, wrinkled and sticky); and as dried blocks. I think the fresh are the best, but many of the nutrients are concentrated when the fruit is partially or wholly dried.

- Eat fresh or semi-dry dates whole, as they are, or stone, chop and add to fruit or vegetable salads, muesli, yogurt and so on.
- Fill whole stoned dates with marzipan, nuts or cream cheese and serve as hors d'oeuvres or petits fours.
- Add pieces of whole or block date to bread, cakes, biscuits and puddings. There are a wealth of such recipes in the English tradition.
- Use whole dates in meat stuffings, or in North African or Middle Eastern stews.
- Try to eat dates with meat or with foods rich in vitamin C, so that the iron is more easily absorbed by the body (see also Plum).

DILL
Anethum graveolens
Umbelliferae family

NATIVE to southern Europe and Russia, dill is related to fennel, caraway, cumin and coriander. In Ancient Egypt it was regarded as a vegetable, a condiment and a drug. The Greeks used it medicinally and Hippocrates recommended it for epilepsy.

No aromatherapeutic oil is derived from dill. The plant itself, however, contains some 60 per cent carvone. Scientific research has confirmed that this substance is powerfully digestive, stimulating and releasing gastric juices.

Therapeutic Uses

Dr. Leclerc prescribed dill for hiccups: chew the seeds or drink a dill tisane and the hiccups will stop immediately.

Dill is the major ingredient of the gripe water used as a digestive soother for babies. Bruise some seeds and steep in hot water. Strain, then sweeten with a little honey if liked, and give in teaspoonsful to colicky babies. For adult insomnia due to indigestion boil 1 teaspoon dill seeds, 1/2 teaspoon angelica seeds and 2 tablespoons lime flowers in 1 litre (1 3/4 pints) water for 10 minutes. Strain, allow to cool a little, then drink.

If someone tends to vomit too easily, dill is a good remedy. And if you want to stop someone snoring, give them a cup of dill seed and herb tea before they go to bed.

Dill also helps to combat fluid retention. In parsnip soup, for instance, it reinforces the vegetable's diuretic properties, and is therefore effective against cystitis and other bladder infections. The essential oil in dill also acts as a natural cleanser and bactericide, and helps get rid of the infection quickly. Use in leek, celery and potato soup as well.

In the Kitchen

All parts of the plant are aromatic, with a sharp but sweet mint/aniseed taste. The leaves are gentler in flavour.

- Cook seafood with fresh dill or "cure" salmon with dill, sugar and salt for gravlax. Add to any fish marinade and to pickled fish.
- When roasting chicken, push sprigs of dill inside the bird and under the skin.
- Add fresh dill to boiled potatoes or other vegetable dishes, to sauces (good in soured cream, or a white dill sauce similar to parsley sauce). Chicory baked with dill, coarse salt and olive oil is delicious.
- Scatter fresh leaves over cucumber, potato or celery and apple salads.
- Blend with cream cheese for a sandwich filling or dip, or use in a herb butter.
- Add the seeds to bread doughs (along with aniseed, caraway and coriander seeds if you like), or to meat stews, rice dishes, braised cabbage or cooked root vegetables. All will be easier to digest.
- Use when pickling small cucumbers. Dill accelerates the diuretic effect of the cucumber, which is most effective for those trying to lose weight. Try pickled cauliflower with dill as well.

DULSE, *see* Seaweeds

EGGS, *see* Meat, Poultry and Fish

ENDIVE, *see* Chicory and Endive

FENNEL
Foeniculum vulgare/dulce
Umbelliferae family

PRINCIPAL NUTRIENTS
Vitamins: A, B
Minerals: iron, phosphorus, potassium, zinc

FENNEL is native to southern Europe, but has spread to many other parts of the world. The herb and spice fennel is a relative of the vegetable developed in Italy, Florence or bulb fennel *(Foeniculum* var *dulce)*; the leaves and seeds of this plant can also be used as herb and spice. All parts of both plants, apart from the root, have a sweet anise flavour.

Therapeutic Uses

Like its close relative, dill, fennel has long been associated with good digestion. It is often used in gripe waters for babies, and in Indian *paan*. For a digestive and pick-me-up tea, boil 1 coffeespoon seeds per cup of water or milk for 2 minutes, then infuse for 10 minutes. Drink 2–3 cups per day. This tea also benefits ailments such as gastritis and enteritis.

For lack of appetite, general fatigue, fluid retention and bladder infections such as cystitis, macerate 60–80 g (2 1/2–3 oz) bruised seeds in a bottle of good red wine for 10 days. Drink a wineglass of this mixture twice a day or, for fluid retention and bladder infections, after every meal.

After eating garlic, chew 1/4 teaspoon of the seeds slowly to aid digestion, to sweeten the breath, to whiten your teeth and clean your gums. Raw bulb fennel eaten slowly will also do wonders for your gums.

Fennel was believed by the Greeks to be a slimming herb, and herb and bulb are both diuretic. But eat raw fennel with care: it can act as a stimulant in small doses and slow down the heart and respiration in high doses. In small quantities, fennel is good for anaemia and for the heart and muscles— tisanes act as stimulant tonics for athletes and convalescents. They can also help headaches.

In the Kitchen

Grow herb fennel or, less productively, bulb fennel, in the garden—it is very tall—and pluck the leaves when needed; save the seeds after the plant has flowered.

• Fennel is the fish herb *par excellence.* Use in fish soups, and with oily fish such as sardines. Boil crayfish and other seafood with lots of fennel. Use the seeds in stock. Tuck a few dried stalks under fish or meat to be roasted, or burn them on the barbecue. Serve raw fennel bulb as a salad to accompany fish.

- Add sprigs of herb or slices of bulb fennel to salads, soups and cooked vegetable dishes. The flowers can be eaten too.
- Add chopped herb to sauces for vegetables (great with asparagus), or mayonnaise, French dressing, béarnaise and so on.
- Add fennel seeds to cucumber salads, or mix with cream cheese. Eat seeds with cheese to help you digest it.
- Steam or braise fennel bulb (with asparagus, perhaps) and coat in a white or cheese sauce made with lots of nutmeg or parsley. Serve with brown rice.
- Add the seeds to bread and biscuit doughs and to sausage mixtures.
- Toast the seeds and use in meat or poultry curries and Greek-style pork dishes.
- Put seeds in a pepper mill and grind over meat stews, fish or pulse dishes to make them more digestible.
- Add 100 g (4 oz) crushed fennel seeds to 1 litre (1 3/4 pints) vodka and leave in the dark for at least a month, shaking from time to time. Drink as a digestive in a small glass, or add to recipes for cakes, bread or fish.
- Make a soup to treat PMT fluid retention: cook equal quantities of asparagus, parsley and fennel in a mixture of water and milk until soft, then purée. Season to taste.
- Eat fennel with beans, cabbage or turnips to help in their digestion.

FIG
Ficus carica
Moraceae family

PRINCIPAL NUTRIENTS
Vitamins: A, B, C
Minerals: calcium, iron, magnesium, phosphorus, potassium, zinc

THE MANY VARIETIES of fig tree are probably native to eastern Asia. It is a very ancient fruit which has always been grown for eating, but is also used in making wines and liqueurs. In North Africa today, a fig alcohol, which burns the throat, is made.

Figs in Britain are parthenocarpic, which means they can fruit without being pollinated. The best eating variety, the Smyrna, requires pollination by a fig wasp.

Figs can be dried, when their nutrients are concentrated. They have a higher content of calcium, magnesium and potassium than any other dried fruit.

Therapeutic Uses
Plato called figs the philosopher's friend as they are said to strengthen the nervous system and brain. The Greeks also used them for asthma and depression. The famous medical School of Salerno described the fruit as a meal in itself: 100 g (4 oz) fresh figs contain 100 calories; 10 g (40 oz) dried figs contain 213.

Figs are also effective for all respiratory conditions, such as coughs, sore throats and lung problems. They are also a very good intestinal stimulant and remedy for constipation because of the indigestible food fibre they contain, lignin, and the protein-dissolving enzyme, ficin. Dried figs are particularly effective. Leave 6 in warm water to cover overnight. Eat for breakfast in the morning, and drink the liquid.

Mouth ulcers, abscesses, stomatitis and gingivitis can all benefit from figs. This may be related to their high calcium content—ounce for ounce, dried figs contain more calcium than milk.

A tisane made of fresh fig leaves can help bring on a late period and calm menstrual pains. Because of their high iron content, dried figs should be eaten by those suffering from dysmenorrhoea and anaemia.

In the Kitchen
Fresh figs have a very short season, but as seasons vary around the world they can be found most of the time. Eat as often as you can for most benefit, or eat them dried—but beware, for these contain 50 per cent sugar.

- For a healthy fruit juice mix 1 kg (2 1/4 lb) figs, 10 juniper berries, slightly crushed, and 8 litres (14 pints) mineral

water. Let stand for 7 days, then strain, bottle and cork.
Wait for another week before using.

- Alternate fresh figs in season with fresh dates for the
  highest benefit from both fruit.
- Eat figs raw as a dessert with yogurt. Peel only if the skin
  is tough. Alternatively poach gently in sugar syrup or
  wine.
- Use small chunks of fresh figs in salads, or halve or slice
  and serve interlaced with Parma or a similar ham. Garnish
  with salad leaves, rocket or lamb's lettuce.
- Stew figs, fresh or dried, with meats such as duck, or add
  to curries, for their tenderising effect.
- Cook hare and other game meats with figs, wine, juniper
  berries and thyme for a delicious healthy casserole. Eat
  with new potatoes.
- Poach with other dried fruit.
- Make fresh or dried figs into jams.
- Chop dried figs and use in cakes or puddings.

FISH, *see* Meat, Poultry and Fish

GARLIC
Allium sativum
Liliaceae family

PRINCIPAL NUTRIENTS
Vitamins: B, C
Minerals: iodine, iron, magnesium, manganese, phosphorus, potassium, selenium, sulphur, zinc

THOUGHT to have originated in Asia, garlic is now grown all
over the world in warm climates. It was used by the ancient
Egyptians to stave off the recurring threat of epidemic, as it
was later used in pomanders in fourteenth-century Europe to
keep plague at bay. Garlic juice acted as an antiseptic during
the First World War. In the intervening years herbalists,
homeopaths and nutritionists have sung its medicinal
praises, and it is now a frequent ingredient even in British
cookery!

Therapeutic Uses

Garlic is packed full of nutrients, particularly vitamins B1, B6 and C, iron and phosphorus. It also contains sulphur compounds, which are responsible for its distinctive taste and odour and many of its therapeutic properties.

If eaten regularly, garlic can prevent infections such as colds and flu; if you are already infected garlic can help drive them away. Because it helps to loosen mucus it is also very helpful in respiratory and lung disorders; it "cleans" your lungs when you have a cough, bronchitis, hay fever and similar ailments.

Garlic is good for circulatory problems because of its iodine content (utilised by the thyroid gland). It can therefore aid anyone with an underactive thyroid gland, those who suffer from poor circulation, fluid retention and cellulite, and people who are overweight. It also benefits sufferers from arthritis and many rheumatic conditions.

Garlic has recently been undergoing considerable investigation by conventional medicine. A number of studies have shown that it seems to increase the activity of anti-clotting substances in blood, and also to lower blood pressure. Garlic has been put forward as the reason why the French do not suffer from ischaemic heart disease as much as do, say, the Scots.

The smell of garlic cooking stimulates the gastric juices, so it is digestive as well as aperitive. However, many people cannot happily digest it. If you want to benefit from garlic but belong in this category, try crushing two cloves and leaving them in boiled water overnight. Strain and drink the liquid the next morning.

In the Kitchen

Keep garlic in a dark, cool, airy place (not in the fridge) to prevent it drying or sprouting. When it sprouts, the bulk of the sulphur compounds go into the new growth and the flesh in the cloves becomes milder. Any sprouts, internal or external, must be removed as they are very bitter. Cut the clove in half and remove the centre green core.

If you want to lessen the impact of garlic in cooking, keep

it as whole as possible: it is the crushing of the flesh that releases most of the sulphur compounds, and thus the flavour and aroma. Eating garlic raw is the most therapeutic way, but is unattractive to many people. Cooking it destroys some of the nutrients, including the sulphur compounds, which makes cooked garlic much milder in flavour than raw. Diallyl disulphide is excreted in perspiration, and from the lungs, which is why garlic-eaters' breath smells so strong. To sweeten the breath, chew cardamom seeds, cloves, parsley or coffee beans.

- Crush peeled cloves and mix with softened butter or olive oil and chopped parsley and chill overnight (well covered, or everything else will smell of garlic). Spread on slit baguettes and bake to make the familiar "garlic bread", or spread on pieces of wholemeal toast along with more parsley. This makes a good starter and is a delicious way of eating garlic for the most sensitive of stomachs.
- Use the above garlic butter (with the parsley too, if you like) as a garnish for fish, chicken or cooked vegetables, to add both flavour and health. It is wonderful spread on large flat mushrooms, then baked.
- Add crushed garlic to mayonnaise, or mix with yogurt, cream, cottage cheese or cream cheese for dips.
- Sprinkle raw, over cooked vegetables.
- Put crushed or halved garlic cloves in olive oil and leave overnight (or longer). Strain the oil and use in salad dressings and for cooking.
- Bake garlic cloves whole in meat dishes, especially roast lamb.

Garlic Gâteau with Red Pepper Coulis

SERVES 4

3 red peppers
salt and freshly ground black pepper
2 large garlic bulbs (not cloves)
1 medium potato, peeled
600 ml (1 pint) milk (cow's, almond or soya)

3 eggs, beaten
1 large tablespoon cottage cheese
freshly grated nutmeg

For the coulis, halve and seed the peppers, then steam for 30 minutes. Remove the skin and liquidise the flesh for a few seconds. Season lightly.

Preheat the oven to 190°C/375°F/Gas 5. Peel the garlic and potato and steam for 15 minutes. Mash to a purée. Add the milk, eggs, cheese and nutmeg to taste, and mix well. Spoon into individual ramekins, and bake in a bain-marie for about 10–15 minutes or until set.

Pour the cold coulis over the top of the hot gâteau in the ramekins, and serve immediately.

Sage and Garlic Soup

This soup is good for people suffering from joint problems such as arthritis, and can be calming, too, because of the sage.

SERVES 4–6

8 large garlic cloves, peeled
1.5 litres (3 pints) water
100 g (4 oz) vermicelli or millet
salt and freshly ground black pepper
7–8 large fresh sage leaves, finely cut
2 tablespoons extra virgin olive oil
50 g (2 oz) Parmesan cheese, grated

Place the garlic and water in a pan, bring to the boil and simmer for 20–25 minutes. Add the vermicelli or millet, and season to taste. Simmer for a further 10 minutes, then add the sage leaves.

Remove the garlic from the liquid. Crush to a paste with the olive oil. Remove the soup from the heat and stir in the garlic paste. Serve hot, sprinkled with the cheese.

GINGER
Zingiber officinalis
Zingiberaceae family

ONE OF the most familiar of spices, ginger is a tropical plant whose underground rhizomes are the parts valued. Used for thousands of years in cookery and medicine it was introduced to Europe by the Romans. Its peppery, aromatic heat is greatly appreciated in many dishes and cures.

Therapeutic Uses
The essential oils of fresh ginger stimulate the gastric juices and so facilitate digestion. Make ginger tea after a heavy meal instead of coffee. Put a few slices of root ginger into a teapot and pour boiling water over it. Leave to infuse for a few minutes, then serve, with honey if liked, and a mint leaf floating on top.

The oils are also antibacterial, so are useful in a lot of meat and poultry cookery. The pepperiness of ginger is warming, so it is good for winter colds, coughs and sore throats. Boil a few slices of fresh root ginger in water, add some honey, and gargle with the mixture when cold. Use slices of fresh ginger in warming drinks; infuse with marjoram and rosemary for colds and rheumatism.

An extremely hot, strong essential oil is distilled from the rhizomes.

In the Kitchen
The spice is available as fresh root, dried root (this needs to be bruised before use), powdered, crystallised in sugar, pickled and stored in a strong spirit or sherry.

* Use fresh ginger, grated or diced, in meat and poultry curries, stews, vegetable and cheese dishes, stir-fries and soups.
* Include fresh ginger in pickles and jams (add rum, honey and lemon to the latter).
* Use preserved ginger and its syrup in desserts, biscuits, cakes and puddings.

- Use ground ginger in gingerbread, bread, cakes, biscuits and milk puddings.
- Sprinkle ground ginger on fruit dishes such as rhubarb, stewed apple or fresh melon.

GINSENG
Panax ginseng
Araliaceae family

GINSENG, the root of a plant cultivated in Korea, China and Russia, looks like a yellow radish. It has been revered for thousands of years in the East, where it is used as a tonic, an aphrodisiac, and in the treatment of anaemia, diabetes, insomnia and neurosis.

Korean ginseng *(Panax ginseng)* is reputed to be the best. Siberian ginseng, *Eleutherococcus senticosus*, is from the same family but of a different genus. The roots are dried, to be either chewed or ground up to make powders or capsules.

Therapeutic Uses
Ginseng is famed in many ways because it is what has been christened an "adaptogen". Active constituents within the roots act as a stress inhibitor and enhance physical and mental capabilities, apparently through hormonal stimulation. Ginseng also helps combat mental tension and stress, tiredness and fatigue. Simmer roots of Korean ginseng in water in a double boiler for about 6 hours, very slowly, and drink the water in the morning. Alternatively you could steep 2 Korean ginseng roots in a bottle of whiskey (vodka or wine): leave for about 2 weeks and drink a small glass of this when you feel tired—it will energise you right to your fingertips.

Hormone-like substances within the root contribute to ginseng's efficacy when taken during the menopause, but this may also be due to its "adaptogen" property, allowing the woman to adapt more easily to the physical and mental aspects of her new state. Sexual anxiety may be minimised in the same way, which is why ginseng has a reputation as an aphrodisiac (the wine above is good). Interestingly, the

Chinese tend to use ginseng as an aphrodisiac for men; they use angelica root for women.

I also use ginseng in a syrup, taken in hot drinks in winter to prevent chest infections.

In the Kitchen

Ginseng is not eaten except by the Chinese (usually in soup), or in supplement form. I enjoy it, as the Koreans do, in the form of tea, which is stimulating and warming.

Ginseng Soup with Miso

A wonderful combination of ginseng pick-me-up and general tonic, with the nutrition of miso (fermented soy sauce). Have a bowl or cup when you need to concentrate or to top up your energy levels.

SERVES 2

1 medium Korean ginseng root
350–400 ml (12–14 fl oz) still mineral water
a scant tablespoon miso
1 tablespoon chopped parsley, chervil or coriander

VEGETABLE SOUP BASE

25 g (1 oz) each of very finely diced carrot, onion, parsnip and leek
1 teaspoon sesame oil
120 ml (4 fl oz) still mineral water

Put the ginseng in the top of a double boiler with the water and cook very slowly, covered, for 5–6 hours. The liquid will reduce to about half. Strain this "ginseng essence."

Fry the vegetables for the soup base in the oil for a minute or so to brown a little, then add the water and cook until still crisp. Add the ginseng liquid, the miso and chopped herbs, and serve hot.

GRAPE
Vitis vinefera
Ampelidae family

PRINCIPAL NUTRIENTS

Vitamins: B, C
Minerals: calcium, copper, iodine, iron, phosphorus, potassium

THE EUROPEAN grape vine is one of the oldest cultivated plants. There are many varieties of grape, roughly divided into two groupings, wine grapes and dessert grapes. The former are red, black or white, and tend to be smaller than those bred for the table; their skins are tough. Grapes are also dried to produce currants, raisins and sultanas.

Grapes played a huge part in my life, as I was brought up in wine-making country, near Cahors. For us children the *vendange* or harvest was the time for *resinet*: some of the leftover grape juice would be boiled to make a delicate-flavoured and delicious jelly. It was used in both food and drink, and medicinally: we were given a teaspoon of it for a sore throat, and some mixed with hot wine when we had a chill.

Therapeutic Uses

Grapes contain nutrients in small quantities, but some of them, notably iron, are concentrated when they are dried. The vitamin C of the fresh grape disappears, of course.

The principal therapeutic properties of grapes lie in treating loss of energy, tiredness and fatigue; they are one of the best tonic fruits for the nervous system. These abilities are due to a substance called oenocyanine, which combines with tannin, and works with glucose and levulose, to give energy.

Drs Leclerc, Moreigne and Rathery, French phytotherapists, say that grapes should be prescribed for dyspepsia, constipation, haemorrhoids, liver problems, fluid retention, gout, arthritis, allergies, tuberculosis, diabetes, heart problems (grape nutrients nourish the muscles of the heart), and for cleansing and detoxifying the blood.

In the Kitchen

Grapes are rarely used in cooking. It is best to eat them raw, on their own or as suggested below.

- Eat grapes with cheese for a healthy and tasty combination. Walnuts or other nuts go well too.
- Add grapes to salads, both savoury and sweet.
- Use grapes, skinned if possible, to fill a pastry flan case.
- Add currants, sultanas and raisins when baking (no British fruitcake or Christmas pudding can exist without them); plump them up in a little water, fruit juice, tea, wine or spirit first.
- Add raisins or sultanas to salads, to pilaffs of grain, or sprinkle them on yogurt or cereals.
- Eat some vitamin C-rich foods with dried grapes to assist in the assimilation of their iron.
- Eat dried grapes as an energising snack—they contain easily absorbable fruit sugars. These sugars have an alkaline reaction and neutralize the acids formed in the body by other foods such as meat and eggs.
- Use dried grapes as an alternative sweetener.

GRAPEFRUIT
Citrus paradisi
Rutaceae family

PRINCIPAL NUTRIENTS
Vitamins: A, B, C, E, P
Minerals: calcium, iron, magnesium, phosphorus, potassium

THE GRAPEFRUIT is a comparatively new member of the orange family, and after the orange and lemon is the most widely grown citrus fruit in the world. The mineola is a grapefruit/tangerine cross while the ugli fruit is an orange/grapefruit cross.

Therapeutic Uses
The vitamin C content helps all the same ailments as oranges (see page 129). Grapefruit are good for fortifying the

lungs and for detoxifying the body (thus all the grapefruit-based dietary regimes). They stimulate the appetite, releasing gastric juices and bile. Taken in the morning, fresh grapefruit acts as a diuretic and blood cleanser.

In the Kitchen

Do not cut, segment or juice grapefruit too long before use, as the vitamin C content will diminish.

- Eat raw in segments or from the halved skin for breakfast.
- Juice and drink a glass before every meal for maximum benefit.
- Grill a half grapefruit, sweetened with a little honey, for a delicious and healthy starter at dinner.
- Eat grapefruit before or after a meal which contains meat, both to assist in digesting the fat in the meat and to help absorb the iron in it.
- Use segments in fruit and savoury salads (it is particularly good with lettuce and avocado), or in any of the suggestions for oranges on pages 130–131.

GUAVA
Psidium guajava
Myrtaceae family

PRINCIPAL NUTRIENTS

Vitamins: A, B, C
Minerals: calcium, iron, phosphorus, potassium

GUAVAS are tropical fruit of trees related to the clove, all-spice berry and eucalyptus trees. They have a pervasive muskiness which can smell sweet and fragrant to some, but to others as if a tomcat had left its scent!

Inside the thin skins, the flesh is divided into a shell (next to the skin and where the flavour lies) and a pulpy middle full of seeds. All of the fruit is edible, including the seeds.

Therapeutic Uses

The vitamin C content is higher than that of blackcurrants and citrus fruit (250–300 mg per 100 g/4 oz), so it is important for mouth and skin problems, infections, stress and so on.

The tannin-rich skins are very astringent and are used in the Far East to treat diarrhoea; the ripe fruit, conversely, can be used as a laxative. In general, the guava is a fruit that benefits digestive, intestinal and liver problems.

In the Kitchen
Try to eat guavas raw and ripe in order to retain the vitamin C. Eat when the skin gives to gentle pressure.

- Cut ripe guavas in half and eat the flesh with a spoon.
- Add peeled slices to fruit salads.
- Add a few slices, along with a cinnamon stick, to Bramley apples when stewing them or making applesauce or pie.
- Cook in a light syrup and purée to use in soufflés, mousses, ice cream, jams and jellies.
- Add the fruit to a tisane to liven it up. Boil a half fruit with your chosen tisane base. Or boil a small guava and a large pear in 1 litre (1 3/4 pints) still mineral water for 5–10 minutes, then let stand for 1 hour. Drink as a pick-me-up.

HAZELNUT, *see* Nuts

HORSERADISH
Armoracia rusticana
Cruciferae family

THIS PEPPERY PLANT and its medicinal properties have been appreciated since ancient times: the leaves were one of the five bitter herbs that Jews were enjoined to eat at the Passover. To the Greeks and Romans, horseradish was a diuretic and digestive stimulant, and in the Middle Ages it was believed to prevent scurvy.

Japanese horseradish, wasabi *(Wasabia japonica)*, is even stronger than horseradish and is the root of a mountain hollyhock. The bright green flesh is grated and used fresh or dried in cookery.

Therapeutic Uses
For a slow digestion, eat a little grated root as a sauce or garnish. Alternatively macerate fresh sliced horseradish in white wine for a few weeks: drink 1 teaspoon of this liquid

diluted in water for digestive purposes; to avoid coughs and colds, drink 2 tablespoons per day; to counter the fluid retention of PMT drink 1 tablespoon diluted in a glass of mineral water before meals.

Boil chopped peeled horseradish in mineral water for 10 minutes, then leave in a dark place for 24 hours. Drink 2–3 cups between meals to help rheumatic problems.

A very strong essential oil is distilled from the roots.

In the Kitchen
You can occasionally buy horseradish fresh, but often it can be found in the wild (make sure digging is permitted at that particular spot). Peel and grate, preferably in the open air as it is very pungent. Dried horseradish flakes can be reconstituted.

- Mix grated fresh horseradish with cream, yogurt or vinegar for a sauce for meat (especially roast beef) or smoked fish.
- Use young leaves of the plant sparingly in salads.
- Use wasabi (available usually in powder or paste form) when preparing the Japanese specialties sushi an sashimi.

HYSSOP
Hyssopus officinalis
Labiatae family

THIS HARDY green bush plant originated in southern Europe and was introduced to Britain and mainland Europe by the Romans, who believed it could keep plague at bay.

Therapeutic Uses
A tisane of the flowers and young green tops can benefit coughs, colds, flu, bronchitis, asthma and similar ailments. Make a syrup for a sore throat by marinating the flowers and leaf tops in sugar syrup for a few weeks. Take 2 teaspoons per day.

The essential oil is extremely toxic, and has caused deaths in France.

In the Kitchen

Hyssop is aromatic and bitterly minty in flavour. Grow in the garden for its medicinal benefits and its pretty purple-blue flowers, and use fresh.

- Sprinkle leaves in salads. Use flowers in salads and fruit dishes.
- Ad chopped leaves to soft cheese, butter, sandwiches, sauces and dips.
- Use chopped leaves in meat and game stuffings, in stews and soups, and in vegetable dishes. They counteract the fats of some meat and fish.
- Use the syrup described above in fruit dishes.

JUNIPER
Juniperus communis
Cupressaceae family

REMAINS OF juniper berries have been found in prehistoric lake dwellings in Switzerland, and they were referred to in Ancient Egyptian papyri. The Romans valued it as an antiseptic, diuretic and hepatic, properties still attributed to the plant.

Therapeutic Uses

Juniper is tonic, stomachic and sudorific. It is also a blood cleanser, so is good for rheumatic conditions and arthritis. It can help infections of the bladder, and stimulates the liver and gallbladder.

Infuse berries in boiling water and drink 1 cup daily to counter fluid retention, indigestion, and liver and kidney problems.

An essential oil is distilled from fresh ripe berries, preferably from those growing in southerly regions such as Italy.

In the Kitchen

Juniper berries can be bought and used fresh or dried. Always crush them before use so that the essential oils and their spicy, resinous, piney aroma are released.

- Cook the berries with meat and game in a stuffing, sauce or marinade. Ordinary meat can become quite gamey in flavour as a result.
- Use with garlic and crushed rock salt as a wonderful flavouring for fresh cabbage or other green vegetable.
- Use in pâtés and meatloaves.
- Macerate berries in gin to intensify the flavour and add medicinal benefits (juniper is the principal flavouring of gin.) This is good for digestion after a heavy meal.

KELP, *see* Seaweeds

KIWI FRUIT

Actinidis chinensis
Actinidaceae family

PRINCIPAL NUTRIENTS

Vitamins: C
Minerals: calcium, iron, phosphorus, potassium

THE KIWI FRUIT or Chinese gooseberry is thought to have originated in China, but achieved world-wide acceptance after arriving in New Zealand in the 1960s.

Therapeutic Uses

100 g (4 oz) kiwi fruit contain more vitamin C than the equivalent weight of orange or lemon, therefore it is particularly valuable for convalescents and people suffering from anaemia or anorexia. Kiwi fruit contain achinidin, a protein-dissolving enzyme, so they are good for the digestion and have laxative properties as well. They are also said to help clear cholesterol from the blood.

In the Kitchen

Kiwi fruit can keep for up to 6 months if stored in a cool place. When you want to use them, place with other fruit such as bananas, apples or pears—the ethylene gas emitted by these fruit will ripen them.

- Eat raw to enjoy the full vitamin C content. Halve and eat from the skin with a teaspoon.
- Peel and slice into a fruit salad, or use as an edible garnish for savoury or sweet dishes.
- Purée the flesh for an ice cream or pie filling.
- Use as a meat tenderiser, one of the benefits of the enzyme: place puréed flesh over the meat, or simply place the insides of the skins on top of the meat.
- Cut peeled kiwis in half and dip into some very good dark melted chocolate to coat. Grind some hazelnuts and sprinkle over the chocolate before it sets.

Kiwi and Cabbage Salad

This salad is extra-rich in vitamin C, both from the kiwi fruit and from the cabbage. Try to find very mild onions, as they have the gentlest flavour and are easiest to digest.

SERVES 4

1/4–1/2 white cabbage, shredded
4–6 kiwi fruit, peeled and quartered or sliced
150 g (5 oz) stoned black olives, halved
1 medium mild white onion, peeled and sliced
a few tarragon leaves, sliced

DRESSING

salt and freshly ground black pepper
1 tablespoon cider vinegar
4 tablespoons olive oil
a few tarragon leaves, very finely chopped

Make the dressing first. Dissolve the salt in the vinegar and the black pepper in the oil. Mix the oil and vinegar together with the tarragon leaves, and pour into a salad bowl. Mix all the salad ingredients together and place in the bowl. Toss and serve.

LAVENDER
Lavandula angustifolia
Labiatae family

THE FRAGRANT shrub familiar in cottage gardens is a native of southern Europe and has for centuries been regarded as something of a cure-all.

Therapeutic Uses
Make a herbal lavender tea and drink to treat female problems such as cystitis, vaginitis and leucorrhoea. Use a decoction for urinary infections.

Drink this tea also after meals for its digestive properties, for rheumatic problems, and at the first signs of colds and flu.

In the Kitchen
The sweet and musky aroma of lavender can be used, sparingly, in the kitchen.

- Spike meat with the leaves and flowers, as you would with rosemary.
- Mix the dried flowers with other sweet herbs for herb mixtures such as *Herbes de Provence*.
- Eat the young leaves in salads.
- Use the flowers and leaves in herbal oils and vinegars (see page xxiii).

LAVER/NORI, *see* Seaweeds

LEEK
Allium porum
Liliaceae family

PRINCIPAL NUTRIENTS
Vitamins: B, C
Minerals: calcium, magnesium, manganese, phosphorus, potassium, sulphur

RECORDS SHOW that leeks were used in cooking and therapy in Egypt two thousand years ago. Pliny records how the

Emperor Nero would drink the juice and eat the vegetable once a month for the benefit of his singing and speaking voice (leeks are still valued for loss of voice). The School of Salerno prescribed leeks for women who had difficulty having children, and also for preventing nose bleeds—a few drops of the juice up each nostril.

Therapeutic Uses

Leeks are pectoral, diuretic, antiseptic and emollient, and can be useful in treating obesity, kidney trouble, diarrhoea, dysentery and enteritis. For the latter digestive and stomachic problems make a leek broth from 10 leeks per 2 litres (3 1/2 pints) water: drink a cup every 2 hours.

For bladder problems and fluid retention, boil 1 kg (2 1/4 lb) white of leek in 2 litres (3 1/2 pints) white wine until reduced by half. Drink a glass of this every day before a meal.

Leek Soufflé Omelette

This is a delicious way of using leeks, combining them with the protein of eggs in a light, easy-to-digest dish.

PER PERSON

3 small leeks
a little still mineral water
salt
1 egg, separated
1 tablespoon rice flour
1 tablespoon soy oil or olive oil
juice of 1/2 lemon
3 stoned black olives, chopped
5 walnuts, shelled and chopped

Wash the leeks very thoroughly, then slice. Cook in a little salted water until soft, then strain and dry.

Mix the egg yolk and flour together. Whisk the egg white until stiff, then fold gently into the egg yolk mixture. Heat the oil in a small frying pan, pour in the egg mixture, and fry for about 5 minutes on each side.

Put the omelette on a plate and serve the warm leeks on top. Sprinkle with the lemon juice and scatter with the olives and walnuts.

In the Kitchen

Leeks are nicest when small and sweet—they toughen as they grow older and bigger. Always wash leeks well, slitting them vertically and fanning them out, as soil can easily get in between the layers of leaves.

- Slice very thinly and eat raw in salads for a refreshingly sweet oniony taste.
- Steam whole as you would asparagus and serve hot, warm or cold with melted butter, vinaigrette, or a lime or mustard sauce. With a spiced yogurt and hazelnuts, they make a wonderful first course.
- Slice and cook in white wine, vermouth or orange juice.
- Par-cook, then bake wrapped in pastry or bacon.
- Slice and cook in a quiche or flan—delicious with soured cream and cumin.
- Use in stews and soups, the most famous soup being leek and potato or Vichyssoise.

LEMON AND LIME
Citrus limon, Citrus aurantifolia
Rutaceae family

PRINCIPAL NUTRIENTS
Vitamins: B, C, P
Minerals: calcium, copper, iron, magnesium

LEMON AND LIME trees are smaller than their cousin the orange, and less hardy. Both originated, like most of the family, in south-east Asia. They were brought to the West by the Arabs, and taken to the New World by Columbus in the fifteenth century.

Therapeutic Uses

The value of lemons in medicine has long been recognized, and they were classified as digestive and blood-purifying in seventeenth-century pharmacopoeiae. They reached the heights of their fame when issued to combat scurvy in the British Navy in the eighteenth century, and in the twentieth century, when the Nobel Prize winner Linus Pauling described their magical powers as a cold preventative. Lemon is the most antiseptic member of the citrus family.

The juice is also good for rheumatic conditions as it dissolves the toxins and crystals which cause gout and thus helps the sufferer to become more mobile. Lemons contain bioflavonoids (the citrin content, or vitamin P), so are good for vein and capillary problems. Lemons and limes also help the symptoms of PMT and insomnia.

For all these conditions, go on a lemon "cure": drink the juice daily, starting with that from a single lemon, then increasing daily by a half lemon to 10 lemons per day (this should take about 19 days). Then reduce gradually by a half lemon per day (another 19 days). Never take too much in one day—the only sure way to success is the slow way. Make sure that the lemons are ripe and soft, with dark yellow skins (older lemons have more juice).

If you have used untreated, organic lemons for this "cure" preserve the skins and pulp in the freezer. Use them to make a special juice which stimulates the liver and gastric juices. Each night put some lemon skins into a container, pour 600 ml (1 pint) boiling water over them, and cover. The next morning drink this liquid mixed with the juice of a fresh lemon. Children can drink it as a cheap, healthy lemonade substitute: add some more fresh water, and a little honey.

In the Kitchen

Lemons and limes have similar properties. Lemons are simply more widely available, and cheaper than their smaller, greener relatives. The flavour of limes is rounder and tangier.

- Add lemon or lime juice to foods to sour them, to "cook" them (as with fish in ceviche), or to prevent discolouration (as in an avocado guacamole, see page 17).
- Use lemon or lime slices, wedges or halves as a savoury and sweet garnish that is intended to be eaten. The juice

adds a welcome acidity to meat or fish, but, more important, it will help the body absorb calcium and proteins.

- Use lemon or lime juice instead of vinegar in vinaigrettes, and add to marinades where it has a tenderising effect.
- Use the juice in desserts such as mousses, pies (lemon meringue, Key Lime) and sorbets.
- Use lemons or limes in jams, jellies, chutneys and pickles for their high pectin content and magnificent flavour.
- Use the peel of lemons and limes in the same way as you would that of orange (see pages 130–131).

LEMON BALM
Melissa officinalis
Labiatae family

THIS FRAGRANT native of southern Europe has been known and appreciated in medicine since ancient times.

Therapeutic Uses
Make a tea from the fresh or dried leaves as a general tonic and to alleviate migraine and headaches, depression, anxiety, insomnia, PMT and menopausal symptoms. Macerate 50 g (2 oz) lemon balm leaves in 1 litre (1 3/4 pints) good white wine and take a tablespoon when symptoms appear. Lemon balm is also emmenogogic and good for the cardiac system.

An essential oil is distilled from the leaves and tops, and it is classified in France as a narcotic. It must only be used by experienced practitioners, and with great care.

In the Kitchen
- Use the fresh leaves in summer drinks such as wine cups.
- Add young shoots and leaves to stuffings, savoury or fruit salads, sauces and omelettes for the lemony flavour.
- Use to replace lemon or lemongrass in a recipe, especially with fish.
- Infuse in the milk for milk puddings.

LETTUCE
Lactuca sativa
Compositae family

PRINCIPAL NUTRIENTS

Vitamins: A, B, C, D, E
Minerals: calcium, copper, iron, phosphorus, potassium

LETTUCES WERE eaten by the Ancient Egyptians, and offered to their god of fertility; in medical papyri they are recommended as a cure for impotence and recorded as having wonderful aphrodisiac effects. The Greeks and Romans also grew them; one of our three main modern varieties, the Cos, is believed to have come from the Greek island of Kos and to have travelled north with the Romans, who were probably responsible for its name in France and America—"Romaine". The other two main varieties are the cabbage lettuce—butterheads or soft lettuces, or iceberg, Webb's and other crisper, round, hearted lettuces—and the newer loose-leaved lettuces such as oakleaf, lollo rosso and lollo biondo. Other plants used as salad leaves are listed on the next page.

Therapeutic Uses
The vitamin and mineral content of most lettuces is not high, but is at its best when very fresh.

Lettuce is one of the great remedies for constipation and should be eaten daily, with olive oil, in salads. It is also diuretic and therefore helpful in dealing with fluid retention, obesity, cellulite, PMT and menopausal problems. A nervous cough can be cured by a lettuce leaf tisane or soup.

One of the most striking of lettuce's properties is its role as a calmant of the nervous system. It contains a substance called lactucerium, a sort of milky latex, which smells and acts a little like opium but without the side-effects. This narcotic property both relaxes people and cures insomnia (and also explains why the Flopsy Bunnies fell asleep after gorging on Mr. McGregor's lettuces). People who are under stress, or who suffer from heart palpitations or anxiety or cannot sleep easily, should eat at night a large lettuce salad with basil, lemon juice and coarse salt, and their dreams should be sweet. They should also drink the following: boil 60 g (2 oz) lettuce in 1 litre (1 3/4 pints) water for 5 minutes, then let it stand to cool down. Drink 2 cups with a little honey in the evening.

In the Kitchen

For your health, organic lettuces are best. Even bolted lettuce can be used in soups and other dishes, losing none of their therapeutic properties.

Never tear or cut lettuce until you are just about to eat it. When the cells are torn, an enzyme is released which destroys the vitamin C. Do not dress a salad of lettuce leaves until just before serving: the vinegar in particular will "cook" the leaves, turn them limp and brown.

• Eat lettuce salads every day, adding other therapeutics such as chives, parsley, tarragon, basil, onions and garlic. Other salad leaves could be added as well—endive, chicory, lamb's lettuce or mâche, rocket, sorrel and dandelion.

• Make lettuce leaves a base for protein salad ingredients— cheese and eggs (Caesar), meat, fruit and nuts (Waldorf) and fish (Niçoise). Flavour with a variety of dressings.

• Cook lettuces only if you have to: in soup, with other vegetables such as potato; with peas; as a wrapping for other foods (good with fish); or, in one of my favourite dishes for a simple evening meal, 4 lettuce hearts (Little Gem), stewed in a casserole with 2 sliced onions in 1 tablespoon sesame oil (serve with whole rice or millet).

Other Salad Leaves

Many leaves can be used in salads and, if they don't have the same uniquely therapeutic properties as lettuce, are still useful and nutritious.

Dandelion *Taraxacum officinale* This most profuse of European weeds has been used in cooking and therapy for centuries. The roots have been ground as a coffee substitute in times of scarcity, but it is the leaves that are tastiest and most nutritious. They are high in vitamin C, potassium, manganese and iron, and are diuretic (the French name is *piss-en-lit!*), hepatic (increasing bile secretion, thus benefiting circulatory and skin conditions such as cellulite), strongly detoxificant, and blood-cleansing. Dandelion can heal wounds, particularly internal ones such as ulcers. Take a strong infusion of the leaves three times a day for any of the above.

- Eat in salads with other salad leaves—the flavour is quite bitter.
- Mince leaves, mix with minced onion and some olive oil, and serve over freshly cooked new potatoes.

Rocket *Eruca sativa* This is a member of the cabbage, cress and watercress family, so the leaves have a very pungent, peppery, almost meaty flavour. They can stimulate the appetite, act as a general tonic, and are diuretic.

- Add to salads, particularly grated vegetables like carrots, for a good colour and texture combination.
- Stir into pasta after briefly cooking in olive oil.
- Serve raw with shavings of Parmesan and a drizzle of new olive oil.

Sorrel *Rumex acetosa* One of the first green food plants to appear in the spring, it is highly prized in France (as it once was in Britain). It has a sharp flavour due to its high content of oxalic acid (which can inhibit the assimilation of magnesium and calcium), but it is good for anaemia, rheumatism and bronchitis, and as a general tonic.

Hot Dandelion Leaf Salad

A traditional dandelion recipe consists of pouring shreds of bacon and its hot fat over the leaves to wilt and flavour them. This one is healthier!

SERVES 1–2

100 g (4 oz) young dandelion leaves
1 shallot, peeled and chopped
1 large mushroom, chopped
1 tablespoon olive oil
lime or lemon juice

Wash the dandelion leaves and dry them thoroughly. Slice coarsely. Fry the shallot and mushroom in the oil until soft and golden, then pour on to the leaves. Sprinkle immediately with the lime or lemon juice and serve with toasted rye bread.

Sorrel Soup

This light, tasty and nutritious soup makes a good lunch or late dinner dish.

SERVES 4

2 large handfuls fresh sorrel leaves, washed
1–2 teaspoons sesame oil or soya oil
2 eggs, beaten

VEGETABLE BROTH

2 potatoes, peeled
2 carrots, scrubbed
1 parsnip, scrubbed
1 piece turnip or swede, scrubbed
1 large onion, peeled
2 bay leaves
1 sprig thyme
500 ml (17 fl oz) still mineral water

Cut all the vegetables for the broth into small pieces, and put with the remaining broth ingredients into a pan. Bring to a boil and simmer for 30 minutes. Strain, discarding the vegetables and aromatics.

In a separate pan, fry the sorrel leaves in the oil quickly until they wilt. Remove from the heat, mix in the beaten egg, and quickly add to the warm broth. Eat straightaway—it's nicer warm than boiling; it will be a wonderful green colour.

- Use in omelettes and soups.
- Eat raw with cheese, especially Roquefort.

- Wrap leaves around fish before cooking: the acidity helps in the digestion of protein. It makes a wonderful sauce for fish, too.
- Add raw sparingly to other salad leaves, or cook to a purée like spinach.
- Add to spinach, either raw or cooked: the flavours complement each other.

Nettle *Urtica dioica* From spring until June new growth, tops and tender leaves are good to eat cooked in soups or as spinach. Cooking destroys the formic acid which is responsible for the sting. Pick the nettles wearing gloves, though!

Nettles are rich in iron and particularly benefit the blood, so they should be eaten by people suffering from anaemia and women with menstrual problems such as amenorrhoea or heavy periods.

LIME, *see* Lemon and Lime

LINSEED, *see* Seeds

LOVAGE
Levisticum officinale
Umbelliferae family

THIS HERB looks rather like celery gone wrong, and has a very pleasant, heavy smell—a yeasty cross between celery and curry leaves.

Therapeutic Uses
Lovage is well known for its cleansing properties. To detoxify after overindulgence, drink a tisane of the leaves (1 tablespoon in 600 ml/1 pint water). Because of its blood-cleansing properties this drink is also good for the skin, gout and rheumatism. Infuse a little mint in the lovage tea to help the liver as well.

The essential oil is distilled from the roots of the plant.

In the Kitchen
Grow lovage in the garden to enjoy the leaves fresh—but at the back of beds as it can grow to 2 m (6 ft 6 in) in height!

Dried leaves retain their flavour well, and seeds are also available. The stems of the plant are crystallised.

* Use the leaves in soups, stocks and casseroles to add a meaty flavour—this is particularly good for some vegetarian dishes.
* Add fresh young leaves to salads—but sparingly, as the flavour is strong.
* Sprinkle the aromatic seeds over cooked vegetable and meat dishes, or over bread dough.
* Grind the seeds in a mortar along with rock or sea salt to make an aromatic lovage seasoning.

MACE, *see* Nutmeg and Mace

MAIZE, *see* Cereal Grains

MANGE-TOUT, *see* Pea

MANGO
Mangifera indica
Anacardiaceae family

PRINCIPAL NUTRIENTS
Vitamins: A, B, C, E
Minerals: copper, iron, manganese, potassium

MANGOES are the fruit of an Asian tree related to the cashew and pistachio nut trees. Mango trees now grow all over the tropics and there are many varieties and types, the fruits differing in size, shape and colouration: those from Africa are large and round, while many from India are kidney-shaped. A fruit for kings, mangoes must be eaten ripe—otherwise they are fibrous in texture and taste like turpentine! When ripe they are soft to the touch and warmly coloured, with a wonderful aroma and flavour and soft, bright yellow flesh.

Therapeutic Uses
Mangoes are highly nutritious and, because of the yellow flesh, are a rich source of beta-carotene. As a result they are

good for the skin. If eaten unripe or in excess, mangoes can cause diarrhoea. The skins of mangoes can occasionally cause a form of contact dermatitis in sensitive people.

Chicken with Mango

This is a delicately flavoured dish, Chinese in inspiration, which should be accompanied by rice.

SERVES 4

4 chicken breasts, skinned and boned
2 large mangoes, peeled and stoned
juice of 2 limes
a little fresh root ginger, peeled and finely chopped
finely ground black pepper
1 dessertspoon sesame oil or soy oil
2 tablespoons chopped fresh coriander leaves

Cut the chicken and mango flesh into small pieces. Mix the chicken with a quarter of the mango pieces, half the lime juice, the ginger and some pepper, and marinate for about 30 minutes.

Heat the oil in a wok and add the chicken in batches if necessary. Stir-fry until just starting to turn golden, then reduce the heat. Add the mango and remaining lime juice, mix well, and allow to cook together for another 15 minutes or so. Sprinkle with the fresh coriander.

In the Kitchen

The sugars in mangoes act as a natural sweetener, useful in cooking when a food is too hot or too spicy. Cutting into a mango can be complicated, as the stone is so large and flat, and it is always a messy job as they are so juicy!

- Eat simply as they are, peeled and cut into sections, or chop and add to tropical fruit salads.
- Use raw or lightly poached as an accompaniment to rich meats such as duck, hot or cold.
- Purée mango flesh and use in a wonderful sorbet, ice cream or mousse.

- Use unripe, pectin-rich green mangoes to make chutneys to accompany curries.
- Juice mangoes, or purée with apple or other fruit juice for an exotic drink.

MARJORAM AND OREGANO
Origanum spp
Labiatae family

THERE ARE three types of marjoram: sweet or knotted *(Origanum majorana)*, pot marjoram *(Origanum onites)*, and wild marjoram or oregano *(Origanum vulgare)*. Both marjoram and oregano are believed to have originated in Asia, but are now grown all over Europe.

Both plants have been used medicinally throughout the centuries, primarily to aid the digestion and as an antiseptic. Essential oils are distilled from their flowering heads; oregano oil is the most important antiseptic oil in aromatherapy because of its high phenol content (80 per cent in Spanish oregano).

Therapeutic Uses
Both plants are stomachic, expectorant, digestive and sedative, and are therefore useful in treating insomnia, migraines, diarrhoea and chest complaints such as bronchitis. For insomnia before going to bed drink a tisane made with a pinch each of marjoram and dried lime flowers.

As a treatment for mouth disorders such as thrush, inflamed gums or a sore throat, make a decoction from either oregano or marjoram.

In the Kitchen
Oregano is more pungent than the other marjorams, and both are best when used fresh, although they dry well, retaining their flavour, aroma and therapeutic benefits.

- Use either or both in marinades for meat—4 pinches along with the peel of 1 orange and about 400 ml (14 fl oz) white wine per 450 g (1 lb) meat. This will enhance the flavour of the meat and help the body assimilate its minerals.

- Use in minced meat mixtures or stuffings, or meat stews, adding towards the end of cooking if possible.
- Liver and other offal can contain toxins, so cook them with digestive and antiseptic herbs such as thyme, marjoram and oregano.
- Cook sprigs of marjoram or oregano with cabbage or other brassicas, and peas or beans, both fresh and dried, to aid digestion and prevent wind.
- Cook mushrooms with oregano and marjoram to help digest a substance called chitin which is present in all fungi.
- Sprinkle the leaves into salads to accompany strong cheeses: this will make the cheeses easier to digest.
- Oregano is an important herb in Italian cooking—sprinkled on a variety of dishes, pizza perhaps being the most familiar.
- Use both herbs in tisanes after meals to help digestion, as the Swiss do after fondue.
- Use sprigs of either herb in a homemade herbal oil or vinegar (page xxiii).

MARROW AND COURGETTE
Cucurbita pepo/Cucurbita pepo ovifera
Cucurbitaceae family

PRINCIPAL NUTRIENTS
Vitamins: A, B, C
Minerals: potassium

MARROWS AND COURGETTES are very closely related members of the botanical family which includes squashes, pumpkins, cucumbers and melons. All share similar characteristics: they are climbing and trailing plants with fruits which, although variable, are mild in flavour and consist mostly of water.

Therapeutic Uses
Both vegetables are diuretic and laxative, and good for the adrenal glands, according to Dr. Leclerc. He recommended them also for piles and high blood pressure. Both flesh and

seeds are supposed to be soporific, so serve in the evening as a good sedative for the nervous system.

In the Kitchen

Courgettes, essentially, are marrows picked very small and young, when nutrients and flavour are at their best. To have any flavour at all, a vegetable marrow should not be any longer than 30 cm (12 in); after this the seeds develop and the fibres become coarse and stringy.

- Thinly slice or grate raw baby courgettes and add a simple olive oil dressing. Also use them in a mixed salad to take most advantage of the vitamin C.
- Sauté sliced, chopped or grated courgettes quickly in a good olive oil or butter, perhaps flavouring them with garlic, lemon, orange or lime juice, or soy sauce.
- Deep-fry chunks or slices of courgette in a light batter as part of an Italian *fritto misto*.
- Braise chunks of larger courgettes briefly in a flavouring liquid (perhaps with aubergines, tomatoes, onions and peppers as in ratatouille); or cook and serve with a Parmesan cheese sauce; or halve, hollow out, stuff with a tasty filling and bake.
- The flowers of both marrows and courgettes can be "stuffed" and eaten (in many elegant restaurants, chefs serve the courgette and stuffed flower still attached to each other). Stuff, then steam, braise or deep-fry. Or add chopped flowers and courgettes to a risotto.
- Cook peeled chunks of marrow in a minimum of water and dress with something to give it flavour—lots of chopped herbs, or a cheese or tomato sauce.
- Cut a marrow in half, remove the seeds, and fill the hollow with a flavourful stuffing before baking, wrapped in foil.
- Use marrow in jams, pickles and chutneys.
- Do not throw away the marrow seeds; dry them and eat them as a snack. They are rich in therapeutic oils.

MEAT, POULTRY AND FISH

THESE FOODS are important because of their plentiful and complete protein. Vegetarians, however, can find ample protein by eating a balance of grains and pulses (particularly soya, the nearest thing to complete protein in the vegetable world).

Meat, poultry and fish are not aromatic in themselves, but it is in concert with them that most aromatic foods are used, and when they can work most effectively. None of these protein foods is ever eaten on its own, even if the aromatic addition is only salt and pepper—without these, the flavour and texture would be boring.

The flavouring benefits are obvious, then, but the health benefits are less so. If protein is eaten on its own, we are unable to digest it properly. Aromatic substances, however, can help break down the food in the gut more quickly so that it can be assimilated more easily. The citrus juice of the orange served with duck actually cuts through the fattiness of the meat; the same is true of the apple served with pork.

Another health consideration involves the potential toxicity of meat, poultry and fish. What we buy is dead. There were already toxic bacteria within the live flesh, but these can proliferate once the animal has been killed. In the West our joint, bird or fish will have been dead for some days when we buy it. Modern refrigeration notwithstanding, it must then be cooked very thoroughly to make it safe to eat, and adding aromatics is one way of doubly ensuring this. The spices in Asian curries serve a practical purpose as well as adding flavour. When I was living in Oman, I bought some fresh tuna from fishermen on the coast. By the time I got home, a mere half-hour drive, the fish was off and the smell was noxious. (I later learned that if I had wrapped the fish in papaya leaves it would have survived the journey better.)

In fact tuna, as well as mackerel, can cause what is known as scombroid poisoning. Another bacteria that can thrive on meat, poultry and fish is salmonella (also present in eggs). A parasitic roundworm, trichinella spiralis, is found in pork and the flesh of other animals that eat meat. In addition, many meats contain antibiotics or growth hormones, and many fish can be affected by pollutants in the water.

Another consideration is the manner of slaughter and the mode of transportation and "storage". Fear in animals produces chemicals akin to the adrenaline produced by humans under stress, which are toxic to the flesh on the carcass. Finally, the conditions in which carcasses are processed are not necessarily as hygienic as we might wish them to be.

For all these reasons a considerable number of undesirable substances can find their way into our own bodies.

Whether you eat meat or not is a purely personal matter. I have described the drawbacks merely to explain the traditional ways of coping—cooking all animal flesh with the essential oils of aromatic herbs, spices, fruit and vegetables, to render them both safer to eat and easier to digest.

MEAT

PRINCIPAL NUTRIENTS

Vitamins: B
Minerals: iron, potassium, phosphorus, zinc

BEEF, lamb and pork contain plentiful B vitamins; in fact animal flesh is the only source of B6 and B12. They are also a rich source of iron in particular, as well as potassium and zinc. They are, however, rich in saturated fatty acids which contribute to high cholesterol levels in the blood and make us put on weight. Fat between meat fibres contributes to the flavour when it is cooked—it contains much of the essential meat flavour and melts, lubricating the meat—but any excess should be cut off before cooking.

Roast joints of beef with aromatics—salt and pepper, mustard or curry powder spread or sprinkled over before cooking—and serve with horseradish or mustard, and aromatic vegetables. Dot lamb with garlic and rosemary before roasting, and serve with mint sauce and redcurrant or other tart fruit jelly. Cook pork very thoroughly indeed, and serve with a tart sauce to counteract its fattiness. If you think a steak or chop might be tough, tenderise (and cleanse) it with an aromatic fruit—fig, pineapple, kiwi or papaya, for instance. Marinating meat in a herb-scented alcohol can also tenderise and purify (see pages 184–185). Cook meat stews with lots of garlic, onion, carrots and other aromatics to make the meat more tender, palatable and healthy.

Offal

PRINCIPAL NUTRIENTS

Vitamins: A, B, D
Minerals: iron, copper, potassium, phosphorus, zinc

Liver, kidneys and sweetbreads are animal organs, and they, like meat, contain good quantities of the B vitamins as well as iron, copper, potassium, phosphorus and zinc. Liver is the single most concentrated source of vitamin A, the fat-soluble vitamin that is actually stored in the liver, and also contains vitamin D. The iron content of liver is particularly high, and 100 g (4 oz) fried liver could supply the complete recommended daily allowance of a healthy adult female, some 10 mg. Sweetbreads contain vitamin C.

Liver and kidney, both excretory organs, are high in purines, chemicals which can produce uric acid within the body, and which exacerbate gout in particular. Soaking them in milk before cooking will leach out some of these toxins. (Liver, interestingly, does not need to be coated in flour before being cooked if it has been soaked in milk.) Cook too with aromatics—garlic, onions, marjoram, oregano, sage and thyme, for instance.

Poultry

PRINCIPAL NUTRIENTS

Vitamins: B
Minerals: calcium, iron, phosphorus, potassium, zinc

ALL DOMESTIC birds are high in good-quality protein, and contain more unsaturated fatty acids than meat. To eliminate as much fat as possible, cut the skin off a bird after cooking. Poultry contains B vitamins, iron, potassium and zinc, but can also harbour the salmonella bacterium, inside and out-side. (Kitchen hygiene is vital when working with poultry.) "Wash" the outside down with lemon juice, insert herbs under the skin, and place pieces of onion, wedges of lemon and sprigs of herbs inside both cavities before roasting. Cook all poultry very thoroughly and serve with suitable aromatics. Chicken often has a sage stuffing, as does turkey; duck is served with an orange or apple sauce.

Eggs

Poultry eggs are high in fat and cholesterol, but can supply good amounts of vitamins A, B and D as well as calcium, iron and phosphorus. The proteins of eggs are very easily digestible, but, like poultry, they are highly susceptible to salmonella.

FISH AND SHELLFISH

PRINCIPAL NUTRIENTS

Vitamins: A, B, D
Minerals: calcium, fluorine, iron, iodine, phosphorus, potassium, selenium

THESE ARE a good source of complete protein, offering vita-mins A, B and D. Fish are divided into two main groups, white and oily. In white fish like cod, the fish oils are con-centrated in the liver rather than the flesh (thus cod liver oil); the flesh, therefore, is very much less rich in fat than oily fish and meat. In oily fish the oils are dispersed throughout the flesh, which makes them higher in fatty acids, but the major-ity of these are unsaturated. Shellfish contains more choles-terol than fish. Both fish and shellfish are rich in minerals.

What are known as omega-3 fatty acids occur in saltwa-ter fish oils. These are an important nutrient, acting in much the same way as the EFAs to boost prostaglandin action (see page 232). They are said to reduce cholesterol in the blood-stream and alleviate inflammatory diseases such as rheuma-tism and arthritis. Oily fish from cold waters—herring, salmon, sea trout and mackerel—contain the most omega-3 fatty acids, but farmed fish contain less than wild.

Buy fresh fish and shellfish if you can, although frozen fish are of good nutritive value. Many canned fish, like salmon, anchovies and sardines, have significantly higher amounts of calcium because of the little bones, which are also eaten. I make a lobster (shrimp or prawn) butter by leaving the shells overnight in lemon juice. They can then be cut or processed easily and mixed with butter. Serve on toast with some shrimps or other shellfish meat on top. Always buy shellfish from a reputable source, as they can thrive even in polluted waters and unpleasant substances can be taken up by their flesh.

Cook fish and shellfish as soon as possible after buying, and use plenty of aromatics: fennel, dill, onion, garlic, parsley and lemon are all excellent. "Wash" the flesh with lemon juice, or put slices of lemon inside the cavity of a whole fish before cooking. Poaching a large fish in court-bouillon (a fragrant light stock) with lots of aromatic herbs is traditional, adding flavour as well as ensuring safety; the lemon juice or vinegar used, being acidic, quickly set the protein within the fish flesh, sealing in the flavour and nutrients. Always cook fish and shellfish thoroughly—although they take much less time than meat—to ensure that any bacteria and micro-organisms are destroyed. Serve with aromatic accompaniments: a dill sauce for gravlax, a garlic or herb mayonnaise for salmon, a tart gooseberry sauce for mackerel, horseradish with smoked fish and pike, and a stuffing, wrapping or sauce of sorrel for trout.

Shellfish such as oysters and mussels are often implicated in food allergies. These can be dangerous, and some people end up in hospital.

MELON
Cucumis melo
Cucurbitaceae family

PRINCIPAL NUTRIENTS
Vitamins: A, C
Minerals: potassium

THERE IS a huge range of melons available, and they differ enormously in size, colour and shape. There are three basic classifications: the musk or netted melons (which include the Galia and what the Americans call cantaloupe), the cantaloupes (among them Ogen and Charentais), and winter melons (principally honeydew). All have sweet flesh: sugar provides 5 per cent of the weight, water accounting for the rest!

Therapeutic Uses

The orange- and yellow-fleshed varieties are rich in vitamin A, so can benefit us in many ways, including regeneration of flesh and tissue. Melons are very rich in fruit sugar, so are often recommended for anaemia.

The fruit are diuretic and laxative, and are useful in treating gout, rheumatism, piles and fluid retention (thus their inclusion in a number of weight-reducing diets, despite that high sugar content).

In the Kitchen

Make sure that any melon you buy was properly ripe when picked: away from the parent plant it will only soften, not ripen or sweeten. A melon will virtually separate itself from the plant when it has ripened to saturation point, so it will show no scar at the stem end; if the stem end shows damaged or cut tissue, the melon was unripe when picked. The skin at the stem end should give to slight pressure, and the scent should be intensely aromatic.

- Eat raw as a breakfast dish, starter or dessert, in wedges or halves, depending on type, with the seeds removed (but kept—see below).
- Mix chunks of flesh into fruit salads.
- Fill hollows in half melons with other fruits—whole or chopped, depending on type—or with sorbet, ice cream, sweet wine or champagne.
- Serve halves or segments of melon with Parma or a similar dried ham.
- Make melon flesh into a purée to make sorbets or ice cream (Charentais is good for this).

- Sprinkle melon to be eaten raw with a sweet spice—ginger is often used.
- Save the oily seeds—they consist of 35–40 per cent fat—and dry them to eat as a snack, as done in many parts of Europe.

MILK, *see* Dairy Products

MILLET, *see* Seeds

MINT
Mentha piperita
Labiatae family

THERE ARE many varieties of mint including water mint, corn mint, horse mint, eau de cologne mint and the familiar spearmint.

Their main aromatic constituent is menthol, a white crystalline substance which causes a sensation of coldness in the mouth.

Therapeutic Uses
Mint is a good blood cleanser because it is antiseptic and antibacterial. Drink mint tea often if you have a skin problem such as acne; this is also effective in countering nausea. Add 2 tablespoons chopped fresh leaves (or 1 tablespoon dried) to 600 ml (1 pint) boiling water. As an expectorant treatment for coughs and colds, and for bad catarrh, add some eucalyptus to this mixture.

Mint is good for the nervous system, and is sedative. Drink as a tea or use in cooking.

The most commonly used essential oil is steam-distilled from peppermint (thought to be a hybrid of water mint and spearmint). Others are distilled from spearmint, pennyroyal, and eau de cologne mints. Mint oils should be used with very great care.

In the Kitchen
Mint is a herb that is used all over the world for its fresh aroma and flavour. It is rarely cooked.

- Use in the traditional sauce for lamb.
- Add sprigs of mint to new potatoes or peas during cooking, and sprinkle with more when serving.
- Chop mint and add to salads, salad dressings, or the famous Middle Eastern bulgar wheat salad called tabbouleh (see below).
- Use mint in fresh chutneys or relishes with yogurt, garlic or coconut.

Tabbouleh

This fresh, refreshing and vitalising salad can be served as a starter, main course or salad accompaniment. It's detoxifying because of the onion, mint and tomato, and nourishing because of the wheat. Use as much mint or parsley as you like, but mint should predominate.

Some bulgar wheat needs minimal cooking first, so check on the packet.

SERVES 2–3

100 g (4 oz) bulgar wheat
a handful of mint leaves, chopped
1/2 handful of parsley leaves, chopped
3 small mild white onions, peeled and chopped
3 medium tomatoes, seeded and chopped
juice of 2 lemons
4 tablespoons olive oil
salt

Put the bulgar wheat in a shallow platter and cover with a little water to allow it to swell. Leave for about 10–15 minutes. Strain if necessary, but it shouldn't be. Mix in all the remaining ingredients, add salt to taste, and chill before serving.

MOOLI, *see* Radish

MUSHROOMS

PRINCIPAL NUTRIENTS
Vitamins: B
Minerals: calcium, cobalt, copper, iron, magnesium, phosphorus, potassium, silica, zinc

MUSHROOMS are fungi, simple plants that grow on dead, living or decaying matter which they use as a food source.

The edible types have long played an important part in many cuisines and many pharmacopiae—they were known to the Greeks and Romans, and the shiitake mushroom was cultivated in Japan in the first century AD. In many countries wild mushrooms are an important food "crop" and are sought enthusiastically in fields, woods and other damp places in autumn.

Many mushrooms are dried, when they intensify in flavour and aroma. A few pieces of dried cep—the *fungi porcini* of Italian cooking—added to a soup or sauce of cultivated mushrooms will improve the flavour greatly.

Therapeutic Uses
Mushrooms contain a variety of nutrients, but not much of any except the vitamin B group, phosphorus and potassium. They are quite rich in protein for a vegetable and are high in essential amino acids—lycine and leucine. They also contain glutamic acid, the sodium salt of which is the flavour enhancer monosodium glutamate. Glutamic acid has a relationship to brain activity, and I find that mushrooms stimulate cerebral activity. I also find mushrooms good for digestive problems, as they seem to help in the assimilation of food. They assist in remineralising the body after illness, and rid it of accumulated toxins and mucus.

In the Kitchen
If you are lucky enough to obtain wild mushrooms they require careful preparation and cooking (primarily because of the expense!), so follow a reliable cookery writer. Otherwise

the general information below relates to the three types of cultivated mushroom—buttons, cups, or flat or open.

Wipe mushrooms clean if you can, rather than washing them. (Dried will need to be soaked in water; cook with this, strained, as it is rich in flavour.) Try not to peel the cap, as this is where the glutamic acid, and thus the flavour, is concentrated. Slice them only if necessary, as they will brown and lose some of their B vitamins. These are not destroyed by heat, but will leach out into the cooking liquid; use this in sauces and stocks if possible.

- To gain the most nutrients, eat mushrooms raw. Slice, and immediately toss in a salad with a dressing.
- Add fresh chervil, parsley or coriander, onion or garlic to mushroom dishes; the oils in these foods help the digestion of a substance called chitin which is found in the cell walls of fungi, which many people find difficult to digest.
- Do not cook mushrooms in too much oil or other fat as they will be less easy to digest.
- Cook mushrooms whole in meat, poultry and fish dishes to enrich them and to ensure good digestion and efficient elimination of toxins.
- Use sliced mushrooms in sauces for protein, rice or pasta dishes, in soups and stir-fries.
- Bake mushrooms whole with a little garlic butter.

MUSTARD
Brassica spp
Cruciferae family

THREE VARIETIES of mustard plant produce the seeds used to make the condiment: black *(Brassica nigra)*, brown *(Brassica juncea)* and white *(Brassica alba* or *Sinapis alba)*. All have been used in cooking and medicine for thousands of years.

Therapeutic Uses
Mustard leaves and seeds are aperitive and stimulant (of the stomach and pancreas), and act as an intestinal disinfectant. The seeds contain 30–35 per cent oil, which is released

when they are crushed and macerated in warm water. These oils, which are hot and peppery, help you to assimilate foods better, particularly fatty ones like meat, and stop intestinal fermentation. Mustard's traditional meat-accompanying role is probably due to its ability to mask or counter spoilage.

An essential oil is distilled from the crushed and macerated seeds. It is very strong, and can burn the skin if used in the wrong proportions.

In the Kitchen
Grow white mustard seeds with cress (see pages 177–178) for a nutritive fresh herb. White and brown mustard leaves are edible too, and contribute a peppery flavour to salads: the greens of the Deep South of America developed from an African variety of mustard plant.

- Use bought made mustard or home-prepared mustard in sauces, matching the pungency of the mustard to the ingredients of the main dish, as an accompaniment to meats, and as a coating for them (see below).
- Use whole mustard seeds, slightly crushed, in Indian cooking (which also uses mustard oil).
- Macerate crushed mustard seeds in oil for a very hot oil to use in cooking and dressings.

Rabbit with Mustard and Olives

Wild rabbit, like many game animals and birds, contains less fat than red meat and domestic poultry. It can be dry, though, and so the addition of bacon may be necessary. The meat is high in protein; and mustard will add flavour, some protection from the heat and dryness, and also digestibility.

SERVES 4

800 g (1 3/4 lb) rabbit pieces
salt and freshly ground black pepper
coarse-grain mustard
4–5 rashers streaky bacon (optional), rinded and cut
    into the appropriate number of pieces

juice of 2 lemons

GARNISH

a mixture of chopped parsley, thyme and mild sweet onion

Preheat the oven to 180°C/350°F/Gas 4. Season the rabbit pieces with salt and pepper, then coat each piece generously with the mustard. Place in an ovenproof dish, cover each piece with bacon, if using, and sprinkle over the lemon juice. Bake for 40–45 minutes. Serve with a salad or steamed rice, sprinkled with the parsley, thyme and onion mixture.

NASTURTIUM
Tropaeolum majus
Tropaeolaceae family

PRINCIPAL NUTRIENTS
Vitamins: C
Minerals: iron

THE SEEDS of this familiar garden plant were brought to Europe from South America in the sixteenth century. Its leaves are peppery in flavour, sometimes even hotter than watercress.

Therapeutic Uses
The leaves and flowers have a tonic, cleansing and antiseptic effect. For acne, drink a decoction of 1 heaped tablespoon of leaves to 300 ml (10 fl oz) water, boiled for a few minutes.

In the Kitchen
Wash flowers and leaves well before use, for nasturtiums are very attractive to blackfly!

- Mix in a salad with mâche, lamb's lettuce or rocket, and dress with extra virgin olive oil and lemon juice.
- Chop or shred leaves and mix with soft cheese for sandwiches, or add to scrambled eggs or omelettes.

- Shred the flowers and add to a risotto, or mix with some good olive oil or butter to top a pasta dish.
- Use the flowers as an edible garnish for many dishes.
- Use fresh or dried leaves for a tisane.
- Pickle the seeds and use like capers—particularly good with fish. (Pick as soon as the flowers fade, before the seeds harden.)
- Crystallise the flowers to use as cake or pudding decorations.
- Make a nasturtium vinegar, using leaves, flowers and seeds (see page xxiii).

NECTARINE, *see* Peach and Nectarine

NETTLE, *see* Lettuce

NUTMEG AND MACE
Myristica fragrans
Myristicaceae family

THESE TWO SPICES are the products of a large tropical evergreen. Yellow flowers are followed by large, yellow, apricot-like fruits which split open to reveal a black seed (nutmeg) with a lacy red covering (mace). The spices are dried separately, and both are available whole or ground.

The School of Salerno in the Middle Ages recorded the "poisonous" effects of nutmeg: one of the constituents of oil of nutmeg, myristicine, is narcotic, hallucinogenic and toxic if taken in quantity. (Malcolm X, for instance, used nutmeg as a drug when in jail.)

Therapeutic Uses
Mace is tonic and stimulant, helping overcome fatigue. It is also digestive, benefiting those who cannot assimilate food easily and who suffer from wind. It is effective in preventing menstrual pain.

Nutmeg is tonic, good for the heart, and beneficial for convalescents and those who are over-tired. In Malaysia it is used in cooking towards the end of pregnancy to tone the muscles used in contraction, but use it with care as it is also believed to cause abortion.

In the Kitchen

Use both spices whole if possible, as their aroma, flavour and therapeutic benefit can vanish very quickly when they are ground. Mace is impossible to grind at home, but nutmeg is easy to deal with in its whole form.

- Use mace in cakes and sweet dishes, and in sausages and curries (to preserve them and make them easier to digest).
- Macerate whole pieces of mace in the milk for rice and other milk puddings, to aid digestion and to stimulate the nervous system: it is wonderful for convalescents. Sprinkle nutmeg over the top to add colour, flavour and extra benefit.
- Add ground mace to the eggs for omelettes along with some tangy herb like coriander. Nutmeg would be good too.
- Sprinkle white- or cheese-sauced vegetables with freshly grated nutmeg before grilling to brown, or add lots to mashed potatoes and other root vegetables.
- Sprinkle freshly grated nutmeg on to hot chocolate drinks—this could act as a quick pick-me-up.

NUTS

PRINCIPAL NUTRIENTS

Vitamins: B, E
Minerals: calcium, copper, iron, magnesium, phosphorus, potassium, zinc

THESE ARE the fruits or seeds of certain plants, usually trees, and the inside of the hard shell is often known as the kernel. Nuts are a concentrated food source, containing many nutrients. They are high in protein, although they generally lack certain essential amino acids such as lysine. (If nuts are eaten with pulses the protein becomes complete, so they are particularly valuable for vegetarians.) Nuts are also very rich in oil—Brazils, for instance, contain up to 68 per cent. This oil is polyunsaturated, though, and many of the nut oils, such as groundnut, walnut and hazelnut, are healthy to use in cooking. Buy the latter two nut oils in small quantities as they go rancid quickly.

Nuts are an important element in the diet because of their vitamin and mineral content. Most contain good quantities of the various B vitamins and of vitamin E. None contain any A, C or D. They are also extremely good sources of calcium, iron, potassium, magnesium, phosphorus, copper and zinc. Some also contain selenium (walnuts and Brazil nuts) and iodine (Brazil nuts and peanuts).

Nuts can be eaten fresh from the shell as a snack food, and can be cooked in various dishes. They are easily digestible and supply plenty of energy, which is vital for children and people who get tired easily. All nuts are recommended for those who suffer from hypoglycaemia or diabetes. Some people can react badly to nuts, though, with the symptoms of food allergy, and nuts have been implicated in attacks of cold sores.

Always buy nuts in their shells, but make sure that the shells are whole. Once the oils have gone rancid the flavour is affected, and bad nuts can also be dangerous to eat. Store shelled nuts in the freezer or in an airtight container.

See also **Seeds.**

ALMOND
Prunus amygdalus
Rosaceae family

A relative of the peach and apricot, the almond tree is native to the Mediterranean. There are two types, sweet and bitter, and it is almost always the sweet one that is eaten. Almonds contain high amounts of vitamins B and E and, apart from the other nutrients listed, fat and an important enzyme, emulsine.

Therapeutic Uses
People have long been advised to chew almonds slowly to soften the throat, to fortify the stomach and lungs, and to

clean and freshen the intestines. The high quantities of phosphorus—550 mg per 100 g (4 oz)—may benefit the brain: phosphorus is responsible for growth, repair of cells and production of energy. Phosphorus promotes hormone secretion, and therefore the quick release of energy necessary for muscle contractions, especially of the heart, and nerve impulses. This is particularly useful for athletes and young children. Phosphorus also helps the absorption of B group vitamins. Almonds are useful for pregnant women as they benefit the health of the fetus.

Almond oil is extracted from the sweet nuts and used as a base oil in aromatherapy as well as in baking and confectionery. As a natural purgative first thing in the morning take a teaspoon of the oil with lemon juice, followed by a glass of boiled warm water. It is also good as a cure for gum infections: as soon as you get up in the morning take a large tablespoon of oil and hold in your mouth for at least 10 minutes, then spit out and gargle with fresh water and lemon juice. This will draw out toxins that have accumulated during the night, and will lubricate the gums and tooth enamel.

In the Kitchen

Almonds are so marvellous, you shouldn't spend a day without their energy-boosting properties: take some to work and put some in your children's packed lunches.

- Eat almonds as a dessert after a heavy meal especially if a lot of wine has been drunk, to remedy any subsequent discomfort.
- Eat 6–20 almonds per day, either by themselves or added to your breakfast cereal, salads of watercress, lettuce, spinach or chicory, or to rice, millet or quinoa dishes (these are delicious accompanied by a mixed salad). The almonds will help you digest the grains, assimilate the phosphorus and fix the calcium.
- Toast almonds for a different flavour.
- Use them ground in curries, stews and baking.

Almond Milk

A variant of this delicious drink is popular in the Mediterranean and Middle East.

1 1/2 tablespoons fresh shelled almonds
1 coffeespoon runny honey
150 ml (5 fl oz) still mineral water

Liquidise together for 5 minutes, then drink. For an even more nutritious drink add a ripe banana. If you don't have fresh almonds, replace with dried, but soak in warm water for 1 hour before liquidising.

BRAZIL NUT
Bertholettia excelsa
Lecythideae family

WHAT WE KNOW as the Brazil nut is actually the seed of a South American rainforest tree. The seeds grow inside three-sided shells which are packed together like sections of orange inside a large hard woody outer covering.

Brazil nuts contain up to 65 per cent oil and 20 per cent protein, so are very nutritious. They contain good quantities of all the minerals, particularly magnesium, phosphorus and zinc, and can be extremely high in selenium and iodine.

Therapeutic Uses
Brazils are energising, as are all nuts. In addition their high zinc content can alleviate a number of skin complaints including acne, herpes and varicose ulcers. They can prevent and reduce the symptoms of colds, and they help anorexics and bulimics.

CHESTNUT
Castanea spp
Cupuliferae family

THERE ARE several varieties of sweet chestnut tree, but *Castanea sativa* is the one that has been cultivated in Europe for thousands of years, bearing prickly capsules which split to release the nuts within.

Fresh chestnuts are extremely nutritious, containing a lot of potassium and reasonable amounts of B vitamins, iron, sulphur, magnesium, calcium and zinc. They have the highest content of vitamin B6 of any nut, and, together with green walnuts, are the only ones to contain traces of vitamin C. Chestnuts differ from other nuts in that they are very low in fat and very high in carbohydrate. If you gather them yourself, let them mature for a few days to enable the carbohydrate to convert into sugar and improve the flavour.

Therapeutic Uses
The minerals in chestnuts stimulate the glands and are a good nerve tonic. They are also a great help for varicose veins and haemorrhoids.

In the Kitchen
Chestnuts form a vital part of a vegetarian diet as they can be used as vegetable, meat substitute and pudding. Christmas in Britain or France would not be the same without a turkey stuffed with chestnuts, and if you have an open fire you can use a special slotted pan to roast slit chestnuts directly over the flames.

• Cook chestnuts and serve them with green vegetables, particularly Brussels sprouts.
• Cook them with rice (see page 45).

COCONUT
Cocos nucifera
Palmae family

THE COCONUT palm grows all over the tropics and has many uses: food, medicine, sugar, drink, alcohol, fibre, timber, thatch, domestic utensils and so on. The coconut is not a nut but a stone fruit. The fresh flesh contains a little (incomplete) protein, rather more fibre, a good quantity of the B vitamins, iron, potassium, phosphorus and magnesium, and a great deal of fat (a good third). This fat is saturated—unusually for a vegetable fat—so the oil extracted for cooking should be avoided. Also unusually for a vegetable fat source, coconuts contain virtually no vitamin E.

Therapeutic Uses

The oils in the flesh act as a natural emulsifier and thus help digestion.

- Use fresh grated coconut flesh in curries, cakes and breakfast cereals (where you could also use dried flakes). Coconut creams or milks can be made at home or bought, and are delicious in curries and other spicy dishes or puddings. Eat chunks of fresh coconut in the hand, or add to salads, or shave over salads and other dishes. Use the flesh (or desiccated coconut, which has double the nutrients of fresh) in baking or in ice cream.

HAZELNUT
Corylus spp
Betulaceae family

VARIOUS TYPES of hazelnut tree are found in Europe, Asia and America. Cob nuts or filberts, grown in Southern Britain, are similar to imported hazelnuts but not identical.

All these nuts are extremely nutritious, rich in potassium and vitamin E, and with good levels of calcium, phosphorus, iron, magnesium and zinc. They have a higher content of manganese and biotin than any other kind of nut. They are fairly low in carbohydrate so can be eaten by people who have a tendency to put on weight, although, as with nearly all nuts, the oil content is fairly high. Coarsely ground or ground as flour, they are used in some Continental cakes and nougats, and they are said to be more easily digestible than almonds.

- Use delicious (but expensive) hazelnut oil in salad dressings.
- Add chopped or whole nuts to fruit salads, muesli or porridge.
- Cook nuts in vegetarian dishes with rice, millet and other grains.

PEANUT
Arachis hypogaea

A MEMBER of the *Leguminosae* or legume family—therefore strictly speaking a pulse rather than a nut—the peanut is also known as the monkey nut and groundnut (the latter because it buries its seed pods in the ground to ripen.) It has become an important world crop, rich in oil and protein: a single 25 g (1 oz) serving supplies 6 g protein, about 10 per cent of an adult's daily needs. It also contains about 40 per cent fat, up to ten times as much as other pulses and twice that of the soya bean. The zinc and iodine content of peanuts is also very high.

The protein content of most nuts is considered incomplete because it lacks some of the essential amino acids; peanuts, because they are pulses, contain these, particularly lysine, and thus are very nutritive, particularly useful when a quick burst of energy is needed. Don't eat too many, though, otherwise you could become constipated!

Peanuts in any form can be fatal to those who are allergic.

In the Kitchen

- Add to salads.
- Make into peanut butter, which is extremely valuable for children.
- A sauce for Indonesian satay can be made with peanuts.
- Use the oil, which is polyunsaturated and bland in flavour, in cooking.

PISTACHIO
Pistacia vera
Anacardiaceae family

THIS SMALL TREE is related to the cashew nut and the mango. The fruit is a green nut seed in a thin-shelled capsule, which gapes open when dried. Containing over 50 per cent oil and 22 per cent protein, they are known for their abilities to calm and revive.

In the Kitchen

- Eat pistachios just as they are, along with salted melon and sunflower seeds as they do in the Middle East.
- Use as garnish, both sweet and savoury.

- Add them to salads or stuffings, rice or other grain dishes.
- Make them into a delicious ice cream.

WALNUT
Juglans regia
Juglandaceae family

WALNUTS were introduced to Britain in the fifteenth century. The whiter the shell, the better the quality of the nut. Most walnuts are plucked from British trees when they are still green, before the shells harden, to be used in pickles.

Low in carbohydrate, walnuts are interesting because of their unique vitamin C content, present only in the green nuts. They are rich too in certain minerals such as potassium, magnesium and zinc, and have a very high copper, selenium, folic acid and pantothenic acid content.

Therapeutic Uses
The magnesium is useful in gynaecological problems as it has a tranquillising effect and can detoxify and decongest the nervous system. It is also of use in PMT, menopause and urinary infections. The zinc content dynamizes the assimilation of all the vitamins, copper, iron and so on.

The leaves can be used for making herb tea to treat liver deficiencies, lymphatic and rheumatic conditions. Boil 60 g (2 oz) leaves in 1 litre (1 3/4 pints) water for 15 minutes. Drink a few cups daily.

In the Kitchen
- Eat the nuts as a snack, or add to salads and cooked vegetable dishes.
- Sprinkle them over the white sauce coating broccoli and cauliflower, to enrich the flavours and textures.
- Try my grandmother's hors d'oeuvre: a mixture of chicory, bananas, raisins, lamb's lettuce, cooked French beans and lots of walnuts. Dressed with a little lemon juice and walnut oil (expensive but very delicious) it is healthy and energising.

OATS, *see* Cereal Grains

OFFAL, *see* Meat, Poultry and Fish

OLIVE
Olea europaea
Oleaceae family

PRINCIPAL NUTRIENTS
Vitamins: A, E
Minerals: calcium, copper, iron, magnesium

THE OLIVE, a spreading tree, is extensively cultivated in the Mediterranean region, North Africa, California and elsewhere. Its small fruits are pickled or salt-cured, or pressed to extract their oil.

Olives have been valued for centuries and are among the longest-living of trees. Some are believed to have lived for a thousand years. An olive twig was carried by the dove to Noah, and thereafter the tree became sacred. In ancient times the tree was claimed to have multiple purposes—to shelter, to warm, to feed and to heal.

Green olives are unripe, violet ones nearly ripe and black fully ripe. All olives are brined and are therefore very high in sodium.

Olive oil is pressed from ripe olives, and the first cold pressing—with no heat involved—is what produces the best oil, extra virgin, which has the least acidity (oleic acid content).

Tapenade

This pâté of black olives from the South of France is delicious as a spread or a dip for crudités. Olives can sometimes be a little bitter, but the walnuts "sweeten" them.

The pâté has all the nutrition and therapeutic properties of the walnuts and olives, and it would benefit the brain, the liver and anyone who is feeling low.

100 g (4 oz) shelled walnuts
100 g (4 oz) stoned black olives
1/2 onion, peeled and minced
1 garlic clove, peeled and crushed
juice of 1 lemon
60 ml (2 fl oz) olive oil

Crush the walnuts and olives together in a mortar, then mix in the onion, garlic and lemon juice. Slowly mix in the olive oil, and your pâté is ready. Serve on toast or biscuits, or inside chunks of celery.

Therapeutic Uses

The olive and its oil are rich in minerals and vitamins A and E. The oil is richer in E than the fruit.

Many French doctors recommend olives and olive oil for diabetics, for those who suffer from liver trouble and for constipation. They can also help during the menopause or in cases of PMT, anxiety due to liver disorder, and high blood pressure. For the latter, boil a few olive leaves in a cup of water for a few minutes, then drink with honey.

A similar tisane was given to us in France when we had a temperature as children. Cut 25 g (1 oz) olive leaves into small pieces, add 500 ml (17 fl oz) cold water and bring to the boil. Allow to infuse for 20 minutes, then drink a small cup between meals.

Olives are beneficial in a number of ways, if a little fattening, but the monounsaturated oil that they produce is one of the healthiest to use in cooking or otherwise. A tablespoon of oil in lemon or orange juice every morning keeps you well, supple and healthy, and is particularly good for the skin.

An unusual olive oil remedy popular in France is as a hangover preventative. Before drinking alcohol or eating heavily at a wedding or dinner, swallow a tablespoon of oil to coat your stomach lining and prevent the alcohol reaching your bloodstream too quickly.

In the Kitchen

This is my favourite culinary oil. I remember coming home from school as a young child and getting a piece of toasted *pain de campagne* rubbed with a garlic clove and doused with fresh olive oil. Nowadays a variety of olive oils is available, ranging in colour from bright yellow to bright green and in flavour from spicy and peppery to new-mown grass. New oils, available from November, are wonderful.

Always protect olive oil from air, heat and light, keeping it preferably in containers other than glass. Because it is high in unsaturated fatty acids, olive oil can turn rancid quite quickly.

- Use olive oils in vinaigrettes for salads; use olives in them, too, as in a Salad Niçoise.
- Use olive oil in mayonnaise (for a milder flavour use half olive and half sunflower or grapeseed oil). Add crushed garlic for an aïoli.
- Brush olive oil on to meat, poultry or fish to be grilled or roasted. Potatoes and other vegetables roasted in olive oil have a wonderful flavour.
- Add olive oil to mashed potatoes instead of butter.
- Sprinkle oil over soups, sliced tomatoes or other salad vegetables, using it as a seasoning as they do in parts of France and Italy.
- Use olive oil lavishly in pasta sauces—in Italy oil is the main ingredient of a simple sauce, with added herbs or garlic or chillies.
- Bake olives in bread doughs, or use to top pizzas.
- Make a black olive pâté (see the following two recipes). This can make a meal on its own spread on a piece of toasted country bread and accompanied by a green salad. Add grapefruit segments and some tarragon and basil leaves for a health bonus.
- Make your own flavoured olive oils by adding garlic or herbs, chillies or a mixture.
- In many Italian restaurants a saucerful of home-flavoured olive oil is offered as a canapé, with chunks of good bread to dip in it and sop it up. See page xxiii.

Black Olive Pâté

There is another olive pâté, which I like to serve on top of halved hard-boiled eggs accompanied by a salad of sliced tomato and cucumber. Another treat is to spread it on top of a rye pancake, or on or in blinis. You could substitute a halved croissant, and serve it with a nourishing salad.

250 g (9 oz) stoned black olives
1/2 fresh chilli, seeded and very finely chopped
1 garlic clove, peeled and crushed
a few rosemary and sage leaves
3 juniper berries
olive oil

Put the olives into a measuring jug, and measure their volume. Put the olives and all the remaining ingredients except the oil in a food processor and then measure in the oil—it should be half the volume of the olives. Blend to a coarse or smooth purée.

ONION
Allium cepa
Liliaceae Family

PRINCIPAL NUTRIENTS

Vitamins: B, C
Minerals: calcium, iodine, iron, magnesium, manganese, potassium, silica, sulphur

THE ONION is thought to have originated in Central Asia, but is now grown all over the world. Related to lilies, asparagus and tulips, the genus *Allium* includes onions of all types—maincrop, Spanish, red, Welsh, shallots, spring and chives, as well as leeks and garlic (see separate entries). All are bulbs which grow underground, singly or in clusters. Shallots are superior in flavour to onion, and do not have the overpowering smell. The pickling, silverskin or cocktail onion is a maincrop onion, picked when the bulb has just formed, before growth proper starts; spring or salad onions (scallions in the USA) are maincrop picked even earlier, before the bulb has formed properly. Even chives form tiny bulbs, but it is their shoots or stalks which are eaten.

Onions have been used in cooking and medicine for thousands of years. Bouquets of onions were left beside sarcophagi at Ancient Egyptian funerals, while in Roman times Pliny praised the onion's effectiveness as a suppository in the treatment of haemorrhoids. In the Middle Ages, the School of Salerno described it as a food vital to counter all winter virus infections.

Therapeutic Uses

Onions are very highly therapeutic, so should be eaten as often as possible, preferably raw.

They are tonic and stimulant, particularly to the nervous system and the liver. Many French doctors recommend eating onions in the spring to waken and detoxify a system tired after winter. Onions are also good in the treatment of anaemia and general tiredness and fatigue.

Onions are also very strongly diuretic, so are good for obesity, glandular imbalance, swellings and fluid retention. A good diuretic recipe for the kidneys and bladder, which will also keep viral infections at bay, is inspired by Dioscorides: add the juice of 4 large onions to 1 litre (1 3/4 pints) of boiled mineral water and leave to macerate for 2–3 hours. Drink 4 glasses of this throughout the day. You could also add 300 g (10 oz) minced onion to a bottle of white wine along with 100 g (4 oz) honey. Leave to macerate in an airtight container for at least 48 hours, shaking from time to time. Filter back into a bottle and take 2–4 tablespoons a day. (You could also use this as a meat or fish marinade base.)

Onions are highly antiseptic. They were always eaten during epidemics, and are still very useful for preventing colds, flu and bronchial problems (they are expectorant in action). Macerate minced onion in hot water overnight and drink first thing in the morning with lemon juice. If you lose your voice because of a cold or bad chill, cook onions in the oven with olive oil, eat with other vegetables, and your voice will return.

Onions are digestive, too, but many people find that eating them raw, when they contain most therapeutic properties, has the opposite effect. Instead, add 1 minced onion to 3 tablespoons olive oil and leave to macerate for at least 30 minutes. The strained oil will contain all the onion minerals and nutrients—use it in a salad dressing. Once your tolerance starts to improve, you can add minced raw onion to soups and steamed vegetables. When cooked, onions lose quite a lot of their active ingredients, although they are still valuable.

Onions eaten raw are stimulant and antiseptic for the urinary system, so are effective in treating cystitis. The wine above is good, too.

In the Kitchen

I have hardly a meal which does not include onion. I add them to soups, pasta dishes, sauces, omelettes, pies, meat and fish dishes, rice, lentils and beans. They are an essential flavouring at the same time as doing you so much good.

- Add sliced mild raw onions (Spanish, shallot, spring onions or chives) to salads, sandwiches or a simple "ploughman's". They all help you to digest fatty foods, cheese and other dairy products.
- Mix raw minced onion with olive oil, spread on toast and eat with a green salad.
- Sprinkle chopped chives or spring onions as a last-minute flavouring garnish on almost any dish you care to name. Onion shoots can be used in the same way, as they contain all the onion flavour and nutrients.
- Cook chopped onion as a foundation vegetable in stews, curries, risottos, pilaffs, quiches and so on. When gently sautéed, the natural sugars of the onion caramelise and brown, giving a wonderful flavour.
- Bake large onions whole, or stuff with a savoury filling.
- Stir-fry whole spring onions.

- Use in sauces like *soubise*, which will help the digestion of the meat it will accompany (traditionally, pork and lamb).
- Cook in soup, which is great in the winter when colds and flu are about, and helps to disperse a hangover!
- To get rid of oniony breath, chew a few coffee beans, cardamom, anise or fennel seeds, or whole cloves, or some fresh parsley or mint.

ORANGE
Citrus sinensis
Rutaceae family

PRINCIPAL NUTRIENTS
Vitamins: B, C, P
Minerals: calcium, magnesium, phosphorus, potassium

THE GENUS CITRUS includes many evergreen trees and shrubs known for their fruits—the orange, mandarin, lemon, lime, citron, grapefruit and so on. The ancestor of them all was probably the bitter or Seville orange, still used today for marmalade.

Oranges were first brought to the Mediterranean by the Arabs, probably from China—hence their botanical name—and it was the Moors who cultivated them in Spain, around Seville. Columbus took them to the New World, and oranges are recorded as growing in Florida, now one of the world's major orange-growing areas, as early as 1539.

Therapeutic Uses
Oranges are stomachic, antispasmodic and digestive. Because of their high vitamin C content they also reinforce the immune system (making them good against infections) and act as a natural blood cleanser (therefore good for the skin and healing wounds); and because of their B and bromine content they act as a sedative for the nervous system. The natural sugars in the fruit are easily assimilated by diabetics.

One of the major benefits of the orange is its content of bioflavonoids (in the citrin and sometimes known as vitamin P, a sort of super vitamin C), which are well known for fortifying the capillaries and vascular system. Scientific tests have demonstrated beneficial effects, particularly on varicose veins.

Mandarin oranges contain more bromine than other types of orange, and therefore have a superior calming effect on the nervous system. They are very good indeed for insomnia, so to ensure a good night's sleep eat several mandarins after a hard day, or when your nervous system is still overexcited with work.

Eating nothing but oranges for a couple of days to a week would be a good way of detoxifying the system after overindulgence.

In the Kitchen

The peel and pith of oranges are actually richer in vitamin C than the flesh, so try to use these in some way—but only if they are unsprayed and untreated. The peel contains most of the aromatic oils of the fruit, and it is this which is expressed for the essential oil.

- Eat raw at least once daily.
- Juice and drink daily, preferably first thing in the morning.
- Cook with the juice for superlative flavour—the acidity can cut the oiliness or fattiness of many foods—but of course you will lose a proportion of the vitamin C. Eating oranges or some other vitamin C fruit with many meats enhances the body's uptake of iron.
- Use orange slices or segments as garnishes for fatty meats such as duck.
- Include segments and juice in fresh or dried fruit salads.
- Use the juice as a flavouring in many sweet dishes—delicious in the batter for pancakes—or with chocolate, a very happy marriage.
- Zest an untreated orange to add intense flavour and colour to salads, cake mixtures and so on. This along with parsley and garlic, is a constituent of gremolata, the Italian garnish for osso buco.
- Cut the peel into very thin julienne strips and use to garnish a simple orange slice salad.

- Crystallise or candy orange peel strips.
- Use orange peel in marinades, sauces and bouquets garnis to add orange flavour.
- When Seville (bitter) oranges come into the shops (usually in January and February), use them to make marmalade.

OREGANO, *see* Marjoram and Oregano

PAPAYA OR PAWPAW
Carica papaya
Caricaceae family

PRINCIPAL NUTRIENTS
Vitamins: A, C
Minerals: potassium

THE PAPAYA is the fruit of a Central American shrub or tree first cultivated by the Carib Indians, from whose language the name comes.

Therapeutic Uses
The flesh of ripe papayas is orange to pink in colour, therefore rich in vitamin A; it is also richer in vitamin C than the average orange. The flesh contains a protein-dissolving enzyme called papain, which means it is digestive and can be mildly laxative. Papayas are said to have a beneficial effect on gallbladder and liver complaints. In 1977, a post-operative infection in a kidney transplant patient was cured by the application of papaya.

In the Kitchen
To prepare a papaya, cut in half lengthways and scoop out the seeds and strings. Keep the seeds, and wash and eat them if you like—they have a peppery flavour similar to cress.

- Eat raw from the skin with a dash of lemon or lime juice—a popular breakfast in the West Indies.
- Dice or slice into fruit or savoury salads.
- Serve halved and peeled, rather as you might a melon, perhaps with Parma ham.

- Purée the flesh to use in mousses, fools, ice creams and juices.
- Use the flesh or the inside of the skins to tenderise meats. In the tropics, meat is wrapped and cooked in papaya leaves for their tenderising effect.
- Make unripe papayas into chutneys, as you would green mangoes.

Tuna Fish with Papaya

The papain in papaya tenderises fish as well, especially tuna, which has very dense flesh.

SERVES 4

400 g (14 oz) fresh tuna, in a slice about 2.5 cm (1 in) thick
salt and freshly ground black pepper
1 large papaya or 2 small
1 large garlic clove, peeled and halved
1 tablespoon sesame oil
juice of 1 lime or lemon
a sprig of fresh thyme

Cut the tuna into 4 equal pieces and season with salt and pepper. Halve the papaya(s) lengthways, and remove and discard the skin and seeds. Slice the flesh into strips.

Rub the garlic halves over the inside of a wok, and then add the sesame oil. Heat until very hot, then sear the tuna on all sides to seal and brown. Reduce the heat and add the papaya, lime juice and thyme. Cover and simmer for at least 20 minutes.

Serve with basmati rice or a salad—white chicory is good.

PARSLEY
Petroselinum sativum/crispum
Umbelliferae family

Perhaps the most familiar of culinary herbs, parsley has important therapeutic powers which are undervalued today—it is used more as a garnish than as an important constituent of a dish and its flavour.

There are several types, the two most common being the curly-leaved or moss-curled, and the plain- or flat-leaved, continental parsley. The latter has the better flavour in cooking, but both are equally therapeutic in action.

Therapeutic Uses

Parsley leaves are diuretic, carminative, stimulant, tonic and blood-cleansing, while the leaves and seeds promote menstruation: parsley juice helps to regulate the periods and to bring on late periods. To make a useful parsley decoction boil a large handful of parsley in 600 ml (1 pint) water for 5 minutes. Drink two cups a day. Parsley is also useful for a variety of other women's complaints such as water retention, indigestion, cystitis and PMT.

Parsley is also an effective treatment for constipation. In an old French remedy, though perhaps one that only the French would countenance, a sprig of parsley is used as a suppository. It is said to work wonders!

Dr. Leclerc recommended parsley for sterility because of one of its constituents, apiol. This rebalances a weak system and stirs it into action. The French, yet again, swear by parsley in the same way as the Chinese revere ginseng. Parsley is also used for liver deficiencies, and kidney and bladder infections.

In the Kitchen

Parsley is rich in iron and vitamins A, B and C: 25 g (1 oz) parsley contains marginally more iron than the same quantity of cooked liver, for instance. Use parsley as often as you can, preferably raw, to gain numerous benefits.

• Eat raw in salads. Chop and add raw to sauces such as mayonnaise, and scatter over soups, sauces, vegetable and rice dishes. Use stalks to add flavour to stock. Chop the leaves and mix with butter for a garnish for fish; or mix with butter and garlic, spread on bread and bake briefly.

- Vitamin C is water-soluble, but is not lost when parsley is fried for a few minutes only to crisp it. This makes a good accompaniment to fish such as turbot or to white meats like veal or chicken, also adding considerable flavour.
- Add chopped parsley (and other herbs if liked) to an omelette, which helps you to absorb protein and vitamins. Use one egg per person, 1 tablespoon soya milk and lots of lightly fried parsley.
- Add masses of chopped parsley to mashed potato. Fish and meatballs are good made with parslied mashed potato.
- Chop with garlic and lightly fry as *persillade*, a perfect accompaniment to boiled or grilled meats or fish; or add finely grated lemon or orange peel for the Italian gremolata, traditional with osso buco, but full of flavour with any meat or fish.

PARSNIP
Pastinaca sativa
Umbelliferae family

PRINCIPAL NUTRIENTS
Vitamins: B, C
Minerals: calcium, iron, magnesium, phosphorus, potassium

PARSNIPS were particularly popular in the Middle Ages in Britain because their starch content made them useful on meatless fast days. Due to their sweetness, they were baked in cakes and puddings.

Therapeutic Uses
Dr. Leclerc attributed diuretic properties to parsnips, advising that they should be given to people suffering from conditions such as gout and rheumatism. He also claims they are useful in cases of amenorrhoea, and for fluid retention before periods.

The active principle of parsnips can be extracted in a juice. This is diuretic for use in rheumatic conditions, and to help urinary disorders such as cystitis. It also helps loss of appetite.

Juice 450 g (1 lb) parsnips with 2 large carrots, 1 whole cucumber and lots of parsley. Drink a few glasses each day.

In the Kitchen

Parsnips are usually cooked, but they are also delicious raw—when, of course, their vitamin C content is fully available. They are best in the autumn and winter months, when they are full of flavour (traditionally after frost). During storage, much of the vegetable's starch is converted to sugar.

- Grate raw in a salad with other vegetables such as carrots, sweet potato and asparagus. Dress with olive oil and citrus juice, or walnut oil.
- Grate and mix with horseradish or radish (the small red ones or the Japanese mooli). This is delicious with herring and other oily fish, complementing their flavour.
- Roast in the oven with garlic to make a good accompaniment to meat. (This was the traditional vegetable for meat in Britain before the potato arrived.) Coat in fresh seasoned breadcrumbs first if you like.
- Bake on a medium heat with olive oil, crushed garlic and black pepper.
- Cook in chunks until tender, then purée and garnish with toasted nuts or pine kernels. Or use the purée with walnuts to make a chunky bread that is good with cheese.
- Use in a soup, puréed or in chunks, with potatoes and leeks. Season with thyme, oregano, parsley and a little basil for a wonderfully welcoming soup in the cold winter months. For those not on a diet, add soured cream or live yogurt.
- Bake cooked and puréed parsnip with cheese (Emmenthal, Gruyère or mature Cheddar) in a soufflé. Accompanied by salad leaves dressed with walnut oil, this makes a good evening meal because it is so easy to digest.
- Juice parsnips for an unusual but nutritious drink.

PEA AND MANGE-TOUT
Pisum sativum spp
Leguminosae family

PRINCIPAL NUTRIENTS

Vitamins: A, B, C, E
Minerals: calcium, iodine, iron, phosphorus, potassium, zinc

THE GARDEN PEA was developed from wild plants in Italy in the sixteenth century, and the mange-tout originated about a century later. The garden pea forms in rows within a pod lined with an inedible inner skin which is lacking in mange-touts *(Pisum saccaratum)*. These are grown not for the peas but for the pod, the meaning of the French name being literally "eat-all". Mange-touts are also known as sugar peas, sugar-snap peas and snow peas; sugar-snaps are sometimes a little "fatter" than mange-touts.

Therapeutic Uses
Both peas and mange-touts, being green, contain vitamins A and C in fairly good quantities. Mange-touts supply more of these vitamins, whereas peas contain more minerals as well as iodine. The iron and phosphorus help the absorption of calcium, while the potassium emulsifies and transforms fats. Both vegetables are stimulant and supply energy.

In the Kitchen
Eat peas as fresh as possible for, like sweetcorn (maize), as soon as they are plucked from the parent plant their sugars begin to convert to starch. (This is why commercial frozen peas are often so much sweeter and tenderer than pods bought in the greengrocer's; the large frozen food companies freeze their produce immediately after it leaves the field, while the pea pods may have taken a few days to reach the shops.)

- Eat peas and mange-touts raw for the best flavour and most nutrition—both are wonderful just to nibble.
- Cook very lightly. Stir-frying or steaming are preferable to boiling, as less of the water-soluble vitamins will be lost. Add mint or another fresh aromatic leaf for flavour.

- Steam mange-touts and eat like asparagus, dipped in melted butter, French dressing or hollandaise.

Potage Petits Pois

There aren't many recipes for petits pois, but this soup is delicious and healthy. The almond, used instead of oil or cream, gives a lovely smell and flavour. You could make the purée yourself by grinding about 6 almonds with a little water, or by mixing 1 tablespoon ground almonds with a little water.

PER PERSON

2 small turnips or carrots
250 ml (8 fl oz) still mineral water
salt
a large handful of podded (or frozen) peas
a little almond purée
a pinch of paprika

Peel and grate the turnips very finely, and cook for a few minutes in salted water. When boiling, add the peas and cook for a few minutes more. Liquidise, then stir in the almond and paprika.

PEA, DRIED, *see* Pulses

PEACH AND NECTARINE
Prunus persica spp
Rosaceae family

PRINCIPAL NUTRIENTS
Vitamins: A, B, C
Minerals: calcium, iron, magnesium, manganese, phosphorus, potassium, sulphur, zinc

THE PEACH is thought to have been native to China, and was brought to Europe via Persia (hence its botanical name) by the Romans. There are several varieties, some with white flesh, some with yellow, and there is also a peach without a fuzzy skin, the nectarine *(Prunus persica* var. *nectarina).*

Both peaches and nectarines are dried, when certain of the nutrients, particularly vitamin A, phosphorus and iron become concentrated. The fibre content also increases.

Therapeutic Uses
Both these fruits are rich in nutrients, the yellow-fleshed variety having a good vitamin A content. They are diuretic, a gland stimulant, good for digestion, and recommended for people who have digestive problems due to nervousness or stress. They are an effective remedy for PMT and menopausal problems.

The leaves and blossom can also be used. The latter has a calming effect on the nervous system, and French doctors recommend infusions of them for coughs. The leaves, made into decoctions, are laxative.

In the Kitchen
Peaches will not ripen after picking, but merely soften. The longer the peach is left on the tree, the more will the bitter compounds in the flesh decrease, so late season peaches are often the sweetest. Try to eat the skin as well as the flesh, as the majority of nutrients are just under the skin.

- Eat whole ones raw, or chop them up into a fruit salad (use a citrus juice to prevent browning). Chopped or sliced, peaches or nectarines can be eaten with cream, fromage frais, yogurt or, in a classic way, with champagne.
- Chilled sliced peaches sprinkled with sugar and rosewater are particularly luscious; garnish with powdered cinnamon and fresh mint leaves.
- Serve halved peaches with raspberry coulis and ice cream for a peach Melba.
- Bake, as the Americans do, in a variety of pies, puddings, tarts and cobblers.
- Poach whole or halved in wine or syrup, perhaps with a little sweet spice like a cinnamon stick. Serve with soured cream and grated dark chocolate.

- Use peaches or nectarines in preserves such as chutneys, jams, jellies and marmalade.
- Spice and bake halves for use as a meat garnish.
- Use dried peaches and nectarines in compotes, puddings, cakes and mincemeat and as sweetmeats.

PEANUT, *see* Nuts

PEAR
Pyrus communis
Rosaceae family

PRINCIPAL NUTRIENTS
Vitamins: A, B, C
Minerals: calcium, iodine, iron, magnesium, manganese, phosphorus, potassium, sulphur

THE PEAR is native to Europe and the Middle East and like the apple, needs a winter to give it a dormant period. Pears were grown in antiquity: Homer wrote of orchards of the fruit being cultivated, and Pliny recorded around 40 varieties. Pears were introduced to America in the early seventeenth century.

Therapeutic Uses
The pear is one of my favourite fruits because of its valuable properties. Pears contain natural sugars, pectin and tannins, and it is the combination of potassium, pectin and tannin that has the ability to dissolve uric acid, thus making pears the number one fruit for rheumatic conditions, gout and arthritis. The phosphorus is good for the nervous system, and the sodium for the digestion. The magnesium assists in the utilisation of carbohydrates, fats, protein and calcium. Pears are also good for high blood pressure, lazy intestines, asthma and anaemia.

Juice the fruit for health-giving drinks, and eat the fruits as well. Liquidise 5 pears to get a large glassful, and drink two to three times per day. This can benefit cystitis and bladder problems, and act as a blood cleanser. Pear and guava together make a good pick-me-up.

When dried, pears become very high in sugars and are therefore very energising. Make a wonderful drink by boiling 60–80 g (2–3 oz) dried pears in 1 litre (1 3/4 pints) water for 15 minutes, then leave to stand for 30 minutes. Drink this juice when you are tired, nervous or suffering from premenstrual or menopausal symptoms.

In the Kitchen

Pears bruise very easily when fully ripe, so they are best bought slightly under-ripe and allowed to mature slowly off the tree. When you cut pears, do so at the very last minute as the flesh will turn brown; you can delay this by sprinkling the cut fruit with citrus juice.

Both cooking and dessert pears are available.

- Eat whole pears raw, or chop or slice into fruit salads. Do not peel, as the skin is where the vitamin C is concentrated.
- Slice dessert pears and serve with slices of avocado in a vinaigrette as a healthy and delicious starter.
- Serve sliced raw pears with Parma ham as a starter as you would melon or figs, or with any blue cheese or Parmesan as a dessert.
- Bake pears in tarts with nuts (a good autumn combination), also in cakes, teabreads and puddings.
- Make into sorbets, ice creams, fools and mousses.
- Bake cooking pears with game, or use baked or spiced as a savoury garnish.
- Poach pears whole, with or without their cores, in a compote with a clove, a small cinnamon stick, a little ground ginger and a light sugar syrup or red wine. Serve sprinkled with toasted sesame seeds, mint leaves, fruit sugar, honey or maple syrup.
- Cook pears in chutneys and jams.

Peppercorns
Piper nigrum
Piperaceae family

PEPPERCORNS—green, black, pink and white—are the fruit of a creeping tropical vine. As a spice, pepper has long been valued; it inspired the great voyages of exploration, and great fortunes were made and lost in the spice trade.

Therapeutic Uses

Pepper contains a substance called piperine which stimulates the production of saliva and gastric and pancreatic juices; this spice therefore is a major digestive, especially of fat. (It is sometimes used to coat cheeses, for instance.) It also stimulates the appetite of people who are anaemic or anorexic. If pepper is used in their meals the stomach will *demand* food, and indeed doctors in Germany prescribe peppercorns for just such a purpose. (Never use too much, though, or it could irritate the stomach lining, give you cramps or make you vomit. If you have this problem, drink some soya milk or eat some natural yogurt.) After a shock or stress the salivary glands can function poorly or even fail, and sucking lightly crushed peppercorns can stimulate them into action once more.

For lung and bronchial infections, boil 3 g of crushed peppercorns in 150 ml (5 fl oz) water for 10 minutes, then add to 50 ml (2 fl oz) strong mint tea. This drink brings up phlegm and relieves a cough. Pepper is antiputrefactive, which is why it is so often used and cooked with meat.

An essential oil is distilled from the crushed peppercorns, black and white.

In the Kitchen

Peppercorns are green when immature. If canned or brined at this stage, they become what is known as green peppercorns; if they are dried in the sun, they become the familiar black spice. White peppercorns come from the mature corn after the red husk has been soaked off and the corn dried. Buy whole peppercorns and grind freshly as required, since pre-ground spices quickly lose their aroma, flavour and active properties. Black is a little more aromatic than white.

• Use freshly ground pepper over a variety of dishes, from meats to vegetables and even over a bowl of strawberries.

- Use in savoury stocks and marinades.
- Coat steaks with coarsely ground black pepper before grilling.
- Macerate coarsely ground peppercorns in a good oil and use in cooking and dressings.

PEPPERS

Capsicum spp
Solanaceae family

PRINCIPAL NUTRIENTS

Vitamins: A, B, C, E, K, P
Minerals: calcium, iodine, iron, phosphorus, potassium

CAPSICUM PEPPERS, both sweet and chilli, are members of the same family as potatoes, tomatoes and deadly nightshade. All are native to tropical America and the West Indies—so the sweet peppers of Mediterranean cuisine, the paprika pepper so characteristic of Hungary and the chillies that so heatedly represent Indian curries were not known in the Old World until after the sixteenth century.

Green sweet peppers *(Capsicum annuum)* are immature, and if left on the plant will turn red, yellow, purple or black. Chillies *(Capsicum frutescans)* are smaller and more pointed than sweet peppers; they contain a chemical called capsaicin, which is what gives them their heat.

Chillies are dried and ground to make chilli powder and cayenne pepper. A particular variety of Hungarian sweet red pepper is dried and ground to make paprika.

Therapeutic Uses

Sweet peppers and chillies are particularly rich in vitamins A and C, the red containing about 15 times more betacarotene than the green. Raw chillies have more of virtually every other nutrient than red or green peppers, but who wants to eat chillies raw!

Sweet peppers contain vitamins K and P, which fortify the capillaries and stimulate gastric secretions; they are also an energising and stimulant vegetable. The chilli, particularly when cooked in a curry with other spices, is antiseptic, diaphoretic and sudorific; it can also help those suffering from colds or flu by softening and releasing mucus and phlegm.

Some people find green peppers a little indigestible; if so, eat the riper yellow or red ones instead.

Red Pepper and Carrot Soup

This soup is wonderfully colourful as well as nutritious. You could use pumpkin, another vegetable rich in vitamin A, instead of the carrot.

SERVES 4

2–3 red peppers
500 g (18 oz) carrots, trimmed and scrubbed
1/2 onion, peeled
1 large garlic clove, peeled
a sprig of thyme
500 ml (17 fl oz) still mineral water

GARNISH

chopped herbs (thyme, chervil, parsley), single
cream or natural yogurt

Seed the peppers and chop into small pieces. Chop 300 g (11 oz) of the carrots together with all the onion and garlic. Place in a pot along with the thyme and water, bring to the boil, then simmer for 20 minutes. Liquidise.

Meanwhile, juice the remaining carrots and add to the liquidised soup. Heat through gently, but not to boiling point, in order to retain as many nutrients as possible. Serve sprinkled with herbs, or with a spoonful of cream or yogurt gently swirled on top.

In the Kitchen

To prepare sweet peppers, wash, dry and seed—the seeds may carry some of the heat of their chilli cousins. Remove the seeds from chillies if less heat is required; both seeds *and* flesh contain the hot chemical. Handle chillies with gloves if possible; the capsaicin can irritate the skin, and if you touch your eyes they can be badly affected. Capsaicin does not dissolve in water and cannot therefore be simply washed off, which is why beer or milk are so much more effective than water in cooling a curry-heated mouth.

- Eat green and red peppers raw for the greatest nutritional benefit. Slice as crudités with a dip or salsa, or use in a mixed salad. Use red or green pepper dice as a colourful edible garnish for a variety of dishes.
- Skin sweet peppers by baking in a medium oven for 30 minutes, then putting in a pan with a lid to cool. The "steam" produced loosens the skin and makes it easy to peel off, making the vegetables more digestible. Slice the flesh and dress with a flavourful dressing or simply some wonderful walnut or hazelnut oil.
- Cook peppers gently in a variety of dishes: sweet ones in ratatouille, pipérade, peperonata, goulash and rouille; chillies in curries, hot sauces and salsas; paprika in stews and goulash.
- Stuff whole sweet peppers with savoury stuffing ingredients such as cooked minced meat and/or rice, chopped mushrooms and other vegetables.

PERSIMMON
Diospyros kaki
Ebenaceae family

PRINCIPAL NUTRIENTS
Vitamins: A, C
Minerals: calcium, phosphorus, potassium

THERE ARE several varieties of persimmon: the kaki or date plum of Japan and China; a native North American variety *Diospyros virginiana* (the name "persimmon" is derived from an Algonquin Indian word); and the sharon fruit, a new strain developed in Israel.

Persimmons look like large orange tomatoes. Kaki and the American variety have large inedible seeds and the flesh must be very soft before it is eaten—otherwise the flavour is very astringent due to the tannin content. The sharon fruit, on the other hand, is seedless and can be eaten skin and all while still firm, as it is very sweet.

Therapeutic Uses

These fruit have been used in Chinese medicine for many years, principally as a remedy for stomach complaints. Because of the astringency, I think they are a very effective (and pleasurable) laxative! The bright yellow-orange flesh also indicates a high vitamin A content, so there are many other benefits too.

In the Kitchen

- Eat ripe persimmons or sharon fruit raw like apples or spoon the flesh from the skin.
- Chop or slice the flesh and use in sweet fruit salads or savoury salads—good with slices of avocado or melon, or with Parma ham. Dress with lemon juice or vinaigrette.
- Use the pulp in mousses, sweet purée sauces, sorbets, ice creams, fools or jellies.
- Bake in bread, cakes, pies and puddings, as did the early American settlers.
- Sprinkle slices with sweet spices such as ginger, nutmeg, mace and cinnamon.

PINEAPPLE
Ananas sativus
Bromeliaceae family

PRINCIPAL NUTRIENTS

Vitamins: B, C
Minerals: calcium, copper, magnesium, manganese, potassium

THE PINEAPPLE, native to eastern South America and the West Indies, was first encountered by Columbus in 1493. It has been grown in hothouses in Britain since the eighteenth century: evidence of its popularity can be seen in the pineapple-shaped finials of many wrought-iron gate posts and railings of the period.

Therapeutic Uses

Pineapples contain the digestive enzyme bromelin (similar to the ficin in fresh figs and the papain in papayas), and is therefore excellent as a stomach tonic. In North Africa pineapple juice is used as a preventative and remedy for food poisoning and virus infections. It is also given to women who suffer from amenorrhoea.

Pineapple takes away the pain of a sore throat and is a decongestant. Drink the fresh juice slowly, leaving it for a few seconds in the mouth before swallowing.

Pineapple Sorbet

This would be particularly popular with children suffering from a sore throat. You could make it look splendid by cutting the flesh very carefully out from the shell of the pineapple, and serving the sorbet in the hollowed-out shell.

SERVES 4

1 large pineapple
100–175 g (4–6 oz) caster sugar
juice of 3 large oranges

Peel the pineapple and cut the flesh away from the core. Cut into small pieces and then liquidise. Sieve and measure out 250 ml (8 fl oz) of the juice into a pan. Add the sugar, and boil to a syrup.

When cool, add the remaining pineapple juice and the strained orange juice, and place in a suitable freezing tray (or a sorbet or ice-cream machine). Freeze, removing from the freezer a couple of times during the process, and stirring hard, until it has reached the right consistency.

In the Kitchen

Many fruit and vegetables, when stored, become sweeter because their starch converts to sugar. Pineapples have no starch content, and since they get their sugar from the plant they will not sweeten once they are picked. So choose large, juicy, ripe fruit.

The bromelin content prevents gelatine from setting, so if you are making a pineapple jelly gently cook the fruit first to inactivate the enzyme.

- Eat pineapple raw as the ideal dessert because of its effect on the digestion.
- Mix chopped pineapple with other fruits in a fruit salad. Serve in the hollowed-out shell of the pineapple if you like.
- Use chunks or slices as meat or fish garnish.
- Cook pineapple gently in stews of pork or other meat for its tenderising effect.
- Stir-fry with slivers of meat or vegetables in Chinese-type dishes.
- Coat in a light batter and deep-fry as a pudding.
- Put rings of pineapple on the base of an upside-down cake or pudding.
- Make into jam, or crystallise.
- Pineapple rings can be dried.
- Juice pineapple and drink often.

PINE KERNELS, *see* Seeds

PISTACHIO, *see* Nuts

PLANTAIN, *see* Banana

PLUM
Prunus domestica
Rosaceae family

PRINCIPAL NUTRIENTS
Vitamins: A, B, C

Minerals: calcium, iron, magnesium, phosphorus, potassium

THE PLUM FAMILY includes many types of differing colours, shapes and flavours, including the greengage and damson. The stones of sloes and bullaces, other close relatives, have been found in the ruins of Bronze Age lake dwellings in Switzerland.

Therapeutic Uses

Fresh plums are fairly low in nutrients, including fibre, but when the fruit is dried to become prunes the vitamin A is concentrated and the fibre content becomes high, as do the iron, magnesium and potassium. Both fresh and dried fruit are high in sugar and carbohydrates, which makes them energising; they are diuretic and laxative, and can benefit sufferers from constipation, piles, many rheumatic conditions, arteriosclerosis, anaemia and asthma. They are also good for the nervous system, particularly when one is over-tired.

Steep some prunes overnight in boiled water; next morning eat the fruit and drink the liquid.

In the Kitchen

Most members of the plum family can be eaten whole and raw, but damsons and sloes, which can be found both wild and in gardens, usually need to be cooked with sugar because they are too tart. For sloe gin, prick ripe sloes with a needle several times, immerse in gin with some sugar and leave, turning occasionally, for several weeks. Making spirits is the principal use to which many types of plum are put in Europe—the quetsch and mirabelle eaux de vie, for instance.

- Eat ripe raw plums for breakfast or as a snack. Halve them to add to breakfast cereals or fresh fruit salads.
- Stew plums gently in water or orange juice, remove the stones and skins, and serve with crème fraîche or yogurt.
- Cook fresh plums in sauces (there's a good Chinese one for duck), in flans and tarts, in steamed puddings and jam or chutneys. Use cooked flesh in mousses, soufflés and fools.

- Soak prunes in water if necessary, and eat on their own at breakfast (the bane of many a British childhood), or with porridge or cereal.
- Include cooked prunes in a compôte or dried fruit salad.
- Use prunes in soup (the Scottish cock-a-leekie, for instance), in stuffings for pork, duck or goose, or in meat stews.
- Always try to eat prunes with meat or a food rich in vitamin C in order to increase the absorption of iron by the body. Meat makes the stomach more acid, which enables iron to be absorbed more easily, and C changes the plant iron to a more readily absorbed form (ferric to ferrous).
- Slice dry prunes into green salads along with walnuts and almonds. Nibble them as a snack.

POMEGRANATE
Punica granatum
Lythraceae family

PRINCIPAL NUTRIENTS
Vitamins: B, C
Minerals: potassium

THE APPLE-SHAPED pomegranate is the fruit of a small tree found in North Africa, the Mediterranean and subtropical Asia. The botanical name means "apple of many seeds"; and from *granatum* came the name of a small "seeding" bomb known as the grenade, the British Grenadiers, and Granada in Spain, where the Moors cultivated many pomegranate orchards.

Therapeutic Uses
Pomegranate, whether eaten as a fruit or drunk as juice, is a good heart tonic and is used in tropical countries to treat dysentery and asthma. The Chinese let the fruit dry, and then suck the skin as a remedy for fever.

In the Kitchen
The outer and inner skins of the fruit are inedible; the only edible part comprises the glistening red crystal seeds, the

sweet (but often sour) pulp surrounding the bitter, tiny black inner seeds.

- Eat the whole red seeds raw, use them as a pretty garnish for meat dishes, or add to fruit salads.
- Juice the seeds. Put them in a muslin-lined sieve and squeeze or press, but not too hard in order not to crush the bitter black inner seeds.
- Add the juice and seeds of pomegranates to a duck or chicken dish—as in the famous Persian *faisinjan*.
- Use the sour-sweet juice in sauces, in marinades, to sprinkle over fish as you would lemon, or to drink fresh.
- Make into a jam or preserve—the fruit is good mixed with cranberries.

POPPY SEEDS, *see* Seeds

POTATO
Solanum tuberosum
Solanaceae family

PRINCIPAL NUTRIENTS
Vitamins: B, C
Minerals: calcium, magnesium, phosphorus, potassium, zinc

THE POTATO originated in South America and was brought back to Europe by the Spaniards in the mid-sixteenth century. Sir Walter Raleigh is believed to have introduced it (as well as tobacco) to Britain, and he was certainly the first to grow it, on his Irish country estate, around 1590.

The newcomer was at first viewed with great suspicion throughout Europe. Because of its rather scabby appearance it was thought to be a probable cause of leprosy. There was an element of logic in this because potatoes contain solanine, an alkaloid which is a nerve poison and can cause a skin rash, an early symptom of the disease. Eventually the hostility was overcome and the new vegetable became a staple food for the Irish, whose population was as a result decimated in the horrific famine of 1845–6 when the potato blight struck.

Therapeutic Uses

Potatoes contain many minerals, principally potassium—there are 630 mg per 100 g (4 oz), flesh and skin, of a baked potato—and because they are eaten in bulk they make a major contribution to the daily diet in terms of protein, fibre, thiamine and niacin (B vitamins). Potatoes provide a fifth of the UK daily intake of vitamin C.

Because of the high carbohydrate content potatoes are good for diabetics. They can energise, remineralise and detoxify the blood, and help high blood pressure, catarrh, fluid retention and kidney and bladder problems, as well as pulmonary and digestive problems. It's interesting that we tend to eat more potatoes in winter, presumably because of the filling carbohydrate. But we also tend to eat richer food in the winter, and potatoes help to emulsify their fats and make them more digestible.

Potatoes are helpful for those who suffer from insomnia and other nighttime problems such as nervous leg cramps, neuralgia or coughs. This is because they contain slightly narcotic properties, the remnants of the solanine (now mostly bred out), which is strongest on or near the skin. The word solanine actually comes from the Latin for comfort or consolation, and substances such as atropine from the potato's relative deadly nightshade are used in both conventional and alternative medicine as calmants.

In the Kitchen

Because the potato grows underground, it is under a great deal of attack from rain-leached chemical fertilisers and insecticides. To avoid ingesting these undesirable chemical constituents, it is best to buy organically grown potatoes.

Potatoes consist of starch, which, during storage, turns to sugar. The starch needs to be cooked to render it palatable, which is just as well, as cooked potatoes contain more nutrients than raw. Store potatoes in a cool dark place to prevent spoilage, greening of the skin and sprouting; all these processes increase solanine, which is not destroyed by cooking.

Potatoes divide roughly into floury and waxy, maincrop and new. Maincrop are waxy when "new" in the autumn, but become floury through storage as the starch develops. Floury potatoes are the ones to mash, waxy or new the ones to fry and use in salads.

Do not keep cooked potatoes for long, as a toxic substance will develop which can be dangerous.

- Baked potatoes are the most nutritious, containing valuable dietary fibre as well as all the other nutrients. Scrub the skin well, using only potatoes that are undamaged, with no greening or sprouts. Eat with a filling or topping of your choice, but remember it is often these that are fattening rather than the potato! (Potatoes contain only 22 calories per 25 g/1 oz when plainly boiled.)
- Eat the skins only of baked potatoes, with a thin layer of flesh, as a snack or starter, perhaps deep-frying them and then serving with soured cream flavoured with spring onions or chives. Use the remaining potato flesh as a thickener in soups, or mash with other root vegetables.
- Lightly scrub new potatoes and steam in their skins. Many of the nutrients are just under the skin, and steaming destroys fewer of these than boiling. The flavour of freshly dug, organically grown new potatoes is incomparable.
- Mash maincrop or floury potatoes with milk, butter and seasonings, or mix with soured cream, a beaten egg, some grated nutmeg and grated Gruyère or Emmenthal cheese. This makes a delicious accompaniment for meat or fish. (Do not try to keep mashed potatoes warm but serve immediately as they lose their vitamin C.)
- Cook potatoes and serve just warm, dressed with an aromatic vinegar, as an accompaniment for herring or other oily fish.
- Add cooked waxy potatoes, again just warm, to a salad of spinach and lettuce. Or toss cooked new potatoes with a vinaigrette and then dress with mayonnaise, adding celery, chives and other items for a potato salad.

- Layer potato slices in a casserole with cheese, garlic and onion. Add herbs to taste, half cover with milk, milk and water, or stock. Bake until soft and the starch of the potatoes has absorbed all the liquid and the flavourings.
- Make potatoes into rissoles, potato cakes, rösti and bubble and squeak, or use them in soups.

POULTRY, *see* Meat, Poultry and Fish

PRUNE, *see* Plum

PULSES

PRINCIPAL NUTRIENTS
Vitamins: A, B, C (when fresh and sprouted), E
Minerals: calcium, iron, potassium, magnesium, zinc

LIKE GRAINS, pulses have been staple foods for thousands of years. They are the dried seeds of members of the Leguminosae family—peas, beans and lentils. They are very nutritious because, again like grains (and seeds), they contain everything for the next generation of plants. One of their principal advantages is that they can be stored throughout the winter, providing nourishment when fresh foods are scarce or non-existent.

All dried pulses are rich in protein and so can take the place of meat for vegetarians. This protein is incomplete, though, in all pulses but the soya bean (see page 158). The best way of eating pulses, therefore, is with grains, whose amino acids will balance those of the pulse. Pulses contain no cholesterol and very little fat (apart, again, from the soya bean). They are good sources of the B vitamins, particularly B6 and folic acid, and calcium, iron, potassium, magnesium and zinc. Eat them with C-rich foods to maximise the absorption of the iron.

Pulses contain toxic substances which inhibit digestion and assimilation. These are inactivated by cooking, so be sure to boil pulses such as red kidney beans for a good 10 minutes first before continuing the cooking, generally very slowly. Pulses also contain fibre, which causes flatulence in many people; certain elements in the pulse are not digested in the small intestine and reach the colon, where they are attacked by intestinal bacteria which produce gas. One way of alleviating this problem is to discard the water in which pulses have been soaked, which could contain some of the indigestible matter. And, of course, aromatherapeutic plants could be added to the cooking water to help this problem as well—savory is the most famed, known in Germany as the "bean herb".

All pulses—apart from lentils—should be soaked in water at least overnight to rehydrate them. They should then be covered with fresh cold water, brought to the boil and boiled for 10 minutes before a longer, slower cooking takes over. This timing will vary according to the type of pulse and its age (how long since it was dried and put in the packet). The older the pulse, the longer it will take to soften. Never add salt to the water when you cook pulses, as it hardens their skins.

Pulses can be sprouted (see Seeds): mung beans produce, for instance, the familiar Chinese beansprout. All are very nutritious.

Broad Beans
Vicia faba

Known as the Windsor, field or fava bean in the United States, the broad bean has been cultivated in Europe and Asia for thousands of years. The seeds which are dried as a pulse are also commonly eaten fresh in season, cooked minimally (out of their pods), after which the central bright green "kernel" can be popped out of its greyish skin. When fresh, of course, these beans contain good levels of vitamin C. Favism is a type of anaemia brought about in people susceptible to a toxin in the broad bean plant's pollen, or in undercooked beans.

In the Kitchen

- Accompany fresh beans with butter, garlic, bacon, parsley or savory.
- Cook or serve dried beans with bacon or sausages, and enhance them with herbs such as thyme and marjoram.
- Ful medames are a variety of small broad beans found in the Middle East, particularly Egypt, where they are cooked with garlic, lemon, parsley and hard-boiled eggs.

CHICKPEAS
Cicer arietinum

THE CHICKPEA, also known as Bengal gram, is native to the Middle East. It has long been cultivated in India as a food crop, being used whole or mashed in curries, or dhals, or ground as a flour for savoury pancakes and breads. It features in much Middle Eastern cooking too—the Mediterranean hummus, for example, is a chickpea paste flavoured with garlic, lemon juice, tahina or sesame paste, and olive oil. Chickpeas are used in many "poor" meat and vegetable stews, notably couscous in Morocco, and feature in Arab, Spanish and South American cooking.

Therapeutic Uses

According to many French doctors, chickpeas help to regulate menstruation and to bring it on. They are a wonderful cleanser of the urinary tract, helpful in treating bladder infections. Make a diuretic soup by cooking chickpeas with barley, parsley and garlic. Chickpeas are also good for nervous disorders and for tiredness.

In *The Cook's Encyclopedia* Tom Stobart reports that the plants exude so much oxalic acid that pickers' shoes can be damaged, and they have to wear gloves to protect their hands.

Chickpea Pâté

This nourishing and filling pâté, a meat substitute, could actually be made with any pulse or mixture of pulses. As the pulse will have been cooked twice it will be easier to digest, and it is helped even more by the parsley, basil and onion. This is an energising and delicious dish when eaten with toast or salad as a starter or light lunch.

SERVES 4

2 cups cooked chickpeas
3 cups froment (toasted wheatgerm, available in
    health food shops)
1 cup chicken stock or broth
1 1/2 cups finely chopped onion
sesame oil
1 cup finely chopped mushrooms
1 1/2 cups chopped parsley
1 tablespoon chopped basil
1 tablespoon tamari or soy sauce
1 ripe red pepper, seeded and cut into thin strips

Soak and cook the chickpeas at least a day in advance. Then process them to a purée. Preheat the oven to 180°C/350°F/Gas 4. Mix the froment and stock together in a bowl, and let stand for about 10 minutes. Cook the onion in a little oil for a few minutes until it starts to brown, then add the mushroom. Cook for a few minutes more. Add to the froment in the bowl the onion and mushroom, the puréed chickpeas and all the remaining ingredients except for the red pepper. Mix well.

Turn half the mixture into a suitably sized bread or pâté tin, grease with a little more oil, then arrange the red pepper strips in a pattern on top. Cover with the remaining mixture and bake for 30 minutes. Eat hot or cold.

KIDNEY BEANS
Phaseolus vulgaris

THERE ARE hundreds of varieties of the basic kidney or common bean, among them white, red and black kidney, cannellini, haricot, flageolet, lima and its larger relative, the butter bean. The plant was originally native to the Americas but has now spread all over the world, and numerous new varieties have been developed. White beans are the seeds of edible bean pods such as green, French and runner beans.

Kidney beans are used in a number of ways around the world, usually in casseroles, slow cooked with aromatics characteristic of the area or country—with chilli in the Mexican chilli con carne, for instance.

LENTILS
Lens esculenta

THERE ARE various types of lentil: the continental which is brownish green, the Puy which is greeny turquoise to black, the red (usually split), and others from India and the Middle East which come in a variety of colours and are known as dhal (both the pulse itself, and the dish made from it).

In the Kitchen
Lentils are very nutritious and are particularly useful for children, old people and pregnant women. They do not need to be presoaked, but do wash them well first.

- Eat hot, simply cooked with herb and vegetable flavourings such as onion, garlic or thyme.
- Leave to get cold and eat as a salad (especially good with red cabbage, chicory, endive or lettuce).

Spiced Lentils

This dish, served hot, makes a good winter meal. Alternatively it could make a deliciously protein-rich salad in the summer.

225 g (8 oz) continental lentils
5 tablespoons olive oil
1 medium onion, peeled and finely chopped
1 large garlic clove, peeled and finely chopped
1 tablespoon coriander seeds, lightly crushed
1/2 tablespoon dry English mustard powder

1/2 teaspoon cumin seeds
1/2 teaspoon freshly ground black pepper
salt
a handful of fresh parsley, coriander, chervil or
    tarragon

Wash the lentils, then cook in enough water to cover them by about 2.5 cm (1 in) until they are soft—this will take about 25 minutes. Leave in their water.

Heat the oil in a large pan, and fry the onion and garlic for a few minutes. Add the coriander, mustard, cumin and pepper, mix well, and cook for a few minutes before adding the lentils and their cooking water. Season to taste with salt, then simmer for 12 minutes. Serve hot, sprinkled with the chopped green herb, or leave to get cold, when it is delicious served with potatoes.

PEAS, DRIED
Pisum arvense

THE PEA that is dried as a pulse is the seed of the wild field pea, probably cultivated since the Stone Age. The purpose of cultivation was to have a dried vegetable to last throughout the winter, a vital staple throughout Europe. Dried peas may be whole or split, bright or dull green, or yellow. They make wonderful soups and purées, and are particularly good with ham, pork and sausages. Mushy peas are a British specialty, often served with fish and chips.

SOYA BEANS
Glycine max

THE SOYA BEAN plant has been used in the East for the last four thousand years and spread throughout Asia, it is thought, due to the vegetarian doctrines of Buddhism. It was not introduced to Britain or America until the beginning of the twentieth century. It is now the principal cash crop in America and is mainly processed for oil; the protein-rich mash left over is fed to cattle.

In the East the bean is used as food, eaten fresh or dried as a pulse, as sprouts, dried and ground into flour, made into bean curd, tofu, tempeh or TVP (textured vegetable protein), or fermented for soy sauce, miso, tamari and so on. Yellow soya beans are made into a drink which replaces cows' milk in the diet of many Asians, and now elsewhere in the world. This is highly nutritious, bacteria-free and easily digestible, ideal for babies and invalids who react to cows' milk products; it contains no cholesterol, no milk sugar (lactose), no milk protein (casein) and very low quantities of saturated fat. Soy flour is useful for those who react to wheat proteins, as it contains no gluten or gliadin.

Soya beans are as near to a complete protein as a vegetable food can be, approaching the amino acid balance of red meat. The oil is high in polyunsaturates and contains many acids (oleic, linoleic, stearic, and palmitic among others) and traces of chlorophyll. The French particularly value soya oil: they believe its linoleic acid content helps to lower blood cholesterol levels.

Soya beans and the foods obtained from them are a good source of all the nutrients of pulses. The beans also contain lecithin and vitamin E. A useful tip is to use soy sauce as a seasoning instead of salt.

PUMPKIN
Cucurbita maxima
Cucurbitaceae family

PRINCIPAL NUTRIENTS
Vitamins: A, B, C, E
Minerals: iron, potassium

THE FAMILY to which pumpkin belongs includes the courgette, marrow, cucumber, melon and watermelon. All consist mostly of water. The first Europeans to taste pumpkin were probably the Pilgrim Fathers, and pumpkin pie is still served at Thanksgiving. In Britain pumpkin is hollowed out for Halloween lanterns, and the succulent flesh and nutritive seeds are usually discarded.

Therapeutic Uses

Ripe pumpkin flesh is bright orange-yellow in colour because it is packed with betacarotene, which converts into vitamin A. The flesh is pectoral, diuretic and laxative, good for inflammation of the urinary system, the kidneys and glands. Dr. Leclerc prescribed pumpkin for patients suffering from haemorrhoids.

The seeds are highly nutritive, containing unsaturated oils, vitamins E and B, phosphorus, iron and zinc. In France the seeds are used to treat insomnia as they have a calming effect on the nervous system.

In the Kitchen

To prepare a pumpkin, wash and dry it well, then cut into smaller pieces, taking out the seeds and stringy parts and discarding the latter. Peel only if you intend to boil the pumpkin. Wash the seeds and dry them.

- Grate very ripe pumpkin raw in salads, when you will benefit most from its diuretic properties.
- Bake pumpkin pieces in their skin, then detach the flesh to eat it. This is better than boiling, when the flesh will absorb water. Purée to accompany meat dishes, as the basis of a soup (see pages 142–143), or sweetened as a pie or tart filling.
- Bake the seeds in the oven or stir-fry in a little oil to brown and crisp them.

QUINCE

Cydonia oblonga
Rosaceae family

PRINCIPAL NUTRIENTS

Vitamins: A, B, C
Minerals: potassium

A RELATIVE of the pear and apple, quinces have a yellow downy skin when ripe. The flesh is hard and acidic with many seeds, and normally has to be cooked, when it turns pink.

Therapeutic Uses

Quinces have long been famed for their wide-ranging properties. The fruits contain a lot of pectin as well as tannins and malic acid, a very strong astringent which can help neutralise acidity in the blood. Quinces were and still are used to stop haemorrhages and to make the blood more fluid. Heart patients in particular could benefit from quinces—as good daily as the half aspirin now recommended—as would women with difficult periods.

Intestinal health, too, is helped by quinces. This is a good nutritive drink for diarrhoea, colitis, enteritis and piles. Cut 3 quinces into small slices, bring them to the boil in 1 litre (1 3/4 pints) of water, and simmer slowly for 30 minutes. Cool, and add sugar or honey to taste.

The quince is also good for the nervous system because of its vitamin B content.

In the Kitchen

Imported quinces can be found in season in Greek- and Turkish-owned greengrocers. Unfortunately, since they have to be cooked the vitamin C content is always diminished.

- Wash, core and chop, then stew in a sugar syrup or simply water. Eat as a compote—with cream to counteract the acidity—or purée to use in soufflés, ice creams, mousses and other sweet dishes.
- Use some slices of raw quince in pear or apple pies or tarts. Just a little adds enormous flavour.
- Cook chunks of quince with meat and gamebird stews, as in the Middle East and North Africa.
- Quinces make wonderful jams, jellies, "butters" and "cheeses" because of their high pectin content. (Quince was the original fruit used in the preserve that was to become marmalade: when a Mrs. Keiller of Dundee was given unfamiliar Seville oranges in 1700, she substituted them for quinces, made a preserve and called it after the Portuguese word for quince, *marmelo*.)
- Make a quince sweetmeat or paste—known as *cotignac* in France and *membrillo* in Spain.

- To make a delicious and unusual fruit liqueur put 2 grated quinces, peel, core and all, into a litre (1 3/4 pints) bottle, add about 50 g (2 oz) sugar, then fill the bottle with vodka, rum, gin or brandy. Leave in a dark place for at least 2 months, then strain.

QUINOA, *see* Cereal Grains

RADISH
Raphanus sativus spp
Cruciferae family

PRINCIPAL NUTRIENTS
Vitamins: B, C
Minerals: calcium, iodine, iron, phosphorus, potassium

THERE ARE many types of radish: the small red and the larger white and pink ones that grow in rows in gardens; the black, supposedly from Spain; and the large white radishes known as mooli or daikon in the East *(Raphanus sativus* var. *longipinnatus).*

Therapeutic Uses
All radishes are antiscorbutic and pectoral thanks to their high content of vitamin C, and help in the treatment of bronchitis, colds and flu. The essential oils in the flesh possess natural antiseptic properties and detoxify the liver and kidneys as well.

In the Kitchen
Use radishes as fresh as possible, although daikon keeps well in the fridge for a week or so. Wash and cut just before eating.

- Eat raw, whole, sliced or grated (according to size) in mixed salads.
- Eat raw and whole as an hors d'oeuvre as they do in France or Italy, with coarse salt and butter or cheese.
- Use as a crudité, with a dip.
- Grate or shred daikon and use as a garnish for Eastern-style soups or in a fresh Eastern-type pickle.
- Juice radishes with celery and apple for an energising drink.

RAISINS, *see* Grape

RASPBERRY
Rubus idaeus
Rosaceae family

PRINCIPAL NUTRIENTS

Vitamins: A, B, C
Minerals: calcium, iron, magnesium, phosphorus, potassium

RASPBERRIES belong to a large family, said to have originated in Asia, which includes the loganberry and blackberry. The fruits consist of a multitude of seeds, each in its own little "fruit packet", joined together as one. This means that raspberries can be frozen rather more successfully than other summer fruit.

Therapeutic Uses
Raspberries and their relatives contain a lot of fruit sugars which are easy to assimilate, so they are good for diabetics. Their salicylic acid gives the fruit a wonderful perfume which stimulates a sluggish system: they are also good for poor circulation.

Raspberries are prescribed for people with rheumatic conditions such as gout, and for those who retain toxins: the fruits seem to activate the elimination of toxins, and with their tiny seeds, which are eaten, are particularly good for constipation. Raspberries are also prescribed for fevers and bladder infections.

The leaves are useful as well, in a tea which can help many of the above ailments. Boil 1 large tablespoon leaves per 600 ml (1 pint) water for a few minutes, then leave to infuse for 10 minutes. For a decoction—which is good for relieving a sore throat or mouth thrush—boil the leaves as above, but for 20 minutes, then leave to stand. Use as a gargle.

In the Kitchen

Raspberries are very fragile and do not travel or pack well. Look out for tell-tale leaks on the undersides of punnets, and there will undoubtedly be one or two mildewed fruit. A few raspberry canes in your garden would be a nicer way to obtain the fruit, but they are very invasive and may take over! A good "pick your own" farm is perhaps the best solution.

- Eat fresh and raw, with cream, crème fraîche or fromage frais.
- Use raw and fresh with cream as the filling for a cake, meringue, flan, tart or pancake.
- "Cook" only by pouring a hot sugar syrup over them.
- Purée to use in fools, mousses and a dessert sauce or coulis. Push through a plastic or nylon sieve rather than a metal one.
- Use with other summer fruits in an English Summer Pudding.
- Make into jams and jellies: they have a good pectin content.
- Make into raspberry vinegar (see page xxiii).

RHUBARB

Rheum rhaponticum
Polygonaceae family

PRINCIPAL NUTRIENTS

Vitamins: A, B, C
Minerals: calcium, magnesium, potassium

THE ROOTS of rhubarb, a leaf stem rather than a fruit, had been used as a purgative for thousands of years by the Chinese before the plant reached the West. Even then, for many centuries it was the roots that were used in Europe, still as a purgative, and then the leaves—a rather dangerous pursuit as they are poisonous, due to their high oxalic acid content. Not until the late eighteenth century were the stalks used as food, and then only by the French and English.

Therapeutic Uses

Rhubarb is still considered purgative—a gentle laxative tonic for the stomach. It stimulates the liver, pancreas and intestines. Its calcium content is largely unavailable to the body because of the action of the oxalic acid (which is what gives the stems their bitter, astringent flavour). It should not be eaten by those prone to forming kidney stones. Rhubarb also has calming properties.

In the Kitchen

The younger and pinker the rhubarb, the sweeter its flavour. As the stalk grows in size and matures, the skin becomes tougher and stringier and the flavour more acidic.

- Lightly poach chopped stalks with sugar and eat for breakfast or for dessert. Flavour with orange juice or with ginger or angelica for further health benefits.
- A simple rhubarb compote is used as a sauce for pork in Scandinavia. This would also be good with duck or goose.
- Bake rhubarb in pies and tarts.
- Make into jams.

RICE, *see* Cereal Grains

ROCKET, *see* Lettuce

ROSEMARY
Rosmarinus officinalis
Labiatae family

PERHAPS the best known of aromatic herbs, rosemary is native to the Mediterranean; its name comes from the Latin *rosmarinus*, "dew of the sea". To the Greeks and Romans it was symbolic of both love and death. It was highly regarded in all culinary and medical treatises in the Middle Ages, and an infusion of the herb was used for drinking, washing and burning as an antiseptic during times of plague.

Therapeutic Uses

Rosemary's principal property is bactericidal. It is also stimulant, antispasmodic, chologogic (benefiting the liver) and diuretic. It helps rheumatic and respiratory conditions, stimulates a sluggish system and fortifies the nervous system, banishing depression, mental and physical tiredness and migraines. Drink a tisane made from 50 g (2 oz) herb to 1 litre (1 3/4 pints) mineral water four times a day. Or use wine instead of water and infuse the herb in it for 3–4 days, shaking every so often: this is good for tiredness, fluid retention and migraine, as well as for those suffering from shock. Drink a small glass 20 minutes before a meal. A little cup of rosemary tea can help after an epileptic fit, and can bring back memory to people suffering from amnesia. Drink a cup of rosemary tea in the morning to combat nervous depression.

Add a handful of rosemary leaves to runny honey, leave for a week and then eat on bread or toast. This is particularly good for a sore throat, but it is also a delicious general stimulant of good health.

Essential oils are distilled from the flowering tops and the stems and leaves. The former is the best.

In the Kitchen

Rosemary contains a great deal of oil in its leaves and therefore dries well, retaining many of its active principles. When using in cooking, chop very finely or use in a sprig that can be removed before you serve the dish: the spiky leaves can be irritating and can get caught in your teeth!

- Add to bouquet garnis, or use whole sprigs in meat marinades, stews and casseroles. The antiseptic essential oils protect against possible meat putrefaction, and help you to digest fat.
- Use small sprigs of rosemary and slivers of garlic to stud a piece of lamb or mutton for roasting. The rosemary alleviates the "woolly" taste, of mutton particularly.
- In Italy rosemary is used in rice dishes; in France it is associated more with ham.
- Add rosemary flowers to a salad of spinach, chicory, lettuce, apple and a few almonds, both for their fragrance and for their therapeutic benefits.

- Crush a lot of dried rosemary with salt and pepper in a mortar. Keep in an airtight jar in the fridge and sprinkle over vegetable, grain, pulse, meat and fish dishes.
- Infuse sprigs of the fresh herb in oils and vinegars to be used in salad dressings (see page xxiii).
- Add sprigs of rosemary to a jar of caster sugar as you would pieces of vanilla pod, or infuse in the milk for milk puddings.

RYE, *see* Cereal Grains

SAGE
Salvia spp
Labiatae family

THERE ARE many types of sage, but two in particular are used in cooking and medicine: *Salvia officinalis* is the common garden herb, while *Salvia sclarea*, or clary sage, is used primarily for one of the best of aromatherapeutic oils.

Sage has been valued for centuries as a medicine, since the time of the Ancient Egyptians. It was highly valued in the Middle Ages as a cure-all, and it can still help in every cycle of our lives from babyhood to old age. Sage is the supreme remedy for almost all ills.

Therapeutic Uses
In twentieth-century French medicine the sages have been shown to be of great use in treating gynaecological problems. They are emmenogogic and help to combat frigidity, congestion of the ovaries and all problems associated with menstruation and the menopause. Sage, in brief, helps to promote and normalise the female cycles. Eat it raw to treat rheumatic problems, catarrh, haemorrhage, excessive sweating and puffiness, particularly when associated with PMT and menopause.

Clary sage is an all-round panacea, helping to fight fatigue and depression, liver congestion, sore throats, mouth infections and headaches, among many other complaints. Make the leaves into a tisane whenever you are feeling low.

A decoction of sage or clary sage is good for mouth ulcers, and as a gargle for sore throats. Add 15 g (1/2 oz) sage leaves, fresh or dried, to 1 litre (1 3/4 pints) water and boil for 5 minutes. Drink slowly.

Many people find the taste of sage too strong, so I always add orange juice to an infusion. The combination is not bad.

Essential oils are distilled from both sages mentioned above. *Salvia officinalis* contains thujone, a dangerous compound, so it is safer to use the oil of *Salvia sclarea*.

In the Kitchen

Sage is best eaten fresh but, because of the strong flavour and aroma of the essential oils, it dries well, losing few of its active principles.

- Make a seasoning from freshly dried sage. Grind it to powder in a mortar, then add some crushed coarse salt. Store in a jar in the fridge and sprinkle over salads, vegetable, meat and fish dishes.
- Store freshly dried sage leaves in honey, a sweet way of gaining its properties. Add to tisanes or use in sweet dishes.
- Add sage raw to salads, soups and stuffings for rich meats such as pork and goose to ease digestion.
- Add sparingly to egg, tomato and cheese dishes.
- Cook veal, liver, ham and chicken with sage, both for flavour and to help fix the iron of the meats.
- Deep-fry sage leaves briefly as a garnish for meats. Clary sage fritters—deep-fried in a light batter—make a delicious starter (see below).

Beignets

These fritters are delicious and crisp, and if they are made with a herb or flower of therapeutic value, then so much the better. Use new, scented flowers, and only the tender tips of tougher herbs such as rosemary or thyme.

If you are feeling nervous, for instance, you could use orange, borage or rosemary flowers; if lacking in energy, rose petals; if you have lung or throat problems, violets. If you just want to show off, use white chrysanthemums which look spectacular! Serve these with pâté before a meal, or after the meal with a sorbet or fruit salad.

Unsweetened beignets of sage or basil, or any other sturdy leafy herb, can be used as a garnish for meats and fish, and broccoli or cauliflower florets and spring onions could also be deep-fried as an accompaniment. Use this batter also to deep-fry slices or chunks of fruit in batter—bananas, apples and pineapple are traditional— as a pudding.

chosen flower, herb or fruit
lemon juice
fruit sugar
ground cinnamon
soy oil for deep-frying

BATTER

(makes 300 ml/10 fl oz)
100 g (4 oz) plain flour
1/2 teaspoon salt
1 tablespoon olive oil
200 ml (7 fl oz) water
2 egg whites

Sift the flour and salt together into a bowl, and make a well in the centre. Add the oil and gradually mix in the water. Rest at room temperature for about an hour.

Meanwhile, for the flowers only, macerate them in some lemon juice for about an hour, then sprinkle with a little fruit sugar to taste and a little ground cinnamon.

Just before using the batter, whisk the egg whites until stiff and fold them in. Dip the flower heads, herbs or fruit into the batter and then deep-fry in the hot oil until crisp and golden. This will take a few seconds or minutes, depending on what you are

frying. Drain well, then serve sprinkled with lemon or
lime juice.

SAVORY
Satureja spp
Labiatae family

THE TWO SPECIES—*Satureja hortensis*, summer savory, and
Satureja montana, winter savory—are closely related na-
tives of the Mediterranean. Throughout the centuries savory
has been used both for stimulating the sexual senses and in
cooking stews of meats and vegetables.

Therapeutic Uses
Savory is emmenogogic, carminative and stomachic. Using
it in cooking helps dyspepsia, flatulence, diarrhoea caused
by virus infections, and enteritis. A seventeenth-century
French surgeon claimed huge successes in curing mouth and
throat ulcers with savory.

Savory steeped with some sugar and Angostura bitters in
a bottle of good port or Madeira makes a wonderful aphrodisiac. Some added angelica or sage and a few black peppercorns also help bring back sexual appetite. The savory
contains natural hormones which stimulate the sexual
glands.

The essential oil, distilled from the leaves (and occasionally from the flowers as well) is high in phenols, like
oregano and thyme, and is therefore very antiseptic.

In the Kitchen
Summer savory is less strong and coarse in flavour than
winter, both of which are not too dissimilar to, but more bitter than, thyme. The herbs dry well.

- In Germany savory is known as *Bohnenkraut*, meaning
  "bean herb", and it is the best herb to use in pulse dishes
  to preempt flatulence and to stimulate digestion and the
  assimilation of the pulses, vitamins and minerals.
- Use savory in meat stews and marinades, especially of
  game.

- Savory was once used as a wrapping for certain French cheeses, and the marriage was a happy one, for savory plus sage mixed into soft cheeses, whether cow, sheep or goat, gives them a wonderful aroma and makes them taste much more subtle.
- For those on a salt-reduced or salt-restricted diet, savory is very useful because its strong peppery flavour makes further seasoning unnecessary in many dishes.
- Make an aromatic vinegar for salad dressings by steeping savory leaves, a few juniper berries and some chopped onion or shallot in wine vinegar for a few weeks.

SEAWEEDS

PRINCIPAL NUTRIENTS
Vitamins: A, B, C, D, E, K
Minerals: calcium, copper, iodine, iron, magnesium, potassium

SEAWEEDS are algae and are found along shorelines all over the world. They are rich in nutrients, and should be appreciated more for their nutritive and therapeutic properties. They have been valued in the East for hundreds of years, primarily as food.

They can be used fresh, but many varieties are dried in the East and these can now be bought in the West. Reconstitute first by soaking in water, then follow the cooking instructions on the packet. In cooking I use seaweeds mainly as a seasoning (see Wakame) in salads or in sauces for fish (a seaweed and caraway sauce for herring or other oily fish is wonderful).

Because of their rich mineral and vitamin content, seaweeds should be eaten as often as possible. They are excellent for the digestive system, for enteritis, constipation and inflammation of the intestines. They can help calm down a digestion suffering the after-effects of a strong curry or other spicy dish. Because of the iodine content and bromine, seaweeds are recommended for glandular deficiencies and nervous disorders. They are also good for the respiratory system.

AGAR AGAR
Gelidium spp

ALSO KNOWN as Chinese or Japanese moss, or as *kanten* in Japan, agar agar is a seaweed of the Far East, where it is used as a foodstuff (it is available dried) as well as being made into a vegetarian alternative to gelatine. It is processed into white or red sheets, strips and sticks.

In the Kitchen

- Use in soups (it is a constituent of a "false" Chinese birds' nest soup giving the soup a similar gelatinous quality to the original), as a vegetable and in salads.
- Use as a gelling agent for desserts (use 5–10 g/1/4 oz per litre/1 3/4 pints milk). It is the setting agent most commonly used in the jellied sweets of Thailand and the Philippines, because once it sets it does not melt or lose shape.

CARRAGHEEN
Chondrus crispus

ALSO KNOWN as Irish moss, carragheen grows on the Atlantic coastlines of America and Europe and is most prized in Ireland. Carragheen is rich in vitamins A and B, and iodine and potassium. It has long been used as a health food in Ireland, and during the famine of 1840–3 was virtually the only food available in coastal areas.

In the Kitchen

- Use as a gelling agent: an Irish dish called carragheen moss is a milk jelly (30–60 g/1–2 oz seaweed to 1 litre/1 3/4 pints boiled milk) served at breakfast or as a dessert.
- Use also as a thickener in vegetable soups or stews, giving them body and texture, or raw or reconstituted in salads (1 teaspoon per person).

DULSE
Rhodymenia palmata

THIS SALTY, TANGY SEAWEED grows on Atlantic coastlines and is rich in potassium and magnesium. It is available fresh or dried.

In the Kitchen

- Cook with potatoes in the Irish hash-like dish called dulse champ.
- Eat it raw in salads with something like cucumber, and a dressing.

KELP
Laminaria spp

IN BRITAIN kelp is commonly known as oarweed and divided into four classifications—tangles, cuvie, sea belt and furbelows. Sweet oarweed *(Laminaria saccharina)* can be collected, washed and dried, then deep-fried in squares for an appetiser, rather like potato crisps.

The kelp most widely used as food is the giant sea kelp *(Laminaria japonica)*, known as *kombu* or *konbu* in Japan. This is an essential element in Japanese cooking, used to flavour *dashi*, the stock that forms a base for most savory dishes. It is "processed" and marketed in various ways, and used in soups or as a wrapping for other foods. *Kombu* strips can make hard foods soft, and so are often used in pulse dishes.

LAVER/NORI
Porphyra spp

THIS SEAWEED is highly nutritious—rich in protein, iodine and vitamins A, B, C and D. Available fresh or frozen, it is highly valued in Wales particularly, where it is made into laverbread. The seaweed is washed, boiled to a purée, then spread on fried bread or rolled in oatmeal and fried as a "cake" to be served for breakfast with bacon. It can be used as a spread with other seafood, or in a seafood sauce or stuffing.

Laver is known as *nori* in Japan. It is mainly sold in dried sheets, to be used as a wrapping for sushi, or for small fish or fillets of fish. It is also shredded and added to soups, or it can be made into "nests" by deep-frying. It is available as a shredded condiment as well, but you can make this yourself at home (see Wakame). Toast *nori* very briefly before use to bring out its subtle flavour, either over a flame or in a hot oven, then crumble over salads, vegetable dishes or soups. Or briefly moisturise to soften.

Nori is actually farmed in Japan in huge "paddy fields". Shallow lakes are closely dotted with bamboo stakes, some of them conjoined with nets; spores of the algae which will become the weed cling to nets and stakes, and grow until the right size for harvesting.

Wakame
Undaria pinnatifida

This Asian seaweed is used mainly in Japanese cookery, and can be bought dried. After reconstituting it becomes very tender and is simmered in soups and stews and used in salads. I crush it and mix it with coarse sea salt (as I do other dried seaweeds) to sprinkle on noodles, soups, rice or vegetables.

SEEDS

PRINCIPAL NUTRIENTS

Vitamins: A, B, C (when sprouted), E
Minerals: calcium, copper, iron, magnesium, phosphorus, zinc

These miracles of nature contain complete genetic instructions as well as latent energy for the next generation of plants. That energy consists of protein, fat, carbohydrate, vitamins and minerals, and seeds are highly nutritive eaten just as they are: the vitamin B content is particularly high, as is the E, although generally speaking there is no vitamin C. There are high levels of calcium, phosphorus, magnesium and iron. The magnesium content of seeds is the highest of all foods. The fats are unsaturated.

Perhaps the greatest advantage of seeds is that they can be eaten raw, cooked and dried, and their nutritive and energising values do not change substantially. They can also be sprouted, when, eaten raw, they possess more nutrients than any other natural food (see page 177 for how to sprout seeds).

The larger seeds such as melon, sunflower and pumpkin can be eaten as a snack and have become very popular as protein food for vegetarians. Seeds are often used as a seasoning—among them anise, caraway, celery, cumin, dill, fennel, lovage, mustard and poppy (for information on seeds not specified on page 178, see the individual entries). They can be sprinkled on soups, salads, casseroles, sauces, vegetables, breads, cakes and all sorts of foods.

Another advantage of seeds is that they have a long shelf life, so long as they are kept away from humidity. If you store them in an airtight container in the fridge, they will not become rancid and toxic to eat.

LINSEED
Linum usitatissimum
Linaceae family

THE PLANT which produces linseeds also yields the fibre flax, which is spun into linen. The seeds contain 30–40 per cent fixed oil which is reputedly good for constipation; in Swiss health centres they mix it with muesli. Linseeds also contain a natural oestrogen which, when the seeds are sprinkled on cereals, fruit and yogurt, can help the symptoms of the menopause.

PINE KERNELS
Pinus spp
Pinaceae family

THE PINE KERNEL or pine nut consists of the kernel or seeds from the cone of a pine tree (usually, in Europe, the stone pine, *Pinus pinea*). They are creamy white in colour, softly nutty in texture and faintly resinous in flavour. Rich in nutrients, they contain vitamins A, E, some B and, uniquely for seeds, a trace of C; they have good quantities too of magnesium, phosphorus, iron, copper and zinc. They are also high in fat and carbohydrate.

They have been prescribed for respiratory illnesses and chest problems. They are most delicious toasted first, in an oven or dry frying pan. Sprinkle on cereals, fruits or yogurt, or on to savory salads. They also add texture and flavour to puréed root vegetables such as parsnip.

POPPY SEEDS
Papaver somniferum
Papaveraceae family

THESE ARE the seeds of the opium poppy. Although in theory the opium alkaloids (contained in latex in the pod) are not present in the ripe seeds, traces remain which I find mildly relaxing and sedative. Use the seeds in baking, sprinkle on vegetable dishes, or add to curry sauces for a thickening effect.

Poppy Seed Salad Dressing

If you have been to the theatre, or want a light meal before you go to bed, this dressing should help you relax and sleep. The lettuce you use it on is soporific too, of course. Use a 150 ml (5 fl oz) cup as a measure.

SERVES 1

1/2 cup newly sprouted poppy seeds
1 coffeespoon fennel seeds
1/2 onion, peeled and roughly chopped
1 coffeespoon minced parsley
1 coffeespoon olive oil
1 cup natural yogurt
a pinch of salt

Put all into a blender or liquidiser and blend until smooth. Use to dress lettuce or other salad leaves, and serve with brown bread.

SESAME SEEDS
Sesamum indicum
Pedaliaceae family

THE SEEDS of the tropical sesame plant contain about 50 per cent oil, which is polyunsaturated. Sesame contains very little betacarotene or vitamin E, but more than makes up for this by its high content of B vitamins (B1, 2, 3, 6, pantothenic acid, folic acid and biotin). The seeds are also very rich in calcium, phosphorus, iron, lecithin and amino acids, and are therefore very good for the nervous system.

Toast in the oven briefly or in a dry frying pan to bring out their nuttiness. Scatter on top of cereals, yogurt or fruit, or use in biscuit- and bread-making. Use sesame seeds in the Middle Eastern paste called tahina, or—in small quantities—the sweet halva.

Gomasio

This is a delicious Japanese seasoning to sprinkle on to cooked vegetables, pasta, jacket potatoes, rice, millet, soups and salads. Simply toast the required amount of sesame seeds until lightly browned, then add coarse salt to taste—about one-third salt to two-thirds seeds. Grind together in the blender until you have a powder, then store in an airtight tin.

SUNFLOWER SEEDS
Helianthus annuum
Compositae family

THESE ARE the seeds of the familiar sunflower, native to Mexico and Peru but long cultivated all over Europe as a source of polyunsaturated oil. The seeds contain many vitamins, particularly A and E, and good quantities of most of the minerals, especially iron. They consist of 25 per cent protein.

Bake the husked seeds in the oven lightly until golden or fry in a dry pan or in a little oil.

- Give as a treat to your children to nibble instead of sweets (but not if they are under four because very small children can choke on them).
- Offer them as a canapé with a drink instead of biscuits or crisps.

SPROUTING SEEDS, CEREAL GRAINS AND PULSES

ENZYME ACTIVITY is highest in seeds, grains and pulses just after they have sprouted, and it is believed that this galvanises the body's own enzymes into greater activity. Phytin is an important ingredient in many "seeds", and this, as phytic acid, can bind up calcium, zinc and iron, making them unavailable to the body. When seeds are sprouted, the phytin level is much reduced.

Use a clean wide-necked jar. Put in a handful of rinsed seeds, grains or pulses and cover with a few inches of cold water (spring, filtered or cooled boiled, in preference to tap). Leave overnight in a warm place, then strain. Rinse again with water and strain once more, then cover the top of the jar with a piece of cheesecloth held on with an elastic band. Put into a dark warm place and leave, rinsing and draining morning and night, for about 3 days. The sprouts should then appear—although it depends on the "seed" being used—and will continue to grow if kept damp. They need a little sunlight now, and will soon be ready to eat. Try to eat the husks of the seeds, grains or pulses, as these are good sources of fibre.

Seeds to sprout: Alfalfa, garden cress, fenugreek, white mustard, pumpkin, radish, sesame, sunflower.
Grains to Sprout: Barley, buckwheat, maize, millet, oats, rye, wheat.
Pulses to Sprout: Aduki beans, chickpeas, lentils, mung beans, soy beans.

Mustard and cress seeds can be sprinkled and grown on damp soil, blotting paper or cloth, and are ready in about 2 weeks. "Plant" the mustard 2–3 days before the cress.

SESAME SEEDS, *see* Seeds

SHALLOTS, *see* Onion

SHARON FRUIT, *see* Persimmon

SHELLFISH, *see* Meat, Poultry and Fish

SORREL, *see* Lettuce

SPINACH
Spinacea oleracea
Chenopodiaceae family

PRINCIPAL NUTRIENTS
Vitamins: A, B, C, K
Minerals: calcium, iodine, iron, phosphorus, potassium

SPINACH is believed to have originated in Persia—the name is derived from the Persian word *aspanakh*—and was brought to Europe in the thirteenth century by the Arabs. Regarded as medicinal then, it has continued to be thought of as highly nutritious, as exemplified by the American cartoon character Popeye. In reality, although iron and calcium are high in the plant, the oxalic acid content makes much of these minerals unavailable to the body.

Therapeutic Uses
Spinach contains other important substances: lime for bones and muscles; arsenic; a fortifying mucilage for articulation and the mucous membranes; and iodine which, with the iron, helps the absorption of the minerals. Saponine helps activate gastric juices and thus digestion and absorption of foods and nutrients. The chlorophyll of spinach seems particularly to help those who suffer from being deprived of sunlight (SAD or Seasonal Affective Disorder). Spinach is

good for the heart, for anaemia, for those suffering from nerves, depression, fatigue, or who are convalescent. It is also useful for PMT and the menopause. Eating it raw is good for the teeth and gums.

In the Kitchen

I prefer to eat spinach raw in order to retain all its nutritious and therapeutic values. It can of course be cooked—but very lightly, and only in the water that clings to its leaves after washing, in order to retain the vitamin C content, and to prevent the leaves turning brown.

Wash spinach thoroughly several times in cold water. Take the spinach out of the water rather than running the water away, to ensure that any dirt is left behind in the sink or bowl. Store damp leaves in a bag in the salad drawer of the fridge to crisp them up.

- Eat raw in salads with sliced mushrooms, walnuts, black olives and olive oil. This is a meal in itself. Spinach is good too, with some chopped white onions and garlic and a few strips of red pepper. Banana slices and apple dice are also good additions.
- The taste of spinach leaves can be strong, so mix with other leaves such as lettuces, endives, radicchio and watercress.
- Hot wilted salads are popular. Simply pour a warmed dressing over the leaves and other ingredients to make the leaves wilt slightly.
- Add grilled bacon, strips of cooked chicken or meat, or garlic croûtons to a spinach salad, raw or wilted.
- Cook spinach very briefly, then drain well and flavour with butter (if you like) and lots of nutmeg.
- Spinach can be cooked in soufflés, in egg and cheese dishes, and as a filling for quiches, pancakes and pasta, but its properties are lost, if not its flavour.
- Juice the leaves.

Spring Onions, *see* Onion

Strawberry
Fragaria vesca
Rosaceae family

PRINCIPAL NUTRIENTS
Vitamins: C
Minerals: iodine, iron, phosphorus, potassium

THE PLUMP large strawberries which we know today were developed in the early eighteenth century from American wild strawberries, although Europe had eaten and appreciated its own wild berries, *Fragaria vesca* and *Fragaria moschata* (the Alpine strawberry) for centuries.

Therapeutic Uses
Because of their high content of mineral salts, strawberries are excellent for rheumatic problems. Dr. Leclerc claims that this fruit reduces the level of uric acid in the blood, alkalising it. Strawberries are also wonderful for the immune system, and good for the regulation of hepatic and glandular functions.

A decoction of fresh strawberry leaves can be helpful to people suffering from cystitis and liver problems after eating or drinking too much. Boil 1 handful of fresh leaves (or half a handful of dried) in 600 ml (1 pint) water with a couple of strawberries for 5 minutes. Stand for 10–15 minutes, then drink every 2 hours.

Beware of strawberries if you tend to suffer from food allergies, as they are commonly implicated in classic symptoms such as stomach upset, hives, hay fever-like reactions and swellings of the face.

In the Kitchen
Strawberries are very perishable, so buy carefully. Wash very briefly and carefully *before* hulling—otherwise water can penetrate the hole and spoil the flesh.

- Eat raw as often as possible during their short season—with cereals, muesli or porridge in the morning for a nutritious and delicious start to the day, or with cream, single, double or clotted, or crème fraîche or yogurt.

- Mix raw and whole or sliced into fresh fruit salads, but only at the last moment as they can soften. Alternatively simply sprinkle them with some orange or lemon juice or wine.
- Never freeze whole strawberries as they become soggy when defrosted. Instead, freeze a purée which can then be used as a sauce, the basis of a fool or soufflé, for a dessert soup, or for an ice cream or sorbet.
- Use slices of strawberries in "savory" salads—they are particularly good with avocados and cucumber.
- Make strawberries into jam—but they will need added pectin.
- Make a strawberry-flavoured gin or vodka. Fill a jar or bottle with strawberries, add sugar to come halfway up, then fill with spirit to cover. Leave for at least a month, then strain.
- Use strawberries as a raw "garnish" on tartlets, with cream, or in and on sponge cakes, again with cream.
- Juice strawberries for a wonderfully nutritive daily drink (strawberries, ounce for ounce, contain as much vitamin C or oranges).

SULTANAS, *see* Grape

SUNFLOWER SEEDS, *see* Seeds

SWEDE, *see* Turnip and Swede

SWEETCORN, *see* Cereal Grains (Maize)

TARRAGON
Artemisia dracunculus
Compositae family

THERE ARE two types of tarragon; French tarragon (*Artemisia dracunculus*) is valued in cooking and medicine, while Russian or false tarragon (*Artemisia dracunculoides*) has coarser leaves and flavour. The plant is thought to have been introduced to Europe by returning Crusaders, as the Arabs had long used it in medicine. Their doctors prescribed it for anaemia, to stimulate digestion and appetite and to prevent bad breath.

Therapeutic Uses

Tarragon is stimulant, stomachic, emmenogogic, digestive and laxative. Dr. Leclerc prescribed it for constipation, intestinal parasites and anorexia. A maceration of crushed leaves in a glass of good white wine, drunk before a meal, is strongly digestive. Juice some fennel, adding some tarragon at the last minute, for depression.

Tarragon is diuretic as well; drink an infusion of 2 tablespoons chopped fresh leaves in 1 litre (1 3/4 pints) boiling mineral water. This is good for dysmenorrhoea; drink three or four times per day leading up to the period, after a meal.

An essential oil is distilled from the leaves. Because it contains a dangerous compound called estragole or methylchavicol, it must be used with great care.

In the Kitchen

Tarragon makes a useful alternative to salt for people suffering from heart problems and obesity, since its flavour is so savory that salt is not needed.

- Cook with chicken, a very famous culinary association. Place leaves under the skin or in the bird before roasting.
- Use raw in salads and as a garnish.
- Chop in herb mixtures for omelettes and sauces (tarragon is a major flavouring in béarnaise sauce and good, too, with mayonnaise).
- Macerate tarragon leaves in white wine vinegar for one of the most successful herb vinegars.

THYME
Thymus spp
Labiatae family

NATIVE to Europe, particularly the Mediterranean, thyme has been used in cookery and medicine for thousands of years. The Ancient Egyptians used it in embalming; Pliny recommended it as a remedy for epilepsy; and in the Middle Ages it was used against plague, leprosy and body lice and strewn on floors as an antibacterial.

Therapeutic Uses

Thyme is tonic, stimulant, stomachic, digestive, antispasmodic, pectoral and balsamic. Eat it often, or use in cooking, to counter asthma, flu, colds, coughs, fever and nervousness. If you have a cold and runny nose, make an infusion of thyme and insert a few drops into your nostrils with a dropper half an hour before breakfast. This will dry the mucus and clear a stuffed-nose headache.

Thyme is very good for rheumatic conditions, thanks to the thymol content. Make an infusion of 15 g (1/2 oz) fresh thyme per litre (1 3/4 pints) mineral water. Take 3–4 cups per day after meals (perhaps with some added mint to improve the flavour): it will help the pain and swellings of rheumatism, as well as flatulence, tiredness and depression, PMT and menopausal symptoms.

Thyme is a powerful preservative and prevents meat fats from turning rancid. It has been suggested that thyme could have the same effect on human tissue. Nasty elements called free radicals course through the body, causing it to deteriorate, age and "turn rancid", and they are associated with cancer and other degenerative diseases. Thyme, so it is claimed, acts as an antioxidant, fighting against the free radicals and so helping to preserve human tissue.

This drink is used as a morning pick-me-up in Greece (it's also quite laxative). Place 450 g (1 lb) figs and a large handful of fresh thyme in enough water to cover them about twice. Bring to the boil and simmer for about 30 minutes. Strain and drink.

An essential oil is steam-distilled from the flower tops and leaves.

In the Kitchen

Thyme is one of the major culinary herbs, together with bay and parsley. It is best eaten fresh, but it also dries very well, when its therapeutic properties are undiminished.

- Use thyme in a bouquet garni, in marinades, in stocks and in stuffings.
- Use sprigs of thyme in long-cooked stews and casseroles. Thyme fixes the iron in meat and also helps you to digest it (as well as pulses).
- Use thyme's preservative and antiseptic properties in pies, pâtés, sausages and pickles.
- Add fresh leaves to bread doughs, omelettes and mushroom dishes.
- Mix fresh leaves into butter for a thyme butter to accompany grilled meat or oily fish, or to rub over a meat or fish that is to be grilled, baked or barbecued.
- Macerate fresh thyme in herb oils and vinegars.

Meat Marinade

With this number of aromatics, primarily the thyme, the meat has no choice but to be palatable and healthy!

1 bottle white wine
25 g (1 oz) fresh thyme
a sprig of fresh savory
4 garlic cloves, peeled and halved
4 shallots, peeled and halved
2 bay leaves
4 cloves
15 g (1/2 oz) black peppercorns, lightly crushed

Mix all the ingredients together and leave the meat to marinate for up to 24 hours.

TOMATO
Lycopersicum esculentum
Solanaceae family

PRINCIPAL NUTRIENTS

Vitamins: A, B, C, E
Minerals: iron, phosphorus, potassium

IN A STRICTLY botanical sense, the tomato is actually a fruit. Only known in the West since the discovery of the New World and, like the potato, a relative of deadly nightshade, it was initially viewed with great suspicion. The green parts of the plant do in fact contain the poison solanine, so the leaves and roots must never be eaten and the seeds must never be sprouted for eating.

Therapeutic Uses

The mineral and vitamin contents of raw tomatoes are quite high, so they are very beneficial to health. Even when cooked, tomatoes do not lose their vitamin A, for instance.

Tomatoes accumulate a lot of energy from the sun during their passage from chlorophyll green to ripe red and are therefore very nutritive and dynamising. They remineralise, being particularly good for the blood (as is the iron content) and for the nervous system (stress and fatigue). The acidity of tomatoes helps to eliminate uric acid from the system, so they are good for arthritic conditions, rheumatism and gout. They also help to detoxify, so are good at combatting skin complaints such as boils and acne.

The high vitamin C content is a benefit in many ways, particularly for the skin and the gums.

Spaghetti with Raw Tomato and Basil

This is incredibly simple, but very fresh-tasting and healthy

SERVES 2

2 large ripe tomatoes
salt and freshly ground black pepper
100 g (4 oz) good dried spaghetti
2 tablespoons extra virgin olive oil, or more if wished
6 large fresh basil leaves

Nick the skins with a sharp knife and then immerse the tomatoes in boiling water for 20 seconds. Remove, plunge into cold water for a minute or so, then peel off the skins. Discard the seeds, and cut the flesh into small dice. Put the diced flesh into a colander and sprinkle with a little salt to rid them of extra liquid.

Cook the spaghetti following the instructions on the packet. Drain well, then transfer to a bowl. Add the olive oil and tomato dice. Tear the basil leaves into small pieces and mix in. Add salt and pepper to taste and eat warm.

In the Kitchen

There are many varieties of tomatoes, and the most widely grown and available are often those with the least flavour. Large beefsteak, tiny cherry or plum tomatoes are the best—you could grow an interesting variety from seed at home. A couple of healthy plants can yield an extraordinary number of tomatoes in late summer—and those that are home-grown and fresh-plucked are even richer in vitamin C.

- Eat raw for greatest benefit, sliced or chopped in a salad: tomato slices dressed with a little walnut oil and some fresh torn basil are wonderful. A little finely chopped spring onion or garlic would not go amiss either.
- Tomatoes make one of the best sandwich fillings, particularly with lots of black pepper and some mustard and cress.
- Grill tomato halves for a good accompanying vegetable, or bake them whole or stuffed.
- Tomatoes neutralise the fermentation of carbohydrate or starch in the intestine, and therefore help digestion. So eat them with boiled potatoes, rice and pasta (see below).
- Make tomatoes into pasta sauces or soup, and use them in vegetable curries and stews such as ratatouille.
- Juice tomatoes for a nutritive drink.

Salade Pomme d'Amour

Tomatoes were believed to be an aphrodisiac, hence an old French name for them—*pommes d'amour*, apple of love. Salad can sometimes be boring, but this one is different—a wonderful recipe for when you are tired and don't want to cook anything. It's colourful enough to be served to guests in the summer, and it's packed full of vitamins because of the raw vegetables and their aromatic essential oils.

SERVES 1

1 lettuce heart (preferably Little Gem)
1 large tomato
1 small carrot, 1 small turnip and 1 small parsnip, trimmed
4 black or green olives, stoned
1 mushroom
1 garlic clove, peeled
a little olive oil
salt and freshly ground black pepper

Wash and dry the lettuce. Cut the top off the tomato and scoop out all the seeds and inner flesh. Open out the lettuce heart and put the tomato inside the hollow. Grate the root vegetables and finely chop the olives, mushroom and garlic. Mix all these with enough olive oil just to cohere, and season with salt and pepper. Stuff into the tomato shell. Chill for a while before serving.

TURNIP AND SWEDE
Brassica spp
Cruciferae family

PRINCIPAL NUTRIENTS

Vitamins: A, B, C
Minerals: calcium, iodine, iron, magnesium, phosphorus, sulphur

TURNIPS (large white root vegetables or, at their best, small ones with white flesh and fresh green leaves at the top) and swedes (large purple-skinned root vegetables with yellow flesh) are members of the same family as cabbage and Brussels sprouts. Turnips were cultivated by the Romans for both flesh and leaves, and were one of the staple foods of Europe before the potato. Swedes, or Swedish turnips, are thought to have been discovered only in the seventeenth century.

Therapeutic Uses

The turnip is an important vegetable because of its high calcium content in both vegetable and leaves—267 mg per small cup as compared to 14.4 mg in tomatoes. Turnips, their leaves, and swedes are also a fairly good source of magnesium, potassium and iron.

Both vegetables are very good for a deficient or tired nervous system, and they are detoxificant and blood-cleansing.

Turnip juice is recommended by Dr. Bertholet, a French phytotherapist, to dissolve and eliminate kidney stones.

The respiratory system also benefits: turnips and swedes should be part of the diet of asthmatics, hay fever sufferers and those with colds, flu or sore throats. Boil 100 g (4 oz) turnips per litre (1 3/4 pints) water for 10 minutes, then let this stand for an hour before drinking. Or make a syrup to take as and when necessary. Juice 250 g (9 oz) turnips and mix with the same weight of sugar and 200 ml (7 fl oz) water. Cook in a bain-marie for 3–4 hours, or even longer if possible.

In the Kitchen

Turnips and swedes contain mustard oils which release sulphur compounds when heated. The longer they are cooked the more they will smell, although the smell is mild in comparison with that of cabbage.

- Grate both to eat raw with other grated roots such as parsnips and carrots. Dress with oil and lemon juice, or a mustard dressing of some sort, or add to cabbage in a coleslaw dressing. Add walnuts, herbs and other flavourings.
- Dice and cook the flesh of both lightly and use as a simple vegetable, perhaps glazed with a little butter or honey or flavoured with a nut oil, horseradish or orange rind.
- Bake small turnips whole. or bake larger ones stuffed with a meat mixture.

- Mash cooked swede or turnip with butter or cream as an accompanying vegetable. Mash them with other vegetables such as potatoes.
- Add chunks of maincrop turnip or swede to stews—they are almost a foundation vegetable like carrot, and can absorb flavour wonderfully.
- Cook dice of swede or turnip in a thick vegetable soup, or purée for a "creamed" soup.
- Cook the leaves of young turnips as spinach—lightly and fast.
- Juice the flesh of both.
- Turnip leaves contain the most calcium of all green vegetables and are therefore very valuable for the teeth and bones. When you buy a turnip, keep any leaves and use them in a salad. They are a little bitter, but excellent with a good dressing or sauce and mixed with other therapeutic salad vegetables such as spinach, chicory, lettuce, tomato, carrots, garlic, onion and walnuts. This salad is particularly helpful if you are feeling a little low and depressed.

Turnip Salad

This is a raw turnip salad which is extremely simple to make and good for the nervous and respiratory systems.

SERVES 1

1 large turnip (not a swede), scrubbed and peeled
juice of 1 lime
a small handful of mint leaves, chopped
a few grilled cashew nuts
a few turnip leaves (optional)

Grate the turnip and add the lime juice and mint leaves. Sprinkle the nuts on top and add some turnip leaves if you have them, for more excitement and nutrition. Mince or chop them and sprinkle on top.

Turnip and Potato Purée

This makes a delicious accompaniment to grilled meat or fish. Again, you could top with shredded turnip leaves at the last minute for their peppery taste.

SERVES 2

200 g (7 oz) small turnips, peeled
100 g (4 oz) potatoes, peeled
salt
2 tablespoons fresh cream
a few turnip leaves (optional)

Chop the turnips and potatoes into small, even pieces and cook in a little salted water (preferably still mineral water) until tender. Mash with a fork, and then mix in the cream. Season with a little more salt if necessary.

VANILLA
Vanilla planifolia
Orchideae family

THE VANILLA POD is the fruit of a tropical American vine. The yellow pods have to be "processed" for the full vanilla flavour to be developed: they are alternately sweated and dried until brown/black and pliable.

When Cortés first travelled to Mexico in the sixteenth century he found vanilla pods being used by the Aztecs to flavour a hot chocolate drink taken after meals as a stimulant. Since then the pods have been used as both flavouring and medicine, as they possess a number of therapeutic properties.

Therapeutic Uses
Vanilla is tonic, stimulant, antiseptic and digestive. It helps greatly in the digestion of rich foods, so use it in dessert recipes such as ice cream, milk puddings and soufflés.

A vanilla wine is good for heavy smokers with a bad cough. Macerate 3 split vanilla pods in a bottle of fortified wine (Malaga, sherry or port) or a sweet wine for three weeks, and drink a small glass after a meal.

In the Kitchen

Vanilla is one of the first flavours and aromas that children recognise and appreciate, although nowadays what they are consuming is often artificial. A synthetic vanilline was first made in the late nineteenth century from eugenol, obtained from oil of cloves; other chemical substitutes have since been synthesised, and they are recognisable by their coarser smell and harsh aftertaste. Some vanilla extracts are made from real vanilla, but try and use the real thing whenever you can.

- Store chunks of whole vanilla pod in a jar of sugar for wonderful flavour, and use the sugar in cakes and desserts.
- Macerate whole pods in the hot milk or cream to be used for desserts of all kinds—rice pudding, crème caramel, soufflés, custards, chocolate or coffee puddings, ice cream and so on. After use the pods can be rinsed, dried and re-used, although the flavour will diminish a little each time.
- For the strongest vanilla flavour split the pods and scrape out the pulpy seeds. Use chopped pods and seeds in the milk or cream for ice cream, say, and strain before freezing. Some of the black seeds will remain, but they will flavour the cream wonderfully.
- Use a vanilla pod instead of a spoon to stir a cup of coffee or hot chocolate, or infuse in a pot of coffee or chocolate for incomparable flavour.

WAKAME, *see* Seaweeds

WALNUT, *see* Nuts

WATERCRESS
Nasturtium officinale
Cruciferae family

PRINCIPAL NUTRIENTS
Vitamins: A, B, C, E
Minerals: calcium, iron, manganese, phosphorus, potassium, zinc

NATIVE to Europe and western Asia, watercress flourishes in or near shallow running water.

Buy it from a reputable source, and never gather it for yourself. If the water has been polluted by farm animals, chiefly sheep, the plant may harbour liver flukes which attack the human liver. This danger is, however, avoided if the watercress is cooked.

Therapeutic Uses
Watercress has been known as both food and medicine for thousands of years.

Modern phytotherapists recommend it for chronic bronchitis with mucus, and it is given as a preventative against colds, flu and all such infections. Watercress has an extremely high vitamin A content (as betacarotene), as well as calcium, iron and zinc. Chew and eat raw watercress slowly to help avoid receding gums and gum infections. Or juice watercress and massage it gently into the gums.

In the Kitchen
Watercress does not keep very well, so try to eat it within a day of buying. Store in cold water up to the leaves in a cool place, and wash thoroughly (but do not soak) before use. The stalks should be used as well, as they too contain flavour and nutrients.

- Use raw as a garnish to any number of dishes, and include in salads.
- Serve in a salad with walnuts and slightly warm cubes of cooked beetroot.
- Chop to use with eggs or cheese in sandwich fillings, omelettes, quiches and so on.
- Chop watercress and mix with butter for a herb butter, or make into a sauce; both are good with fish. Or use puréed watercress as a stuffing for fish.

- Add watercress leaves to other dishes made with green leaves for that hot peppery flavour.
- Make watercress into a soup which is delicious hot or cold.

WHEAT, *see* Cereal Grains

YOGURT, *see* Dairy Products

PART TWO

THE SYSTEMS
OF THE
BODY

THE BLOOD AND THE CIRCULATORY SYSTEM

THE HEART is the centre of the circulatory or cardiovascular system, and through it via a vast network of blood vessels blood is carried to and from each organ and tissue of the body. Blood is pumped out of the heart into the arteries; eventually it reaches the capillaries—the smallest blood vessels in the body—at which point the oxygen in the blood is transferred by chemical exchange to the tissues. Carbon dioxide and other waste products are returned to the system (eventually to be excreted), and capillary blood then returns to the heart through the veins.

PREVENTING PROBLEMS

The most serious problems of the circulatory system involve the heart. Atheroma, angina pectoris and coronary thrombosis all involve blockages of the arteries, and although there are many potential reasons for these blockages, faulty diet is often implicated. Other possible causes of artery damage are smoking, obesity, raised blood pressure, lack of exercise and a family history.

In order to prevent such diseases try to avoid smoking, stress and too many fatty foods, which cause fatty deposits to be laid down inside the artery walls, and make the passages narrower. Do positive things like eating sensibly to avoid being overweight and taking gentle but effective exercise.

Eat foods that positively enhance the workings of the

heart and the blood. Green vegetables are good, especially
green beans and spinach. Several foods are helpful for high
blood pressure, among them asparagus, buckwheat, marrow,
courgettes, olives, pears, rice and potatoes. Foods that are
helpful in ridding the body of cholesterol include apples, oat
bran, kiwi fruit and yogurt. Many fruits are actually a heart
tonic: cherries, grapes, pomegranates and almonds are
among them. And garlic and onion, both all-round panaceas,
also benefit the heart and circulatory system.

The blood can benefit, too, from diet. Anaemia is dealt
with below, but some foods actively cleanse and purify the
blood, and these include artichokes, asparagus, celeriac, cucumber, dandelion, potatoes, turnips, swede, onion, citrus
fruit, grapes, pears and quinces. Herbal tisanes can be made
from chervil, juniper, mint, lovage and parsley, and these
herbs should be used in cooking as well.

TREATING PROBLEMS

Aromatherapy cannot prevent or treat the more serious circulatory illnesses, but aromatherapeutic oils—as well as the
oils contained in foods—can stimulate the entire circulatory
system, helping to prevent lesser problems such as cellulite,
haemorrhoids and varicose veins. Circulation and the quality of blood can also be improved by eating aromatherapeu-
tically.

The Heart

A good balanced diet, with plenty of raw or lightly cooked
vegetables and fruit, a lesser amount of carbohydrates, limited protein and very little fat, oil and sugar is best for the
heart and circulatory system. The vitamin B complex and
the antioxidant vitamins A, C and E are good for heart
health, and vitamin E also has anti-clotting properties (cholesterol or fatty deposits can lead to an increase in blood
clotting). Minerals are important as well, particularly magnesium, which research has shown to have a stabilising effect on the rhythm of the heart. Selenium, a micro-nutrient
or trace element which is available from vegetables grown

in selenium-rich soils, is antioxidant in action. Cod liver oil or other fish oils are health food supplements which are increasingly being viewed as valuable for the heart because, like vitamin E, they can decrease the blood's tendency to clot.

I believe that *how* we eat can contribute to heart health too. Large meals can physically stress the system, increasing the workload of the heart as it strains to help the digestion do its job. Eating little and often is much more sensible. And, of course, you must eat slowly and chew your food well.

Palpitations—the sensation of an irregular heartbeat—can be frightening, but they can be quite normal after exercise, or stimulants such as caffeine or nicotine. Many women experience palpitations during menopause. Tisanes made from calming plants such as orange leaves, basil, lemon balm, rose petals, sage and artichoke leaves will help. Garlic, too, is good for the heart, as are apples.

Health writers, doctors and nutritionists have long been debating what is known as "the French paradox". The French seem to eat as much fat and to smoke as much as the Scots, but the figures for cardiovascular disease are strikingly different. The Scots have some of the highest mortality rates, whereas the French have the lowest in the Western world. Wine, particularly red, has been shown in several important studies, some undertaken by the World Health Organization, to play a significant part in these statistics. Among many other benefits, moderate red wine intake actually increases what is known as HDL cholesterol, which helps to clear the body of the harmful, LDL, cholesterol.

Anaemia
This is the most common of the blood diseases, caused by not producing enough haemoglobin—the pigment of the red blood cells which carry oxygen to the whole of the body. Anaemia manifests itself in pallor, dizziness, tiredness, lack of appetite and general malaise among many other symptoms. Iron deficiency anaemia is the type most frequently encountered, because iron is vital for the manufacture of

haemoglobin. Other nutrients needed for red blood cell health are vitamins B6, B12 and folic acid.

Iron

Many foods contain iron: liver and kidney are particularly good, as are most red meats. Duck and game also contain fair proportions. Iron is found too in most fish and shellfish. Since fish is a source of healthier "oils" than meats, they should form a major part of our protein intake—try tuna, mackerel and sardines, all cooked simply and served with lots of fresh vegetables and salads. Many vegetables and fruit contain iron: dark green vegetables such as watercress and spinach, and dried apricots are important sources.

Iron is not very easily absorbed, but is made more available to the body by the action of vitamin C. Eat C-rich foods with, before or after iron-rich foods; drink lots of orange juice, accompany with lots of salad, or follow with a good helping of fruit. Particularly good in both iron and C levels are prunes and plums, figs, avocados, pears, blackcurrants, berries of all kinds, fennel, dates, apples, rhubarb, mushrooms, nuts and melons. A good way of taking in iron consists of mixing dried fruit (in which minerals are concentrated) with grains for a home-made breakfast muesli.

Some vegetables and herbs have the ability to "fix" iron in foods. The betacarotene of carrots and the essential oil of thyme are particularly effective; eat the carrots raw or very lightly cooked, and pop a sprig of thyme into vegetable cooking water or to the marinade or cooking juices of meat. Seaweeds also contain betacarotene.

The cooking of Baltistan, in Northern India, has recently become popular and Birmingham is the Balti Centre of Britain. The foods are cooked and served in iron pots, and recent research has shown that these foods contain significant traces of iron.

The Vitamin B Complex

B6 and B12 are particularly important: vitamin B6 (pyridoxine) is needed for the use of protein in the diet, and for haemoglobin in the blood; lack of this vitamin can contribute to heart disease. The best sources are liver, kidney, oily fish and red meat, as well as nuts. Wheatgerm and brewers' yeast are rich in B6, so sprinkle them on muesli and cereals and into soups. Sweetcorn, cabbage, Brussels sprouts and many pulses are also good sources.

B12 or cyanocobalamine is found in liver, eggs, white fish, red meat and dairy products. The vitamin does not occur in plants. Lack of it can contribute to a more severe form of anaemia called pernicious anaemia.

A deficiency of folic acid can also cause a form of anaemia, particularly during pregnancy, and folic acid supplementation before pregnancy has proved very successful in preventing spina bifida, a foetal malformation. Folic acid is contained in liver and most green vegetables. Wheatgerm is also a good source.

Helping Anaemic People to Eat

People who are anaemic need to be encouraged to eat, so choose tasty and colourful foods for them. Lightly cook vegetables such as cabbage, fennel, onion and garlic, or serve celery, watercress, apple and so on raw. Use lots of herbs such as savory, lovage, mint, parsley and thyme. A watercress soup made with lemon juice and chicken stock would be a good stimulant for the appetite. A spinach salad, high in iron, could be dressed with a Roquefort dressing; this is virtually a medicine in itself because of the culture used in the making of the cheese.

Make foods for anaemic people bright and attractive to look at. Red foods seem to be especially popular—try tomatoes, beetroot, red peppers (see the soup recipe on page 142), red plums and red apples.

Wine can help stimulate the appetite as well. Cahors red, from the south-west of France, is made from the Auxerrois grape mixed with Merlot and Tannat; it is richly fruity, full of tannin and iron, and contains plenty of vitamin B12. Dr. Maury recommends it in cases of anaemia, haemorrhage, and for convalescents and those going through the menopause.

Broken Veins and Bruises

Small broken veins mostly affect people with fair and delicate skins. The veins and capillaries near the skin are not necessarily broken but weak, so the blood shows through them. The skin has a ruddy look from a distance, but when viewed closely a network of fine red lines is revealed. Bruises result from damage to skin tissue, and the purple colouration consists of blood leaking from damaged blood vessels. In both cases the veins and capillaries need to be strengthened.

Vitamin P or the bioflavonoids, citrin and rutin, are the most effective, as well as vitamins C and E. Eat plenty of C-rich foods such as citrus fruits, and try to eat some of the pith which is where a lot of the citrin is concentrated. Fresh vegetables are good sources too, as is wheat. Sprouted buckwheat (see pages 177–178) is rich in many nutrients useful for the skin. Herbal teas contain a lot of rutin. Vitamin E, perhaps *the* skin vitamin, is contained in wheatgerm, brown rice, oats, corn, dairy products, meat and most fruit and vegetables. Nuts, olives and other foods from which oils are produced are a good source, as are the oils themselves. There are good E proportions in onions, leeks and parsley.

Haemorrhoids and Varicose Veins

Veins may become varicose (swollen) in various parts of the body, most commonly in the rectum as haemorrhoids or piles, and in the legs. Haemorrhoids can be caused by strain exerted on the abdominal muscles through heavy or improper lifting, but are more usually brought on by constipation. Varicose veins in the legs are caused by an interruption of the flow of blood back to the heart. The condition occurs mostly in people who have to stand a lot, for it is movement of the legs that makes their muscles contract and help to pump the blood upwards. Inefficient circulation is the root cause of both conditions.

A good diet, rich in fibre, vitamins A, C and E and the bioflavonoids, is vital. Myrtle berries are particularly helpful for haemorrhoids, as are leeks, which lubricate. Quince and apple are also lubricant because of their high pectin content. Pumpkins contain a great deal of vitamin A, which strengthens veins and capillaries, so eat as often as you can. Other foods which are particularly useful are rhubarb, grapes, cherries, chestnuts, pears, plums, melons, parsnips, marrows, courgettes, turnips and garlic. Chervil is good. Try to avoid hot spicy foods, which exacerbate these conditions. Drink plenty of fluids.

Exercise is very important: walk briskly or jog, take up t'ai chi or yoga, swim or do gentle stretching exercises.

Cellulite

This is another condition caused by poor circulation. High levels of oestrogen encourage the body tissues to retain water; when the fat cells become interspersed with this water, the skin becomes bumpy and orange peel-like. It can also be caused by poor digestion, constipation and bad posture, all of which cause retention of toxins and fluid. Many factors can exacerbate cellulite, in particular smoking, which robs the system of vitamin C and the bioflavonoids.

A good healthy diet virtually devoid of animal fat will prevent the formation of cellulite. Oils are still needed in the diet, but macerate herbs in them to intensify their nutritive properties. Eat plenty of raw fruit and vegetables and avoid foods which encourage fluid retention, such as refined carbohydrates and processed meats. Fibre is all-important, as are fruits and vegetables such as asparagus, dandelion, lettuce and celery (good for elimination) and melons and pineapple. Eat lots of citrus fruits and almonds. Use yogurt or fromage blanc instead of butter. Eat iodine-rich seaweeds to boost your circulation and digestion. Flavour foods with chervil or cumin.

Fluid Retention

Also known as oedema, fluid retention causes swelling or puffiness in the tissues. It usually affects the hands, feet and ankles and the area around the eyes, but can be found in any part of the body. The most serious cause is some sort of kidney disease, but pregnancy, PMT, standing or sitting too long and injury can all cause the body to retain fluid.

Eat diuretic vegetables such as asparagus, green beans, fennel, garlic, onions and potatoes, and use juniper in cooking. Diuretic fruits include cherries, grapes and melons. See also the section on the kidneys and the urinary system (page 218).

Aromatherapeutic Foods for the Circulatory System

Herbs	Spices	Fruit	Vegetables	Other
basil	cumin	apple	artichoke	brewers'
chervil	juniper	apricot	(globe)	yeast
fennel	peppercorns	(dried)	asparagus	cod liver
lemon balm		avocado	bean, green	oil
lovage		banana	beetroot	dairy
mint		cherry	cabbage	products
parsley		currant	carrot	fish
rosemary		date	celeriac	game
sage		fig	celery	grains
savory		grape	courgette	meat
tarragon		grapefruit	cucumber	nuts
thyme		kiwi	dandelion	offal
		lemon	fennel	poultry
		lime	garlic	pulses
		melon	greens	seaweed
		olive	leek	shellfish
		orange	lettuce	wheatgerm
		pear	marrow	yogurt
		pineapple	mushroom	
		plum	nettle	
		pomegranate	onion	
		prune	parsnip	
		quince	pepper	
		raspberry	potato	

Aromatherapeutic Foods for the Circulatory System (*cont.*)

Herbs	Spices	Fruit	Vegetables	Other
		rhubarb	pumpkin	
		strawberry	sorrel	
			spinach	
			swede	
			sweetcorn	
			tomato	
			turnip	
			watercress	

THE BRAIN AND THE NERVOUS SYSTEM

THE NERVOUS system is divided into two parts: the central nervous system which consists of the brain, the brain stem and spinal cord; and the peripheral nervous system which consists of all the nerves that connect from the brain and spinal cord to every part of the body, including the muscles, eyes, ears and skin.

These nerves in turn are divided into several groups. The sensory nerves—those involved in sight, hearing, taste, smell and touch—send messages about what is happening to the brain, after which the motor nerves are mobilised to take the appropriate action. Some motor responses are automatic, as in digestion: when food reaches the digestive tract, the process of digestion starts without the brain consciously telling it to do so. (In fact it is often the sense of smell, so vital in aromatherapy, that is the initial stage of digestion; you smell a food and, without your consciously knowing it, your digestive juices start to flow.)

These involuntary or subconscious motor responses are known as the autonomic nervous system, and are divided into the sympathetic and parasympathetic nerves. These nerves "oppose" each other, controlling most of the body functions and keeping them in constant and fine-tuned balance. They also operate when, for instance, you are frightened or stressed. The brain sends messages through the spinal cord to all parts of the body. The sympathetic nerves stimulate the whole body and prepare it for action: adrenaline is produced and the heartbeat speeds up, the digestion is inhibited, and the pupils become dilated. Once the emergency is over the parasympathetic nerves reverse the process, slowing down the heartbeat, stimulating digestion and constricting the pupils.

Preventing and Treating Problems

The serious diseases which can affect the brain, the spinal cord and the nerves include brain haemorrhage and tumors, epilepsy, motor neurone disease, multiple sclerosis and Parkinson's disease. Lesser ailments which fall within the orbit of the nervous system, such as headache, depression and insomnia, can often be helped by aromatherapeutic principles and as well as by diet.

Most of these minor problems are caused by an imbalance between nerve systems, and by an over-production of adrenaline. Adrenaline is produced to allow the body to cope with physical danger such as the sabre-toothed tiger that would have threatened our ancestors—the "fight or flight" reaction—but stressors nowadays are different, more often psychological than physical, and often continual rather than sporadic. We cannot attack or fight money worries or health problems, or indeed physically run away from them. If there is no proper release, physical and/or mental symptoms can appear: fatigue, headaches, depression, nausea, diarrhoea and insomnia. In extreme cases, stress and anxiety can lead to severe mental illness.

Preventing such problems is usually easier said than done, but try to remove or reduce the stressor(s) if possible. Advice from friends or a professional, or simply a sympathetic ear, could help. Allow time each day to relax your body and mind through exercise, meditation, yoga, by lying in a hot bath, reading a good book or watching TV. This will relax the mind as well. Avoid tranquillisers and antidepressants, which do not remove the underlying causes of the stress but merely disguise them. Alcohol and tobacco, although they can seem relaxing, are dangerous in excess and, like pills, quickly become addictive.

Vitamins, Minerals and the Nervous System

A diet rich in the right nutrients is vital to enable the body to cope with nervous stress, whether physical or mental. Vitamins B and C are needed for the health of the blood vessels in the brain, and vitamin E will help prevent blood clots.

The B complex vitamins are particularly important. These are found in liver, whole-grain cereals, pulses, green vegetables and dairy products, as well as brewers' yeast. B1 (thiamine) works on the oxidation of glucose in the brain and nervous tissue; a deficiency results in a lack of energy, loss of appetite and irritability. B2 (riboflavin) is needed for the proper functioning of the brain. A deficiency of vitamin B3 (nicotinic acid or niacin) can cause deep depression. Pantothenic acid is important for coping with stress, and a deficiency can result in personality changes such as restlessness or irritability. It is also needed by the adrenal glands, so a shortage can cause many nervous system problems. Vitamin B6 (pyridoxine) is vital: insufficient can cause insomnia, headaches, nervousness, depression and an inability to concentrate. B12 (cyanocobalamine) is involved in the function of the whole central nervous system and in the formation of the sheaths surrounding nerve fibres.

Magnesium is often referred to as nature's tranquilliser, so eat foods rich in this mineral—dark green vegetables such as raw spinach, dried fruits (dates are particularly good) and nuts, a very rich source.

Phosphorus is useful too, and is widely available in most types of food. It is involved in the metabolism of many nutrients, particularly in brain and nerve tissue. Fish contains a fair proportion, and some eminent researchers have claimed that, because of our far-distant marine ancestry, fish is the ultimate brain food.

Calcium is required for the health of the brain and nervous system too, and is widely available in food, particularly dairy foods. Other ways of gaining calcium are by boiling up bones—chicken bones for stock or soup, say—or eating marrow bones in a pot au feu or osso buco. You can eat certain fish bones too—there is a lot of calcium, magnesium and phosphorus in canned fish such as sardines, pilchards and anchovies, and in fish which you eat whole such as whitebait. If you think something is too bony, put it in the food processor and then spread on toast.

Many other foods are considered good for the brain, particularly mushrooms, whose glutamic acid content stimulates brain activity. Also useful are seaweeds, grains such as buckwheat, rice and rye, vegetables such as asparagus, celery and onion, fruit such as bananas, avocados, pears and figs, as well as chestnuts and chickpeas.

Stress and Anxiety

In this technological society, we are all subjected to daily stress far beyond what is desirable, and we all cope in different ways. Some people seem to cope with higher levels of stress than others, but this could ultimately manifest itself in high blood pressure. Others can become sleepless, or suffer from headaches, nervous indigestion or even stomach ulcers, at a much lower stress level.

Always eat lightly when under stress, and cook food lightly too. Concentrate on foods which are calming in character such as artichokes, apples, pears, cherries, beetroot, tomatoes, courgettes, marrows, sesame and poppy seeds, lettuce, mandarin oranges, potatoes, pumpkin, nuts and aubergines. Cook with and make therapeutic teas from herbs such as chamomile, basil, coriander, tarragon, lemongrass, fennel, hyssop, lavender, thyme and mint. Ginseng can help calm you down.

Above all, avoid stimulants such as tea, coffee, chocolate, alcohol and nicotine.

Depression

Most of us can get a little depressed at times, but when it becomes impossible to lift it can develop into more serious and more acute disease. There is a winter depressive illness, known as SAD or Seasonal Affective Disorder, which affects some half a million people in the UK alone, chiefly in December, January and February. This is caused by a chemical imbalance in the hypothalamus due to the shortening of daylight hours and the lack of sunlight. A further 20 per cent of the UK population suffer from "winter blues", a milder form of SAD.

I think proper food is vital when you are depressed, or else you may just sink further into the pit. Eat foods rich in vitamins A, B and C; include some meat, nuts (especially peanuts) and lots of green vegetables like sorrel. Wheatgerm is an energiser and contains plenty of vitamin E; scatter it on your breakfast cereal or yogurt. Eat beetroot, dates, apricots, grapes, figs, tomatoes, turnips, swede, cherries, peas, pears, plums and prunes. Cook with and make teas with rosemary, thyme, borage, lemon balm, angelica, clary sage, coriander, cinnamon and vanilla. Spinach is particularly effective in combating SAD. Mushrooms are good too.

Treat yourself to a glass of a good wine: a Puligny-Montrachet or a St. Emilion would be ideal, if pricey. A glass of champagne cheers most of us up.

Fatigue and Tiredness

There are many forms of fatigue: it can be the physical reaction to exertion or heavy exercise, or it can be mental fatigue caused by hard academic or book work, late nights or emotional stress. Hormonal changes too can cause fatigue, so adolescent and menopausal women often suffer.

Sleep and relaxation are essential. Some foods can help

you sleep (see below), while others can perk you up. Dates and dried fruits are wonderful storehouses of energy, as are nuts. Apples and pears, fennel, cherries, plums, rice, onions, chickpeas, tomatoes, turnip and swede are all good vitalising foods. Chocolate is effective too, as are olives—try some biscuits with tapenade, an olive pâté, as a snack (see page 126). Cook with or drink teas made with anise, coriander seeds, cloves, cinnamon, mace, nutmeg, rosemary or clary sage.

Ginseng is very revitalising; drink a small glass of ginseng spirit (see page 77) when tired.

A glass of champagne can make you feel instantly more lively (it must be the bubbles); or add some Cassis for a Kir Royale. Drink only one glass, though, or the effect will be lost.

Insomnia

Most men and women suffer from sleeplessness at some time or another and it's usually through stress of some sort: worrying about the family, health, money, relationships or career. Lifestyle can be a major contributor if you eat meals quickly or skip them; if you're permanently dieting; if you're rushing here and there; not taking enough exercise; smoking or drinking too much; eating too late at night; or not allowing enough time for your body and mind to relax. Sleeping pills should never be the answer—there are many simpler and safer remedies.

Eating lightly in the evening is often the answer to sleeplessness brought on by indigestion. Try to include some lettuce because of its soporific compounds, or eat a citrus fruit, apple or pear as dessert. A glass of red wine could help your digestion and make you relax. Calcium-rich foods would be good as well, and you could have a milky hot drink before you go to bed. Or drink a calming herbal tea—try basil, coriander, chamomile, marjoram, oregano, lavender, lemon balm, rosemary, thyme or mint.

Migraine and Headache

Headaches can be caused by disease, major or minor (colds, flu and neuralgia among others), or by stress or eyestrain. Migraines are severe recurrent headaches, one of the commonest diseases of the nervous system. The latter can be hereditary, and affects more women than men. A simple headache causes temporary distress, but a migraine can severely incapacitate sufferers for several days. No persistent headache should be taken lightly.

Feverfew is a herb which helps control the incidence and severity of migraine attacks. Eat leaves in a sandwich or salad or make into a tisane.

If a headache is caused by the congestion of catarrh, colds or flu, or by digestive problems, eat lightly throughout the day—a soup made with lots of basil, say—or fast, drinking only hot water acidulated with lemon juice. Certain herbal teas can help: try chamomile, lemon balm, coriander, basil, or marjoram, oregano or fennel.

Migraine can actually be brought on by a number of foods, among them cheese, chocolate, citrus fruit, pork, and red and white wines.

Jetlag

This is rather a unique disorder of the nervous system, and has many physical and mental symptoms; fatigue, sleep disturbance, nausea, and aching or swollen limbs. It's all to do with the body clock which, when disturbed by travelling east or west through several time zones, can become completely desynchronised, upsetting many physiological and psychological rhythms. People who travel regularly can be more permanently affected: air stewardesses, for instance, can stop having periods.

The answer, from personal experience, is to take exercise beforehand, eat virtually nothing, drink plenty of water, and then exercise again at the other end. Eat a few citrus fruit and a handful of nuts, raisins and other dried fruit during the flight: this will give you energy. Avoid airline meals, which, even if they are good, only make you feel bloated because you are sitting down for so long. The pressurised cabins of planes are dehydrating, so drink plenty of still mineral water (not alcohol, because that too is dehydrating).

Aromatherapeutic Foods for the Nervous System

Herbs	Spices	Fruit	Vegetables	Other
angelica	anise	apple	artichoke	brewers'
basil	cinnamon/	apricot	(globe)	yeast
borage	cassia	(dried)	asparagus	chocolate
chamomile	clove	avocado	aubergine	dairy
coriander	coriander	banana	beetroot	products
fennel	mace	cherry	celery	fish
hyssop	nutmeg	date	courgette	ginseng
lavender	vanilla	dried	fennel	grains
lemon balm		fruit	garlic	liver
lemongrass		fig	greens	nuts
marjoram		grape	lettuce	pulses
mint		grapefruit	marrow	seaweeds
oregano		guava	mushroom	seeds
parsley		lemon	onion	shellfish
rosemary		lime	pea	wheatgerm
sage		olive	potato	
tarragon		orange	pumpkin	
thyme		pear	sorrel	
		plum	spinach	
		prune	swede	
		quince	tomato	
		rhubarb	turnip	

THE JOINTS, MUSCLES AND THE SKELETAL SYSTEM

THE ADULT human skeleton consists of over 200 bones, all connected to each other by articulated joints. These joints are operated by a complex system of muscles which coordinate all the movements of the body and help to maintain its posture.

Problems of the joints and muscles include osteo- and rheumatoid arthritis, back pain, fibrositis, gout, lumbago, rheumatism, sciatica and slipped disc. All are painful and a number involve swelling, inflammation and stiffness. Some are caused mechanically, for instance by lifting a heavy object badly which leads to lumbago, sciatica, or a slipped disc. Other problems are related to age, such as the wear and tear of osteoarthritis. Gout is related to chemical imbalance in the body, while rheumatoid arthritis is a disease of connective tissue.

PREVENTING PROBLEMS

Injury is a prime contributor to joint damage, so always take care, particularly when lifting heavy weights which impose extra strain on the joints and muscles. Good posture is important, too. Sitting badly for long periods, or consistently standing with your weight on only one hip, can unbalance the body and cause joint problems. Wearing high heels can damage both your back—because of the unnatural position it is forced into—and the joints of your feet, causing bunions.

Being overweight can put unnecessary stress on your joints, particularly those which are weight- or load-bearing such as the hips and knees. Bad muscle tone can also contribute to joint problems. If the muscles are not holding the bones and joints as tightly and supportively as they should, problems can occur; lax stomach muscles, for instance, particularly in people who are overweight, can cause and then exacerbate lower back problems.

Sensible exercise is a good way of keeping joint and muscle problems at bay—but bear in mind that over-strenuous exercise can actually *cause* problems. Gentle exercise such as swimming, cycling or walking keeps many joints in good working order. Weight-bearing exercise helps keep the bones strong—particularly useful for menopausal women, for whom osteoporosis is a threat. Gentle body shaping and conditioning exercises in a gym or exercise class will help good muscle tone.

Diet has a major part to play in a number of ways. A sensible diet will prevent you becoming overweight. A nutrient-rich diet will supply all the vitamins and minerals needed by bones, joints and muscles; lack of some of these nutrients can predispose people towards rheumatic problems. Foods which are cleansing and detoxifying are good, too, as they can help rid the system of toxins which contribute to joint and muscle swelling and pains, particularly gout. Foods rich in calcium and magnesium are particularly important for the formation of synovial fluid, which lubricates the joints. Calcium-rich foods include milk, yogurt and cheese, green leafy vegetables such as spinach and watercress, and nuts, seeds and pulses. Tinned fish which you eat bones and all is especially good, as are whitebait, which are eaten whole. Magnesium-rich foods include nuts and seeds, whole grains, pulses, dark green vegetables and seafood.

TREATING PROBLEMS

Arthritis

Osteoarthritis is to a certain extent the result of the natural wear and tear of living and ageing; rheumatoid arthritis is an inherited disease which can appear in quite young people. Loss of synovial fluid, change in bone structure in the joints, and inflammation all lead to pain and stiffness and, in rheumatoid arthritis, to possible crippling.

Eat a good detoxifying and diuretic diet. Appropriate vegetables include broccoli, cauliflower, green beans, celery, celeriac, asparagus, cucumber, cabbage, leeks, lettuce, radishes, sorrel and tomatoes. Fruit include melons, pears, apples, berries, currants, cherries, bananas, grapes and grapefruit. The minerals contained in many of these fruit and vegetables are lubricant as well.

Try to avoid eating too much protein, as red meats in particular can produce acidic conditions within the body. Fish, though, is good, particularly the oily kind, so eat it at least twice a week. Don't overcook it, and seal it in some way to prevent the protein of the flesh escaping: fry coated in flour or batter, or poach in a liquid containing a little wine, lemon juice or cider vinegar—acid sets the protein. Take fish oils in supplement form: cod liver oil is famed for its lubricating benefits in all sorts of joint problems.

Avoid coffee, tea and most alcohol, and instead drink teas made from apple skins, lavender, lovage and so on. An occasional glass of wine is not forbidden: Dr. Maury recommends diuretic wines that contain less alcohol and are rich in manganese: they include dry champagne, Chablis, Alsace and Pouilly Fuissé.

Gout
This is a joint disease associated with a build-up of uric acid, one of the body's waste products which is usually excreted by the kidneys. The build-up causes crystals to collect in the joints, inflaming them and limiting their movements. Gout often begins in the big toe but may affect other joints, and it can also damage the kidneys.

Gout is associated with high living and over-indulgence, but stress can play an equal part. A simpler diet can help: cut out fat and sugar, eat protein moderately, and avoid offal. The cells of animal organs such as liver and kidney contain elements called purines; these include uric acid, and all are excreted as uric acid. Avoid also other purine-rich foods such as sardines, anchovies, fish roes and yeast extracts.

When eating a protein food such as cheese, eat it with something like celery or apple. Increase your intake of raw vegetables and fruit, particularly those which are detoxifying (see Arthritis, page 214). Green beans, celery, asparagus, artichokes, carrots, tomatoes, radishes and dandelion leaves are particularly good. Some fruit can help dissolve uric acid; pears are best, but apples, grapes, blackcurrants, citrus fruit, raspberries and strawberries are also effective. Drink tisanes of lovage and blackcurrant leaves for the same purpose.

In general drink a lot of liquid—but not alcohol—to prevent a build-up of acids and to speed their elimination. Juice some of the vegetables or fruit listed above and drink a couple of glasses per day: try carrot and celery, or celery and apple. Drink them with water. A light vegetable broth could also be very helpful when you have an attack.

Supplement your diet with vitamins B and E, or eat foods rich in them.

Rheumatic Conditions

Rheumatism encompasses a whole range of complaints such as bursitis, fibrositis, lumbago, sciatica and unspecified aches and pains. In general it means inflammation, with or without pain, which affects the soft tissue, ligaments, tendons and muscles that surround and are attached to the joints.

Eat a good diet (as recommended above) with lots of raw fruits and vegetables, particularly those which detoxify and are rich in calcium and magnesium. Celery is perhaps the best. Seafood and fish oils are good, too. Garlic and onions eaten raw in salads can help dissolve and dispose of many toxins. Some herbs and spices are good in infusion—allspice, bay, lavender, ginger, juniper, horseradish and lovage among them. Infuse cloves in boiling water to help relieve pain. Drinking an early morning glass of hot water acidulated with cider vinegar or lemon juice can make you feel very much more supple.

Aromatherapeutic Foods
for the Skeletal System

Herbs	Spices	Fruit	Vegetables	Other
bay	allspice	apple	artichoke	cider
chervil	clove	banana	(globe)	vinegar
lavender	ginger	cherry	asparagus	cod liver
lovage	horseradish	currant	bean, green	oil
oregano	juniper	grape	broccoli	dairy
rosemary		grapefruit	cabbage	products
sage		lemon	carrot	fish
thyme		lime	cauliflower	grains
		melon	celeriac	nuts
		orange	celery	pulses
		pear	cucumber	seafood
		plum	dandelion	seeds
		prune	garlic	walnut
		raspberry	greens	(leaves)
		strawberry	leek	
			lettuce	
			onion	
			parsnip	
			potato	
			radish	
			sorrel	
			spinach	
			tomato	
			watercress	

THE KIDNEYS AND
THE URINARY SYSTEM

THE URINARY system consists of two kidneys and the bladder, plus the ureters (the tubes which connect each kidney to the bladder) and the urethra (the passage through which urine and, in men, semen as well, passes out of the body). The kidneys are responsible for clearing the blood of poisonous waste products, and keep fluid levels in balance (the human body contains some 60–70 per cent water). Any excess fluid is passed into the bladder from the kidneys, and then excreted through the urethra as urine. The blood is filtered by the kidneys many times per day. People with severe kidney disease have this job taken over by a dialysis machine, or may require a transplant.

The kidneys are also responsible for the production of a hormone which stimulates the production of red blood cells, and for the conversion of vitamin D into its highly active form. In this form it stimulates the absorption of calcium and phosphorus from the intestine.

The most common and treatable problems of the urinary system are cystitis, urethritis and stones, which form in the kidney or bladder.

PREVENTING AND TREATING PROBLEMS

Diet can play a large part in preventing kidney disease. Many foods and flavourings are diuretic, encouraging the excretion of fluid from the body; some also contain essential oils which are disinfectant and cleansing. Drinking a lot is also important. Water is best, and for preference it should be filtered or still mineral water than fizzy mineral water or tap water.

Onion, fennel, asparagus, celery and parsley are all

strongly disinfectant and diuretic and, eaten raw, will keep the system clean and working well. All are good in salads, or you could make a light soup from them. Raw juices are strong in action: asparagus with fennel, say, or fennel, celery and parsley would not taste very good, but they would do you good! Onion is the best food of all; eat it as often as possible, or drink the wine described on page 127 when there is a problem. White wine itself is diuretic and cleansing, according to Dr. Maury.

All green vegetables contain nitre, which is a bladder disinfectant. Other foods include corn (use it in soup, perhaps), dandelion, grapes, juniper berries (crush 3–4 berries in a mortar and add to any tisane), currants, cherries and strawberries. When the last two are in season, eat as many as you can; a tisane of cherry stalks, or blackcurrant or strawberry leaves, is especially valuable. You could actually go on a strawberry detoxifying diet, something that most people would enjoy! Celeriac, dill, leek, potatoes, chickpeas, radishes and raspberries are also detoxifying. If your system is sluggish, galvanise it into action by eating globe artichokes, asparagus or aubergine.

Many of these foods can be strong in action, and different people will respond in different ways to each one. If celery doesn't seem to work at first, try another food. Go slowly, though, and don't overdo things.

Avoid coffee, tea, sugar, salt, spices and spicy foods. Salt makes the body retain fluids while spices can exacerbate kidney conditions. It is probably wiser, if you have kidney problems, to think vegetarian and avoid meat and dairy products; the latter are rich in calcium anyway, but the digestion of proteins and fat can force your kidneys to work too hard.

Stones

Small stones which form in the urinary tract—in kidney or bladder—are themselves formed from an excess of salts in the bloodstream, mostly calcium. Some stones are made of uric acid, which is why gout can play a large part in kidney disease. It is not properly understood why stones form, but when they do they can cause severe problems. Small stones may stay undetected and unfelt but if they grow or move they can cause excruciating pain. A stone which moves from kidney to ureter and is caught there can create a urinary obstruction, and all can lead ultimately to kidney disease.

The best preventative is to drink plenty of fluids (preferably still mineral water) to counteract the potential build-up of the calcifying salts and minerals. There is some evidence to suggest that people who live in hard water areas are more protected from stones (and indeed cardiovascular disease) than those who drink soft water. Exercise can play a part too: mobility reduces the release of calcium from the bones and therefore inhibits stone formation.

Avoid calcium-rich foods such as dairy products and cheese, and avoid offal (see page 104). Eat the foods mentioned above, as well as French beans, turnip and swede. Also eat a lot of chervil.

Cystitis and Urethritis

This bladder infection is caused by bacteria already present there, or which enter the bladder through the urethra. Its symptoms are painful urination and sometimes a high temperature. Women who are on the Pill are more prone to get it because the hormones change the bacterial flora of the urethra and bladder as well as those of the vagina; the same can happen after a course of antibiotics. The enlargement of the uterus that takes place during pregnancy can also press on the bladder and encourage infection.

Urethritis is an infection of the urethra, again caused by bacteria. It can be sexually transmitted, and can be associated with other infections such as thrush. What is known as "honeymoon cystitis" is usually urethritis.

Yogurt may help rebalance the internal bacteria. The best treatment is to drink the cooking water of corn on the cob, cooked with the "silk" still attached to it. (Eat the corn as well, of course.) Avocados prevent the proliferation of bacteria in the bladder, and pears, parsnips, lavender and a tisane of strawberry leaves can also be of benefit. A sage tisane could help the cystitis that often appears during hormonally unbalanced times such as menopause.

Aromatherapeutic Foods for the Urinary System

Herbs	Spices	Fruit	Vegetables	Other
basil	cardamom	avocado	artichoke	cereal
chervil	juniper	cherry	(globe)	grains
dill		currant	asparagus	(maize)
fennel		grape	aubergine	chickpeas
lavender		melon	bean, green	walnut
parsley		pear	celeriac	yogurt
sage		plum	celery	
		prune	courgette	
		raspberry	cucumber	
		strawberry	dandelion	
			fennel	
			leek	
			marrow	
			onion	
			parsnip	
			potato	
			pumpkin	
			radish	
			swede	
			turnip	

THE LIVER

AFTER FOOD has been digested, the liver controls more than five hundred chemical reactions in which the digested food, already broken down into its three main constituents of carbohydrate, protein and fat, is metabolised or further digested. The liver is also a storage, recycling, detoxifying and manufacturing organ.

The following are but a few of the liver's vital functions. It synthesises amino acids (the building blocks of protein): in so doing, it converts them into ammonia, a substance potentially toxic to the body, but this is further converted into urea, a constituent of urine, and excreted by the kidneys. The liver also controls the level of glucose or blood sugar in the blood, and stores glucose in the form of glycogen; this it synthesises from carbohydrate. It manufactures bile (stored in the gallbladder), which is essential for the breakdown of fats; these are not properly digested or metabolised elsewhere in the body.

As well as storing glycogen, the liver stores the fat-soluble vitamins A, D, E and K, also B12, folic acid, and some minerals such as iron and copper. As well as detoxifying and converting ammonia, the liver breaks down and detoxifies harmful substances such as drugs and alcohol. As well as manufacturing bile, the liver makes the beneficial (LDL) type of cholesterol, and plays a part in red blood cell formation.

All of these functions can be disturbed by diseases which affect the liver, and malfunctions of the liver can lead to serious disease elsewhere in the body. Hepatitis is an inflammation of the liver caused by a virus, toxin, obstruction, parasite, or drug (including alcohol). Diabetes is a disease of faulty metabolism; if the pancreas does not produce insulin, a hormone involved in the liver's control of blood sugar levels, the liver cannot do its job properly. Gout is considered a metabolic disorder too (see page 215); and faulty metabolism of fats can ultimately lead to severe diseases such as atherosclerosis. Excessive consumption of alcohol can cause liver damage, perhaps even cirrhosis. Certain drugs can have the same effect: many people who have tried, and failed, to attempt suicide by overdose on paracetamol have suffered severe liver damage.

Liver problems can lead to any number of other problems including fuzzy eyesight, poor hearing, high blood pressure, over-pigmentation of the skin, swelling in the legs, muscle weakness, glandular imbalance, varicose veins and piles, asthma, hay fever, sinusitis and cellulite. Jaundice, a yellow tint to the skin, is the familiar result of liver malfunction.

PREVENTING AND TREATING PROBLEMS

Diet is paramount in looking after the health of your liver. Avoiding excess alcohol is the first consideration. Quite apart from making the liver work too hard in its detoxifying capacity, alcohol metabolism can interrupt the metabolism of other vital nutrients such as carbohydrates and fats, which can result in a low blood sugar level. Some experts say that one to two drinks a day are not harmful, and indeed can generally benefit your health; others claim that, although the liver can cope with the occasional binge, it copes less well with a continuous "drip feed" of alcohol. Perhaps modest drinking with two or more alcohol-free days per week is the best and healthiest approach. Certainly once any liver problems do exist alcohol should be avoided altogether to allow the liver to regenerate—which in the majority of cases it does.

To help the liver in whatever condition eat a diet that does not contain much fat. Avoid too much red meat, poultry and oily fish, and refined cooking fats such as salted butter. White sugar, white bread, cakes, biscuits and sweets are all bad for the liver as well as for the health in general. Eating too much at once is bad, too; medical nutritionists advise patients suffering from liver problems to eat little and often.

Foods that are good for the liver are fresh vegetables, raw

or lightly cooked—the best is raw celery—fresh fruit and nuts, and whole grains. Potatoes, although carbohydrate, are not advised for liver patients but they are good for diabetics. Aromatic substances such as herbs and spices—as well as the onion family and garlic—play a vital role, and actively promote the health of the liver, spleen, pancreas and gall-bladder, stimulating, dynamising and decongesting. They can also promote liver regeneration. Cook any protein that you do eat with those herbs or spices which benefit the liver.

Aromatherapeutic Foods for the Liver

Herbs	Spices	Fruit	Vegetables	Other
bay	clove	apple	artichoke	grains
borage	cumin	avocado	(globe)	nuts
chervil	garlic	blackberry	asparagus	(including
fennel	ginger	(leaves)	aubergine	walnut
lovage	horseradish	cherry	beetroot	leaves)
mint	juniper	currant	cabbage	
parsley	mustard	elderberry	carrot	
rosemary	nutmeg	grape	celeriac	
sage		grapefruit	dandelion	
tarragon		guava	endive	
thyme		lemon	leek	
		lime	onion	
		olive (black)	potato	
		orange	radish	
		papaya	spinach	
		raspberry	tomato	
		rhubarb		
		strawberry		
		(and leaves)		

THE LUNGS AND THE RESPIRATORY SYSTEM

THE RESPIRATORY system is dominated by the lungs, but in fact all the organs which contribute to breathing are part of it—the nose and mouth, and the air passages leading to the lungs: throat, larynx, trachea and the two bronchi. These air passages not only take oxygen to the lungs and carbon dioxide from the lungs, but they also filter the inhaled air, which is why so many respiratory system infections hit the nose and throat: these are in the front line and trap infection before it can reach down to the lungs.

Many viruses and bacteria can attack the respiratory system, but most of the subsequent infections are minor and disappear within about five days. If an ailment lasts longer, medical help should be sought, especially for elderly people or the very young. Allergies are a particular problem for the respiratory system: allergens breathed in can cause many disorders, including asthma and hay fever.

Common problems of the respiratory system include asthma, bronchitis, catarrh, general chest infections, coughs, fever, hay fever, headaches (see page 211), neuralgia, flu, pneumonia, sinusitis and sore throat. Emphysema and cancer of the air passages and lungs are less common.

PREVENTING PROBLEMS

To keep all infections at bay and to build up the body's defence, it is important to eat a diet rich in vitamins A, B, C and D and protein. Vitamin A maintains the health of the respiratory passages; a deficiency increases susceptibility to infections. Research has also shown that there is a correlation between B vitamin deficiency and lung disease. Remember that the B complex should be treated as a whole; it is probably useless to take them separately as supplements. They are all present in natural foods such as green leafy vegetables, brewers' yeast, whole grains and offal such as liver, kidneys and heart. (But note that many B vitamins are water-soluble and may be lost in the cooking water; they can also suffer through oxidation and light.)

Eat plenty of oily fish, and take cod liver oil for its vitamin D, which is very preventative. Eat lots of onion and garlic, which are antibacterial and antiviral and also contain sulphur. Other foods that contain sulphur include almonds, apricots, cucumber, chestnuts, dates, green beans, greens in general, horseradish, leeks, oats, onion, citrus fruit, pears, radishes, strawberries, swede, turnips and wheatgerm. All these contain essential oils which can get rid of bacteria and viruses. If you eat horseradish, for instance, you cry straightaway and loosen mucus, so you are already eliminating and detoxifying yourself. Potatoes and rice fortify the lungs because they detoxify as well. These foods should all be eaten all year round, but particularly in late summer and early autumn, when they will prime the body to resist the infections of winter. Angelica can help you guard against infections, as can ginseng, carrots and guavas.

If you suffer from allergic respiratory problems, steer clear of the particular allergen, be it pollen, dust, mites or whatever, as much as possible.

TREATING PROBLEMS

If you have a mild respiratory infection, stay in bed and keep warm, avoiding damp, pollution and cigarette smoke. Minor problems can easily become major ones in a vulnerable system: a cough could become bronchitis, and bronchitis pneumonia. During a flu epidemic keep away from public places as much as possible, and if you have an infection yourself stay away from others, especially old people and small children. Most respiratory diseases are highly contagious.

Eat as well as you can, depending on how you feel. Soups are good, as they are warming, diuretic and not too stressful on the digestive system: those made with potatoes, celery, onion and leeks are good, especially if you add some rye. Protein is still important because it is necessary for the repair of body tissue. Avoid dairy products, though, as they actually create mucus.

Drink plenty of fluids, but not the stimulants coffee or tea. Expectorant herbal tisanes are best—make them from bay, eucalyptus, hyssop, lavender, lemon balm, rosemary, sage or thyme. Barley water with lemon juice is good, as is lemon juice by itself, with some hot water and honey, for the vitamin C and its detoxifying effect. Expectorant raw juices are beneficial: try cucumber and celery together with the juice of half a lemon. Alcohol isn't out of the question—a little whiskey or brandy in a herb tea will do you more good than harm, and I find *Glühwein*, a German version of mulled wine, good for when I'm feeling sniffy with a cold; heat red wine gently with spices such as cinnamon and cloves, along with lemon peel and honey.

Other foods which are good for the respiratory system include turnips, swede, watercress, leeks, radishes, apples, figs, pears, plums, prunes and redcurrants. Herbs and spices include cinnamon, marjoram, oregano, mint, borage, chervil, bay and sage.

Coughs and Sore Throats

Coughing is a protective response which helps to rid the lungs of irritants, and can be a symptom of a variety of diseases including asthma, bronchitis, the common cold, flu, hay fever and pneumonia. Sore throats can be caused by the cough itself, by many of the same diseases, and by laryngitis and tonsillitis. Tisanes made with expectorant herbs (see above) help, as do drinks made with cinnamon (which is antiseptic for the throat, as well as warming and soothing). A cup of hot water with lemon and honey is the most effective treatment for a sore throat. Foods such as lemon and ginger, for their vitamin C content and warmth respectively, alleviate coughs; avoid hard foods, which could hurt the throat. Soups, particularly those made with a lot of garlic, would be nourishing but not too painful to swallow.

To relieve a sore throat, suck ice cubes made with boiled water, lemon juice and pineapple juice (pineapple clears mucus as well), or eat ice cream or sorbet (see pages 145–146). A syrup made from bilberries (see page 26) is a good antibacterial for laryngitis and tonsillitis; currants, blackberries, raspberries and apricots are good fruits to eat. Vanilla is good for a smoker's cough, and other beneficial foods include olives, potatoes, radishes and sorrel.

Mucus and Catarrh

This excessive secretion of phlegm from the air passages is most commonly caused by colds and flu, although hay fever, bronchitis and sinusitis could also be involved. Potatoes and mushrooms are good foods to eat, and you should drink tisanes made from the expectorant herbs and spices (see above). Chamomile and chervil are good for hay fever, as are carrots.

Foods with hot spices in them can help you breathe—at least you'll be able to taste them! Curry or dishes with mustard, horseradish, peppercorns, ginger, chilli and so on will help.

Fever

You can have an abnormally high body temperature—anything two degrees or more over 37°C (98.6°F)—because of bronchitis, a cold, flu, tonsillitis or pneumonia. Drink lots of fruit juices, mineral water and herb tisanes as above—it's important to rehydrate the body after the loss of liquid caused by a high temperature and the perspiration that accompanies it. Whole or white rice cooked with bay, chervil, thyme or rosemary is nutritious and easy to digest. Raspberries and the red "seeds" of pomegranates are easy to eat, too.

Research has shown that vitamin E can relieve the high temperature of pneumonia.

Aromatherapeutic Foods for the Respiratory System

Herbs	Spices	Fruit	Vegetables	Other
angelica	chilli	apple	asparagus	brewers'
anise	cinnamon/	apricot	bean, green	yeast
basil	cassia	bilberry	cabbage	cod liver
bay	clove	blackberry	(especially	oil
borage	ginger	currant	red)	eucalyptus
chamomile	horseradish	date	carrot	fish (oily)
chervil	mustard	fig	celeriac	ginseng
fennel	vanilla	grape	garlic	grains
hyssop		grapefruit	greens	honey
lavender		guava	leek	nuts
lemon balm		lemon	lettuce	offal
marjoram		lime	mushroom	pine kernel
mint		olive	onion	pine needle
oregano		orange	peas	seaweed
parsley		peach	pepper	wheatgerm
rosemary		pear	potato	
sage		pineapple	pumpkin	
savory		plum	radish	
thyme		pomegranate	sorrel	
		prune	spinach	
		quince	swede	
		raspberry	tomato	
		strawberry	turnip	
			watercress	

THE FEMALE REPRODUCTIVE SYSTEM

THE FEMALE reproductive system includes the ovaries, Fallopian tubes, uterus, vagina, vulva, breasts and nipples. When a girl baby is born her ovaries contain about 1 million cells, which then gradually decrease. At puberty some 300,000 cells remain, and it is then that the reproductive cycle properly begins. Each month for the next 30 to 40 years one of these cells is transformed into an egg for possible fertilisation, so there is quite a lot of wastage! (Only about 400 eggs are released throughout a woman's fertile life; the remainder degenerate.)

If the egg is not fertilised, it and the lining of blood prepared for it in the womb, the endometrium, are shed in the process known as menstruation. After that 30 to 40 years menstruation ceases, the woman's body produces no more eggs, and she becomes infertile during the last part of the reproductive cycle, the menopause.

This whole cycle is controlled by hormones. At puberty a region of the brain called the hypothalamus stimulates the pituitary gland to release hormones into the bloodstream. The first of these is a follicle-stimulating hormone (FSH), which travels to the ovaries and starts the transformation of an ovarian cell into a mature egg. As this develops, the hormones oestrogen and, later, progesterone, are produced. It is an imbalance between these two hormones that is thought to cause many reproductive system problems, and it is the gradual withdrawal of hormones from the bloodstream that heralds and marks the menopause.

Hormonal imbalance can contribute to problems such as amenorrhoea, dysmenorrhoea, premenstrual syndrome or tension (PMS or PMT), fluid retention and cellulite. If the hypothalamus, pituitary gland or ovaries are stressed in any way the finely tuned hormonal balance can be disturbed, and this not only causes malfunctions elsewhere in the reproductive system but it can lead to a diminution in the sense of well-being, to listlessness, fatigue, and a vulnerability to many other potential ills.

PREVENTING AND TREATING PROBLEMS

A good diet is essential. A woman's body requires many nutrients such as vitamins A, B, E and F, together with minerals—in particular, zinc—in order to synthesise the hormones involved in the menstrual cycle. It is because sufferers from anorexia and bulimia nervosa do not ingest anything like the nutrients that their bodies require that their periods cease. Shock, or severe or constant emotional stress, can also interfere with the cycle. It has been recorded recently, for instance, that nurses who served in the Gulf War have been starting their menopause early—another symptom of the Gulf War syndrome.

The conventional medical response is usually drugs such as antibiotics, diuretics or tranquillisers, or hormone "balancers" in the form of the Pill or HRT (hormone replacement therapy). Sometimes these can cause further disturbances to the cycle, and I would always favor a more natural approach using food, herbs and spices.

Many essential oils in herbs and spices are emmenogogic in action, acting to promote and normalise the female cycles. These aromatics include basil, cinnamon, cumin, lavender, lemon balm, mint, nutmeg, parsley, sage, clary sage, tarragon and thyme. A possible explanation for their influence is that certain essences closely resemble the female hormones (sage, for instance, is highly oestrogenic). Other plants and foods containing natural hormones include ginseng and sprouted seeds, pulses and grains. A sensible and nutritious diet which includes these foods—the herbs in cooking and salads, and as tisanes—should keep the system ticking over.

The prostaglandins have been likened to hormones but, instead of being released from and by glands such as the ovaries, as are oestrogen and progesterone, they are resident in and work on individual parts of the body. They are important for all cell growth and regeneration, the health of the skin and cardiovascular system, and benefit women in particular.

To ensure a healthy supply of prostaglandins in turn, the body needs a balanced intake of essential fatty acids (EFAs), often known as vitamin F, which are vital for proper food metabolism. First-pressing oils such as safflower, sunflower, soy and olive contain good levels of an EFA called linoleic acid. Another EFA, linolenic acid, is found in leaf vegetables, linseed, and fish oil (cod liver oil). Gamma linolenic acid is even more special, and is found in plant seed oils such as sesame and evening primrose. The vitamin E of all these oils is good for women—for the skin as well as the reproductive system—so use them as much as possible in cooking and in salad dressings.

Seaweeds are beneficial, so sprinkle them dried on to salads and other dishes. Calcium and magnesium will help with the depression that can accompany PMT or menopause, so eat shellfish, oily fish, canned fish, nuts, seeds and dairy products such as cheese. Choose your cheese carefully, though, as something like Cheddar is very dense and can be too difficult to digest, particularly if you are suffering the symptoms of PMT or menopause. Goat's or sheep's cheese will be easier for the body to assimilate, as would goat's or sheep's milk yogurts. Remember to add suitable herbs and spices to anything that you find difficult to digest, but try to avoid fatty foods, particularly meat, when you feel tired, as they will be more difficult to break down. Parsley and sage are particularly useful in all women's problems.

Menstrual Problems

Amenorrhoea is the absence of periods at any time between puberty and the menopause. Avoid stimulants like tea, coffee and alcohol; instead, drink tisanes made from the oestrogenic herbs sage, chamomile or parsley, or from fig leaves. Eat pineapple, which promotes menstruation.

Dysmenorrhoea is painful menstruation; the pain suffered

each month takes the form of headaches, backaches and, most usually, abdominal cramps. In the days leading up to a period it is sensible to eat foods rich in calcium and magnesium (see previous page), both of which are needed for muscle relaxation. Food rich in the B complex vitamins, particularly B6, are helpful too: liver, kidney, wheatgerm, brewers' yeast, peanuts and oily fish. The liver helps to replace the mineral iron lost during the period, particularly if it is a heavy one.

Herbal tisanes can ease the pains of dysmenorrhoea: try anise, caraway, chamomile, fennel, lemon balm, parsley and fig leaves. Bilberries can help counter heavy periods.

PMT can affect women in a variety of ways: for a few days before a period begins, ankles, hands, stomach and breasts can swell, there can be weight gain, indigestion, constipation, insomnia, headaches and mood swings. Eating sensibly can help avert and minimise many of these symptoms. Eat little and often, which eases the stress on the digestion. Eat foods rich in the tranquillising B complex vitamins and magnesium (see above). Never take stimulants like tea or coffee, or chemical diuretics, to counter fluid retention and swellings, as these can increase nutrient loss from the body: eat foods, and drink tisanes made from herbs and spices, that are gently and naturally diuretic in action: green beans, juniper, cardamom, chervil, fennel, citrus fruits and watercress. Calming foods that are especially helpful for PMT sufferers include chamomile, mint, anise, dried apricots, almonds, pears, peaches, nectarines, lettuce, spinach and thyme.

For all menstrual problems, cook relevant and healthy foods with some of the herbs mentioned above. Evening primrose oil can be an effective supplement.

Genital Infections
The two most common infections of the female genital system are leucorrhoea—an inflammation of the vagina, caused by bacteria and giving rise to a thick discharge, and thrush—a yeast-like fungus which causes itchiness and inflammation, usually in the vagina, and a discharge. Both can occur

following a course of antibiotics, when the body's chemical balance has been altered; both can also be associated with the Pill, pregnancy and menopause (all times, again, when the hormonal balance is changing).

A good preventative diet, rich in vitamins A and B, is essential. Natural live yogurt can help restore the balance of internal beneficial bacteria. Lavender can be useful.

Pregnancy

Kitchen aromatherapy can help boost the mother and growing baby, and alleviate some of the discomforts, major or minor, which a pregnant woman can encounter. First, eat a good diet, rich in nutrients to help the baby. Folic acid is particularly associated with foetal health just before and immediately after conception: a deficiency can lead to spina bifida in babies with a genetic susceptibility. Foods rich in folic acid are wheatgerm, liver, kidneys, dark green vegetables, peanuts, walnuts and cauliflower.

Counter swelling feet and other areas with some of the tisanes and foods mentioned above; also eat a lot of citrus fruits, whose vitamin C content is mildly diuretic. This can also help the blood vessels, preventing circulatory problems such as varicose veins.

Stay calm and relaxed during pregnancy by eating foods rich in magnesium, a mineral known as nature's tranquilliser. Nibble almonds, a rich source, as a snack, and add them to salads and cereal dishes. If you suffer from insomnia eat lettuces and mandarin oranges, and drink calming teas such as lavender. Include buckwheat, carrots, lentils and rice in your diet.

Sexual Problems

Hormonal imbalance, the vaginal dryness and anxiety of menopause, stress and depression in general can all contribute to problems such as frigidity. Aromatherapeutic plants can help in tisanes which are relaxing (chamomile and mint, for instance), or aphrodisiac (ginseng, savory, basil or celery). The herbs could be macerated in spirits or wines (see the aphrodisiac pick-me-up on page 4); some wines are actually reputed to be aphrodisiac in themselves, particularly red wines (Dr. Maury recommends Médoc as well as Pouilly Fuissé and Champagne Brut). Never over-indulge in alcohol, though, as this can depress the central nervous system and lessen desire. Foods which are thought to be aphrodisiac could be tried, among them oysters and caviar. All seafood is reputed to increase sexuality and fertility. Peppercorns are considered aphrodisiac by the French, and ginger has a similar reputation. Boil 1 teaspoon each of peppercorns, savory, hyssop and ginger in 600 ml (1 pint) water for 10 minutes. Drink, and hope for the best! You could add the decoction to a glass of wine, half and half.

Ginseng does have a definite effect on the libido, so you should make the ginseng wine or spirit described on page 77. Drink when needed. You could also add a little of this to a chicken soup, with a little lemon juice, a couple of angelica roots and a further tiny piece of ginseng. This would be a fantastic pick-me-up when you are tired premenstrually or menopausally.

The Menopause

The end of the reproductive cycle is viewed by many women with apprehension in the belief that the loss of their fertility will go hand in hand with loss of sexuality, beauty and youthfulness. The years over which menstruation gradually ceases can indeed bring problems—among them hot flashes, moodiness, itching skin, palpitations and insomnia—but it is a natural process, and many women can actually acquire a new self-awareness and relaxed confidence.

A careful diet could possibly replace HRT in those who are suffering symptoms. Foods that might help are whole rice, dried apricots, almonds, pears, peaches, nectarines, buckwheat, spinach and lettuce. The sprouts of seeds, grains and pulses are particularly effective because they contain natural hormones, as do ginseng and linseeds. Herbs and spices to add to your cooking and use in tisanes are anise, cardamom, chervil, sage and rosemary. A sage and nettle tea is very rich in substances similar to female hormones.

Japanese women do not suffer from menopausal symptoms in the way that Western women do. Research published in *The Lancet* in 1993 revealed that the oestrogenic compounds of traditional foods such as tofu, miso and soya beans had a marked biological effect on women whose own oestrogenic activity had slowed because of the menopause.

Aromatherapeutic Foods for the Reproductive System

Herbs	Spices	Fruit	Vegetables	Other
angelica	anise	apricot	asparagus	brewers'
basil	caraway	(dried)	bean, green	yeast
chamomile	cardamom	bilberry	broccoli	buckwheat
chervil	cinnamon	currant	carrot	cheese
clary sage	clove	fig	cauliflower	cod liver
dill	cumin	grapefruit	celery	oil
fennel	ginger	lemon	lettuce	evening
hyssop	horseradish	lime	parsnip	primrose
lavender	juniper	olive	spinach	oil
lemon balm	mace	orange	watercress	fish (oily)
mint	nutmeg	peach/		ginseng
parsley	peppercorns	nectarine		grains
sage		pear		(sprouted)
savory		pineapple		lentils
tarragon		quince		linseed
thyme				millet
				nuts
				offal
				pulses
				(sprouted)
				rice
				seeds
				(sprouted)
				shellfish

| Aromatherapeutic Foods for the Reproductive System (*cont.*) | | | | |
Herbs	Spices	Fruit	Vegetables	Other
				wheatgerm
				wine
				yogurt

THE STOMACH AND THE DIGESTIVE SYSTEM

IN ORDER to function and stay alive the body needs a constant supply of energy which comes from the food that we eat. The food is digested and divided first into its three main constituents, carbohydrate, protein and fat. This process starts in the mouth, and continues via the alimentary canal to the stomach, and then the intestines, colon and rectum, involving also the liver, pancreas and gallbladder. But between the mouth and rectum lies a system of great complexity that can break down in a number of ways.

The mouth produces saliva, which softens foods and makes them more liquid and easier to swallow. Sometimes the process can start even before anything is placed in the mouth; as an aromatherapist, I must emphasise the importance of the nose and the sense of smell. The aroma of food cooking—spices frying, bread baking, meat roasting or onions browning—can make saliva flow in the mouth, ready for action!

Food chewed and bound with saliva passes down via the

oesophagus into the stomach, where it is churned with gastric juices, primarily hydrochloric acid. This is produced when food is present, but also in response to anger or stress: if it is continual, the acid may eat into the stomach lining and cause a gastric ulcer. In the stomach, protein is partially broken down; carbohydrate and fat are not. After a time the churned food passes into the duodenum, the first part of the small intestine. Carbohydrate foods may leave the stomach after about two hours, protein after about three, while fat may take as long as four hours.

In the duodenum, digestion proper starts. All three constituents of food are further broken down. If acids are not neutralised properly here, a duodenal ulcer can result. Then, in further parts of the small intestine, absorption begins. Protein is absorbed into the blood as its constituent amino acids; carbohydrate is absorbed similarly, as its constituent sugars (principally glucose). Fat is turned into small globules, and bile from the liver starts to break them down. The liver plays an important part in these conversions, with unwanted matter being excreted as urine via the kidneys, and feces via the colon and rectum. Fat is not excreted, but stored in the body.

The commoner symptoms of digestive disorders are abdominal pain, diarrhoea, constipation, indigestion and nausea. The causes can be just as diverse, ranging from eating the wrong foods, eating too fast, infection or food poisoning to more serious matters such as liver malfunction or cancer of the stomach or colon.

PREVENTING PROBLEMS

Most problems of the digestive tract are caused by several factors acting in tandem. One simple factor may seem to be the trigger, but heredity, diet, infection, the immune system, and physical (or indeed mental) blockage may all play their part in bringing about a single disorder. In general, though, most digestive problems are caused by eating the wrong sort of diet—too much refined or fatty food, too little fresh fruit and vegetables—but lack of exercise, lifestyle and stress can also be implicated.

Most plant foods contain essential oils which stimulate the digestive system, helping to galvanise sluggish organs into action; they assist in the assimilation of other foods and are cleansing and antibacterial, rendering many other foods safer to eat. Herbs and spices are particularly valuable, for their oils help break down the food when it reaches the stomach, and intestines. For no matter how nutritious individual foods might be, their nutrients are of little use to the body if they are not released and assimilated properly.

Foods and flavourings that stimulate the digestive system include angelica, aubergine, beetroot, caraway (possibly the best of all), cinnamon, cassia, garlic, ginger, grapefruit and other citrus fruits (which are also detoxifying), onion, pears, horseradish and mustard. Foods and flavourings to help digestion include avocados, celery, buckwheat, fennel, potatoes, peaches, rice, kiwi fruit, lovage, marrow, courgettes, mushrooms, almonds, papaya, savory, spinach and seaweed.

If you do suffer from digestive trouble, there are several precautions you can take. Never overeat, particularly rich and fatty foods. Large meals are bad for any system: eating smaller meals more often is preferable. Don't drink to excess—this can cause a hangover, an acute digestive problem known also as gastritis—or smoke, which can have a harmful effect on the digestive system. Don't eat or drink too fast, which can stress the system: always chew food properly, which is good both for stomach and digestion, mouth and teeth (see page 252). Never eat late at night, or your digestion will be working away while you are trying to sleep: this is the classic time for indigestion. Eat a diet rich in nutrients and fibre, which will keep your system in regular order. Try to avoid diuretics like coffee and tea, replacing them with herbal tisanes. Taking some form of regular exercise is important.

Food hygiene is vital to avoid bacterial and other contamination. Don't cook with aluminum pans: aluminum salts can leach out into the food and interfere with the secretion of gastric juices.

TREATING PROBLEMS

Once digestive problems exist, there are many possible aromatherapeutic treatments depending on the symptoms.

Abdominal Pain

This can be caused by many problems other than digestive ones—by dysmenorrhoea, for instance—but it can result from constipation, gastritis, gastric flu, colic (infant or adult) or food poisoning. If the pain is accompanied by nausea and vomiting, excessive diarrhoea or fever, obtain medical help.

No one feels much like eating when in pain, especially if it is caused by something you have eaten as is usually the case with adult colic, but a clear vegetable soup with some antiseptic thyme in it could be palatable. The heat can be comforting, too. Herbal teas can help: try chamomile, mint, dill, caraway, fennel, anise or lemon balm. Give a colicky baby some chamomile tea, or the water in which fennel and carrot have been boiled.

Diarrhoea

Frequent loose or liquid motions, which may be accompanied by abdominal pain, can be caused by a number of factors—by stress or fear, by drugs, by exposure to unfamiliar bacteria (as in "holiday tummy"), by viruses such as flu, by bacteria or amoebae as in dysentery, or by food poisoning. Inflammations of the bowel, such as colitis, are characterized by diarrhoea.

Particular care must be taken with old people and babies, as they can quickly become dehydrated. Keep any patient warm, and make them drink plenty of fluid—preferably still mineral water or herbal teas such as chamomile. It's best to avoid food until the diarrhoea has eased. Then, simple, starchy, bland food is the most acceptable: boiled or steamed rice or barley, and puréed carrot or pumpkin—these are decongestant and will add bulk to the stools. Cooked leeks can be helpful, as can apples; the pectin in the latter acts as an antidiarrhoeal. Although raw fruit and vegetables should probably be avoided as much as possible for a short while—

they contain too much fibre—raw bananas can be binding. Other foods which help counter diarrhoea are pomegranates, bilberries, currants, guava and seaweed. Caraway is particularly good for the diarrhoea of colitis.

When the attack has passed, and a normal healthy diet is being eaten again, stay clear of dairy products for a while as they can be painful to digest. Also cook food with thyme and bay to take care of any bacteria that might still be lurking in the system.

Constipation

Difficult and infrequent defaecation can cause abdominal pain, tiredness and stress. If long-standing, it can contribute to a number of other problems such as general malaise, a greasy or unhealthy skin, cellulite and haemorrhoids. The most common cause is a diet lacking in sufficient fibre or roughage—the cellulose of vegetable foods. Cellulose forms the main structure of grains, vegetables and fruit, and cannot be digested by the body; it is valuable because it absorbs other waste products of the body, enabling them to pass through the bowel relatively quickly and easily.

The first necessity, then, is to eat a diet rich in this fibre— fresh fruit and vegetables (retain skins and seeds as much as possible) and whole grains and pulses (rye, millet and linseed are particularly good). Some oat or wheat bran, which is virtually pure fibre, can be sprinkled on to foods: mix it into the juices of a fruit salad, into yogurt or cereal for breakfast, or into gravy, where it will be easily swallowed. Some aromatic foods are mild laxatives in themselves, among them cooked or raw fennel, carrot, marrow and courgette. Borage, tarragon and fennel are helpful herbs, and seaweed can be stimulant. Many fruits are good, particularly when dried; try apples, melons, persimmon, raspberries, guavas, cherries, figs, plums, prunes and papaya. A tablespoon of first pressing olive oil in the morning can work wonders. If the oil is used in a dressing for lettuce, one of the great remedies for constipation, the results will be even more miraculous!

Indigestion

This is the more common name for a number of symptoms and problems, medically known as dyspepsia, which include abdominal pain, nausea, flatulence and heartburn. Any of these can be the result of non-digestive factors such as stress or tension, but more usually they are associated with unwisely chosen food and its faulty digestion.

Heartburn is a burning pain behind the breastbone. It is linked with regurgitation, when digestive acids from the stomach flow back from the oesophagus, sometimes right up to the mouth, and cause discomfort. This can be a particular problem during pregnancy. Drinking milk or eating natural yogurt could help, because of the calcium (the principal ingredient in many proprietary antacids).

Wind and flatulence can be the result of distension of the stomach and intestines by gas. This could be swallowed air—we do this anyway, but more when we are nervous. It is, however, more often to do with the fermentation of certain foods in the digestive system, due to bacterial action. Pulses, for instance, possess elements which pass to the colon undigested; there they are worked on by intestinal bacteria, which create gas in the process, producing discomfort. Other wind-producing foods are salad vegetables such as radishes, green peppers and cucumbers, and members of the cabbage family; their sulphur content is to blame. The answer is either to avoid these foods or to cook them with herbs and spices which aid their digestion. These include allspice, anise, basil, bay, cardamom, cloves, horseradish, dill, lemongrass, mace, marjoram, nutmeg, oregano and, possibly best of all, savory. Angelica stems, if chewed after meals, can also help prevent flatulence; herb and spice seeds, such as anise, caraway, cardamom and cumin—included in the *paan* offered after Indian meals—can help digestion as well, and prevent flatulence. Pineapple is a good fruit to eat because of its enzymes, as are figs, citrus fruit, kiwi fruit and papaya.

Some people do not produce the enzymes that digest the

sugar in milk (lactose), which can cause flatulence when dairy foods are eaten. Many babies suffer from a reaction to cows' milk; if so, provide alternatives such as goat or soya. Gluten, the protein of wheat, can also cause allergic digestive problems for many people; if diagnosed as suffering from coeliac disease (usually in infancy) they should avoid all wheat products, as well as other grains such as barley, oats and rye. Rice would be the best alternative grain, or millet or corn, and soya and other flours could substitute for wheat flour.

Loss of Appetite

An unwillingness or inability to eat is usually temporary, the consequence of a minor infection such as a cold or flu, or some mild digestive problem. Anorexia or bulimia nervosa are psychological disorders, but they concern food, eating and lost appetite. If a sufferer reaches a certain stage in her morbid hatred of fatness, and thus of food, the whole body, let alone the digestive system, can break down. Anorexia can be fatal, so restoring an interest in eating is vital. Aromatic herbs, spices and foods are the key to rekindling lost appetite.

If your body simply needs a rest from food after a minor illness, take some herbal teas (see the list below) and wait until you feel hungry again. Then eat small meals of highly nutritious foods which are easily digested. If you want to encourage yourself or someone else to eat, herbal teas such as fennel and anise, perhaps mixed with mint, are good appetisers, as are marjoram, lemon balm and thyme. Aromatics and foods which enhance the appetite and stimulate the digestion include angelica, aubergine, beetroot, cinnamon, cloves, coriander, ginger, horseradish, mustard, parsnips, pears, lemon, lime, peppercorns and sweet ripe peppers.

For anorexics, cook their favourite meals, but serve in small unthreatening portions. There is some evidence that zinc deficiency is associated with a reduction in ability to taste and smell, so foods which are rich in this trace element could be useful; red meats (especially beef), liver, fish, shellfish, whole grains, pulses, cheese, nuts and seeds are good sources. Many wines can encourage the appetite to return. Dr. Maury recommended a glass of Banyuls or Sauternes to be drunk before meals. (See also Anaemia, page 199.)

Aromatherapeutic Foods for the Digestive System

Herbs	Spices	Fruit	Vegetables	Other
angelica	allspice	apple	artichoke	bran
basil	anise	avocado	(globe)	grains
bay	caraway	banana	aubergine	linseed
borage	cardamom	bilberry	beetroot	milk
chamomile	cinnamon	cherry	carrot	nuts
dill	clove	currant	celery	olive oil
fennel	coriander	fig	courgette	pulses
lavender	cumin	grapefruit	fennel	seaweed
lemon balm	ginger	guava	leek	
lemongrass	horseradish	kiwi	lettuce	
lovage	juniper	lemon	marrow	
marjoram	mace	lime	mushroom	
mint	mustard	melon	onion	
oregano	nutmeg	orange	parsnip	
savory	pepper	papaya	pepper	
tarragon	vanilla	peach	potato	
thyme		pear	pumpkin	
		persimmon		
		pineapple		
		plum		
		pomegranate		
		prune		
		raspberry		

THE SKIN

THE SKIN securely wraps and contains the whole body, and its only "break" is at the teeth and gum margin, where enamel meets flesh. The skin is composed of layers: the outer epidermis with its many tiers of skin cells, and the inner dermis, with its network of tough collagen and elastin fibres, and the small capillaries that bring oxygen and other nutrients to the skin and take away the toxic waste products. Sebaceous glands which produce an oil substance known as sebum are rooted in the dermis, but they open to the surface at pores located in the epidermis.

The skin keeps undesirable toxins out of the body, although it can take in and absorb substances (aromatherapeutic essential oils, for instance); sadly, it can let in less desirable substances, through damage to the epidermis such as a cut or burn. It is also an excretory organ, ridding the body of waste substances such as perspiration and sebum. If something interferes with these functions, the skin may suffer.

The skin is a mirror of body health, and its nature is greatly influenced by what is going on in seemingly unconnected systems. For instance, if the principal excretory systems of the body, the liver and kidneys, are not working adequately, the skin often shows this very clearly, being a sort of dumping ground for toxins released from the body. Faulty digestion can show in the skin, as can stress, and a number of skin disorders are linked to hormones—adolescent acne and premenstrual spots, for instance.

PREVENTING PROBLEMS

Total body health is crucial to skin health, and many people have less than perfect skins because of the battle that their bodies wage continually against the twentieth-century lifestyle, with its bad diet, stress, lack of exercise and any number of pollutants.

The nutrients and fibre of fresh fruit and vegetables are vital, as are proteins, but the latter must not be too rich in saturated fats (pork, lamb, bacon and so on), as these can cause an over-production of sebum and lead to blackheads and acne. A conventional current treatment for acne is a low-fat, meatless diet which also cuts out sugar, salt and stimulants such as tea, coffee and alcohol, all of which are detrimental to the skin. Foods which are too hot or spicy, such as strong curries, can exacerbate certain skin conditions.

Vitamins, particularly A, B, C and E, have a very definite relationship with the skin. A lack of vitamin A, a skin nourisher, leads to excessive dryness; a B2 deficiency can lead to blisters and cracking at the corners of the mouth, and to some forms of dermatitis. A severe lack of vitamin C causes scurvy and gum disease. Vitamin E is often known as *the* skin vitamin, and it can help in treatment of the skin disease psoriasis. Vitamin P—the bioflavonoids rutin and citrin—is particularly good for the health of the veins and capillaries that carry blood to the skin.

Cook with and use in dressings cold pressed oils like soy, corn or safflower, which are rich in essential fatty acids or EFAs (vitamin F). The body and skin do need some internal lubrication from beneficial oils, and the oils in nuts, fish and seeds are unsaturated as well as being rich in other nutrients. Lecithin, a source of protein, phosphorus, choline and inositol, is good for the skin; it is naturally found in eggs and soya beans. Magnesium-rich nuts and dates should be nibbled instead of sweets, especially by the young who are particularly vulnerable to skin infections. The calcium of dairy products is valuable, but you must be careful: many cheeses, for instance, can be indigestible, so could contribute to skin problems.

TREATING PROBLEMS

Apart from a nutritionally adequate diet, one of the major things you can do to help your skin is drink a lot. Mineral waters, diluted fruit juices and appropriate herbal tisanes all flush out the system. Some blood-cleansing and detoxifying foods include garlic, onion, borage, lovage, pears, citrus fruit, celeriac, cucumber and tomatoes.

Skin Damage and Infections

Vitamin C foods, particularly citrus fruit, help heal damage to the skin, so if you have a burn or a cut eat them raw and drink their juices. If the skin is cut, blood will produce clotting factors to seal the wound quite quickly, but the main worry is infection. The chlorophyll in green plants is a natural antiseptic and encourages regeneration, so apply raw crushed herbs like dandelion, hyssop, parsley, marjoram, rosemary and thyme just as you would a dock leaf to a nettle sting. Lemon juice is antiseptic as well (although it could sting), as is celery juice.

If you burn the skin, whether on direct heat or in the sun, it's less a case of eating than of *applying* what you might eat. Puréed raw potatoes, carrots or celery—or their juices—applied to the area will be cooling and healing. A calendula or lavender decoction can soothe as well, as can slices of melon, and some natural yogurt.

When the skin's ability to act as a waste disposal unit is disturbed, infections such as abscesses and boils can occur around the sebaceous glands or hair follicles. These and the crusty spots of impetigo (usually in children, on the face, neck and scalp), are caused by an invasion of bacteria such as staphylococci or streptococci. Abscesses and boils tend to appear when the sufferer is run down, but can be symptomatic of hormonal upheaval (as can acne), or certain blood disorders and diabetes; impetigo is usually due to direct infection, such as a child rubbing dirty hands over his or her face. All these infections respond well to antibiotics, but kitchen aromatherapy can help as well.

Flush the system out for at least a day by fasting and drinking only mineral water. Eat lots of raw fruits and vegetables, and only gradually return to a normal healthy diet. Cook with lots of antibacterial fruit, vegetables and herbs.

Cold sores are caused by a viral rather than bacterial infection, that of herpes. Drinking infusions of thyme, savory, borage or chamomile could help. Take multi-mineral supplements and a homeopathic remedy such as oligo elements. Some people believe that taking lysine, the essential amino acid missing from so many plant protein foods, is good for the skin, and therefore can help prevent and shorten attacks of the virus.

Skin Disease

Acne is the classic skin disease, caused by the over-production of oil in the sebaceous glands, and is generally due to hormonal imbalance. The inflammations and spots can become infected by bacteria and turn into boils and cysts. Good diet is paramount (see above), as are cleanliness and hygiene. French doctors use dates to cure young patients of acne.

Both dermatitis and eczema are characterized by inflammation, swelling and itchy rashes, which may lead to blisters and weeping scabs. Many forms of the diseases are associated with inherited allergic tendencies—to dairy products or gluten, say—and some are the contact form, when the sufferer's skin reacts to a "new" substance such as a washing-up liquid or antiperspirant. Both can be exacerbated by stress.

Eat foods that are rich in vitamins and in minerals such as sulphur: artichoke, lettuce, cucumber, celeriac, radishes, onion, garlic, watercress and nuts. Make soups with lots of leeks, potatoes, onions and carrots in them; these are all good blood cleansers, as is asparagus. Light cream cheeses such as fromage frais and Petit Suisse, and yogurt, can be helpful, as can fruit such as grapes, lemons, grapefruit and pineapple.

The specific cause of the skin disease psoriasis is not

known, but it can be inherited. Patches of flaky skin can become so dry that they crack and become infected (see previous page). Diet is perhaps the best approach: eat foods rich in vitamins A, B and E, and lecithin and wheatgerm. Supplements of vitamin E, cod liver oil and oil of evening primrose are good too.

Skin Condition

If you bruise easily—some women do during menstruation, and so do obese and anaemic people—try to eat more vitamin C- and P-rich foods, for these will strengthen the blood vessels. This is also sound advice for people who have broken veins and capillaries, giving that ruddiness in the cheeks so characteristic of Anglo-Saxon skins (see page 202).

An older skin needs a supremely healthy diet, which will help ageing cells work as efficiently as they can. Stimulants such as alcohol, tea and coffee are diuretic and drying, as are cigarette smoking and lying in the sun. Drink lots of mineral water and herbal tisanes. A lettuce tisane can help prevent wrinkles, and thyme should be used in cooking because of its claimed antioxidant effect.

Aromatherapeutic Foods for the Skin

Herbs	Fruit	Vegetables	Other
bay	apple	artichoke	buckwheat
borage	apricot	asparagus	cider
chamomile	avocado	carrot	vinegar
chervil	bilberry	celeriac	cod liver
hyssop	date	celery	oil
lavender	fig	cucumber	dairy foods
lovage	grape	garlic	evening
marjoram	grapefruit	leek	primrose
mint	guava	lettuce	oil
nasturtium	lemon	onion	fish
oregano	lime	pepper, red	lecithin

Aromatherapeutic Foods for the Skin (cont.)

Herbs	Fruit	Vegetables	Other
parsley	mango	potato	linseed
rosemary	melon	pumpkin	nuts
savory	orange	radish	oats
thyme	papaya	spinach	offal
	pear	tomato	oils (corn
	pineapple	watercress	safflower,
			soya)
			pulses
			seeds
			sprouted
			seeds,
			grains,
			pulses
			wheatgerm
			yogurt

THE MOUTH

THE MOUTH could be said to be one of the hardest-working parts of the body, as it is almost constantly in use. It is through the mouth that most substances are introduced into the body, and we use it to eat, chew, talk, drink, kiss and sometimes to breathe. The sense of taste is situated in the mouth, and the saliva which constantly washes its interior marks the beginnings of digestion. The mouth contains the hardest substance in the body—the teeth—but this meeting of enamel and skin is the only break of skin in the entire body, so it is perhaps no surprise that the mouth can be the source of many health problems.

PREVENTING PROBLEMS

Although the main cause of mouth problems is poor hygiene, diet and the health of the mouth are intimately related. In the 1930s an American dentist, Dr. Weston Price, studied various groups of isolated peoples—Eskimos, Australian Aborigines, Polynesians, and people living in remote Swiss and Peruvian valleys—all of whom ate a natural, "whole" diet appropriate to their environment. Although there were obviously racial diversifications, Dr. Price found consistently good jaw structures and healthy teeth. But when he returned a generation later, after Western "civilisation" and its diet (rich in refined sugar, flour and so on) had been introduced, he found degeneration both in the individuals he had studied before and in the children who had been born in the intervening years. There was tooth decay, malformation of jaw structure and overcrowded teeth (which leads to decay). In his book *Nutrition and Physical Degeneration* he attributed this change entirely to the change in diet.

Chewing

This is one of the most important functions of the mouth, and we have largely forgotten how to do it. A lot of modern food does not need chewing, and so our jawbones, teeth and gums are not being "exercised" as they should be. Chewing initiates the flow of saliva, and if foods are not mingled with enough saliva to ease their passage to the digestive organs problems can ensue.

Foods that need to be chewed—raw or lightly cooked vegetables or raw hard fruits—are essential for a healthy mouth. This will help to keep the teeth and gums clear of the bacteria which are the cause of plaque and tartar, and thus of tooth decay, dental abscesses and gum disease. (It is carbohydrates or sugars which these bacteria live on, so sugary foods of all kinds should be avoided.) The essential oils contained in many foods are also disinfectant and antibacterial. The carrot is a typical example; eaten raw and not too finely chopped or grated, its crispness "abrades" the teeth and gums, while its nutritive properties benefit the mouth directly and the body as a whole (it contains vitamins A and C, both vital to body and mouth health).

Chewing properly not only improves the health of your teeth and gums, but can also improve the circulation in your face. When people lose their teeth their faces lose shape and "fall in": if chewing properly helps to prevent that tooth loss, and at the same time exercises the face, then chewing each mouthful a few more times is worthwhile. A lot of people also show tension in the mouth through stress or anxiety, through being in pain, or premenstrually, and these tensions could be relaxed by chewing slowly and deliberately. (I have also seen tension lines around the mouths of those who, for some reason or another, are eating only with their front teeth—usually because they have trouble with their back teeth.)

Chewing slowly and properly is also a very pleasurable occupation. As you chew, the aromatic particles in foods are released and you are given pleasure through your senses of taste and smell. It is also relaxing; a form of "yoga", called *hesychia*, concerning how to relax when you eat, was developed in France in the fourteenth century by a Benedictine monk.

Try *hesychia* for yourself by tasting and chewing some of the following foods, all of which contain strong essential oils.

- Fennel, fennel seeds, anise seeds
- Apples, pears, grapes, peaches
- Raw carrot, parsnip, radishes
- Almonds, hazelnuts, walnuts

Finally, chewing properly can stop you putting on weight. Taking time to chew well will make you eat less anyway. Thorough mastication will ensure that the food is better digested, absorbed and eliminated, all of which will counter weight gain.

Vitamins and the Mouth

Vitamins A and C are very important for mouth health, because a lack of either can affect the collagen or connective tissue, which includes the gums, as well as the enamel of the teeth. The classic C deficiency disease is scurvy, which manifests itself in bleeding gums, and which was the scourge of sailors on long sea voyages until the discovery of the benefits of lemons or limes. The best sources of C are fruit, especially berries and citrus fruit, and raw green vegetables—it is water-soluble, and so can be lost in cooking water. Betacarotene, which becomes vitamin A in the body, is found in green, yellow and orange vegetables and fruit; vitamin A as retinol is obtained from animal and fish liver oils and dairy food, and is not lost in cooking.

TREATING PROBLEMS

If mouth problems *do* occur, many foods can be helpful.

Toothache

While waiting to see the dentist when you are in pain, you could suck a clove, or a piece of cinnamon or cassia, holding it over the site of the pain, for its antibacterial and anaesthetic effect; peppercorns could help too. A clove of garlic would be as valuable in the antibacterial sense, but perhaps not quite so popular with your friends and the dentist! An old folk remedy is to slowly drink the juice of a turnip or onion, both natural analgesics.

Gum Disease

Gum problems can occur at times of hormonal upheaval such as puberty, pregnancy, before a period and at the menopause, as well as being disease-based. Take foods that are decongestant, such as carrots, parsnips and leeks, either eating them raw or extracting and drinking their juice. Sage is also useful.

Raw spinach is very effective for the teeth and gums, particularly the bleeding gums that herald full-scale gum disease, pyorrhoea. This and a degeneration of the pulp of the teeth have become common problems due to habitual use of refined cereals, sugars and other deficient foods. Other aromatic food plants for the gums include apple, bilberry, redcurrants, fig, horseradish, marjoram, oregano, mint, almond and olive oils, raspberry leaves and ginger.

Mouth Ulcers

A mouth ulcer reacts to many foods, so avoid acidic things such as fresh fruit (although some lemon juice applied directly to it could cure it), salt, pepper, vinegar, alcohol and tobacco. Eat foods that are alkaline and soothing—a leek and/or potato soup made with milk, or milky puddings such as crème caramel or rice pudding. (Sweeten dishes with honey or maple syrup.) Make purées of vegetables with milk and eat eggs, meat and fish, as well as seaweeds like wakame. Figs, celery and watercress are good foods, and you could make decoctions of mint and savory to heal and soothe. Sage is good here, too.

Bad Breath

This is often due to digestive problems, but could also be caused by conditions in the mouth. Chew fresh parsley, or coriander, cardamom, dill, fennel or cumin seeds, which contain cleansing and freshening essential oils. Many of the seeds are digestive in action as well, so you could be benefiting in two ways simultaneously. A sucked clove or piece of cinnamon or cassia is breath-sweetening as well.

To Whiten Teeth

Sage leaves were one herbal remedy used in ancient times to keep the teeth white, but I think we could widen that and use a number of plants for their natural chlorophyll content—parsley, chervil, basil, fresh spinach and other green vegetables, all eaten raw—as well as citrus fruit.

The Mouth in General

Liquorice is good for the mouth. Chew a small piece of the root, or, less valuably, eat it in sweet form.

Alcohol is good for the mouth! As well as helping digestion by breaking down proteins, it helps to clean the mouth and acts as a natural bactericide and antiseptic, killing unwanted bacteria. One measure—of brandy, whisky, vodka, red wine, white wine or champagne, drunk in a relaxed way—will do the trick!

Aromatherapeutic Foods for the Mouth

Herbs	Spices	Fruit	Vegetables	Other
basil	cardamom	apple	carrot	dairy
chervil	cinnamon/	bilberry	celery	products
fennel	cassia	currant	fennel	fish
marjoram	clove	fig	garlic	liquorice
mint	coriander	grapefruit	greens	meat
oregano	cumin	guava	leek	nuts
parsley	dill	lemon	onion	oils
sage	ginger	lime	parsnip	(almond,
savory	horseradish	orange	potato	olive)
	peppercorns	raspberry	spinach	seaweed
			turnip	
			watercress	

THE EYES

ONE OF the five main sensory organs and part of the nervous system, the eyes are very sensitive. If you are experiencing unusual symptoms—pain in the eyes, or blurred vision—you should see your doctor, as eye problems can occasionally be symptoms of something more serious.

The commonest eye problems are conjunctivitis (an inflammation caused by virus, bacteria, allergy or a foreign body), redness or irritation (caused by conditions such as hay fever or simple tiredness).

PREVENTING PROBLEMS

Vitamin A is the most significant nutrient for the health of the eyes, as it forms part of the chemical structure of their light-sensitive areas. A deficiency of this vitamin can cause a disease called xerophthalmia, which affects people who are severely malnourished or who suffer from digestive complaints such as coeliac disease. A deficiency can also cause a form of night blindness, as a result of which British pilots were issued with carrots to eat during the Second World War. We should eat lots of raw carrots, preferably old ones, which are rich in betacarotene (the precursor of vitamin A in the body). Other betacarotene-rich foods are dark green vegetables such as spinach, curly kale, spring greens, mustard and cress, watercress and parsley, and orange and yellow vegetables such as pumpkin, sweet potatoes, tomatoes and red peppers. Yellow and orange fruit are useful, too:

dried and fresh apricots are rich in A, as are mangoes, papaya, cantaloupe melons, quinces and guavas.

Foods with plenty of vitamin A as retinol are animal sources such as cod liver oil, liver (fried calf's liver contains 39,780 mg of retinol per 100 g/4 oz), Cheddar cheese and eggs. Milk has some vitamin A, particularly in the summer, as does cream. Human milk contains more A than cow's or sheep's, one of the reasons why babies benefit from being breast-fed.

TREATING PROBLEMS

Some herbal infusions can calm irritated, red or tired eyes: use chervil, lovage, fennel seeds, lettuce, chamomile or walnut leaves.

Just looking at the colour orange seems to be able to calm tired eyes and strengthen them. Sit and look at a bed of marigolds, for instance. And infusions of marigolds or calendula (of the same family), as well as dandelion flowers, can help the eyes in the same way.

Parsley juice can be used on a compress for the eyes, as can grated potato or apple. The minerals within the fruits or vegetables help disperse toxins and swellings. Slices of cucumber, potato or apple can be used as "compresses" as well.

Aromatherapeutic Foods for the Eyes

Herbs	Fruit	Vegetables	Other
parsley	apple	carrot	cod liver
	apricot	cucumber	oil
	(dried)	fennel	dairy
	guava	greens	products
	mango	lettuce	offal
	melon	pepper, red	
	papaya	potato	
	quince	pumpkin	
		tomato	

Aromatherapeutic Foods for the Eyes (*cont.*)

Herbs	Fruit	Vegetables	Other
		watercress	
		spinach	

THE HAIR AND SCALP

THE HAIR on our heads grows out of the scalp, which is a continuation of the skin, one of the five principal sensory organs. The scalp is therefore subject to some of the problems that beset the skin in general. It is sometimes surprising that it is not affected more severely, considering what we do to our hair and scalp—washing frequently with strong shampoos, curling, drying, colouring, brushing, perming and so on.

The hair itself grows out of over one hundred thousand hair follicles in the scalp. When it is developing within the follicles it is living material, so a good diet and a plentiful supply of nutrients are essential. After the hair comes through the scalp it is dead, but its condition still depends on nutrition because, although hairs are constantly being lost, they are also constantly being replaced. The condition of this dead hair is now largely dependent on how it is treated, and many problems come about through misuse of hair products.

A few hair problems are caused by ill health, and loss of hair or loss of colour or condition can all occur after severe illness, after a shock, or after a period of poor nutrition. They can also occur at times of hormonal upheaval, so menopausal women may experience hair thinning and loss; adolescents can suffer from overactive sebaceous glands in the skin (on the scalp these lie alongside the hair follicles) which results in spots, acne, greasy hair and/or dandruff.

PREVENTING PROBLEMS

First, the hair must be treated considerately, without too many chemical treatments such as colouring or perming. Eat a diet rich in nutrients for the hair, the skin, capillaries and circulatory system in general. Protein, particularly fish, is very valuable. Vitamins A, B, C and E, especially the last, are vital. E is available in wheatgerm, vegetable oils (and the vegetables, fruit, grains and seeds they come from), nuts and seeds (primarily almonds, hazelnuts and sunflower seeds), in dark green vegetables, cod liver oil and lobster, liver and heart, and some fruit, most significantly the avocado.

B is useful too, particularly pantothenate or pantothenic acid, which is needed for the adrenal glands (and thus for many stress situations, which can cause a number of hair problems). This is found in liver, kidneys, heart, salmon, peanuts, sesame seeds, raw mushrooms, bran, wheatgerm, cheese (Danish blue is a good source), and also in some other meats, fish, vegetables and fruit.

The diet should be similarly rich in minerals and micronutrients, chiefly calcium, iron, magnesium, cobalt, copper, iodine and zinc. Citrus fruit are good for general scalp and hair health.

TREATING PROBLEMS

A number of foods, either ingested or applied in some form, can be very helpful for hair problems.

Alopecia or Loss of Hair
Alopecia is the term for total or partial baldness. Male pattern baldness is a form of alopecia; in women hair loss can be age-related as well. Alopecia can be caused by stress or, more commonly in women, by maltreatment of the hair.

Massage of the scalp can help stimulate and restore follicle function. Do so with decoctions of nettle, watercress or nasturtium, or use some cider vinegar, which can help with scalp eczema as well. Therapeutic oils to rub into the scalp can be made with rocket or peppercorns.

DANDRUFF

Dandruff is probably the commonest hair problem: the white scales are dead skin shed by the scalp. This is the result of overactive sebaceous glands, and the condition is associated with stress, hormonal imbalance, poor diet and maltreatment of the hair.

Avoid eating fatty, oily foods, although some foods which contain oil are good (olives, olive oil, nuts and avocados). Massage a dry scalp with coconut oil, and eat fresh coconut. Make strong teas of fresh or dried thyme or rosemary, and rub into the scalp between shampoos. Add the juice of a lemon to the teas, as lemon is very astringent and helps clean the scalp.

Aromatherapeutic Foods for the Hair and Scalp

Spices	Fruit	Vegetables	Other
peppercorns	avocado	greens	bran
	grapefruit	mushroom	cider vinegar
	lemon	nasturtium	cod liver oil
	lime	nettle	
	olive	rocket	dairy products
	orange	watercress	fish (oily)
			nuts
			offal
			oils (vegetable)
			seeds
			shellfish
			wheatgerm

APPENDIX I
THE BENEFITS OF WINE

IT MAY seem curious, indeed shocking to some, but in most French families even very young children drink wine. From as early as three or four years of age they eat at the table with their family and friends, and share both food and wine. The wine—diluted considerably with water, of course—is known as a *coupe d'eau*, and the French do not look upon this as unusual in any way.

Wine in France is part of the heritage, part of daily life, and from a very early age my brothers and I were initiated by our father, who was a connoisseur. On birthdays and special occasions such as Bastille Day, 14 July, he would introduce us to a specially chosen wine, teaching us about its origins, its nose, its subtlety and its body, and asking us for our untutored opinions. It was an introduction which none of us ever regretted, and we have been grateful ever since. Even later, at school, the canteen tables displayed bottles of wine as well as carafes of water: my boarding school in Normandy—the home of the cider and Calvados apple—offered strong cider!

The French believe that, far from turning children into alcoholics, wine is something that should be learned about and appreciated from the very beginning. This is not just so that the correct wines can be chosen to accompany the food, but also because wine is looked upon as a medicine. To start with, wine drunk during a meal helps the digestion, but French doctors believe it can do even more. One of these,

Dr. E. Maury, the husband of my mentor, Marguerite Maury, even wrote a book about choosing the best wines for health—it was a national bestseller!

This aspect of wine consumption was also known to me from an early age. I remember accompanying my father to visit my grandmother in hospital after she had had an operation. My father brought her some bottles of champagne to lift her spirits, and the nurses expressed not the least surprise as this was common practise. They even complimented my father on his choice, saying that the patient would be easier to cope with and that it would speed her recovery. When I suffered from period pains I was always given a glass of Banyuls, a sweet wine, to soothe and calm me. It worked. And if any of us children were thought to be a little anaemic—we were from a family of doctors—we were given a glass of red Burgundy for its mineral, especially iron, content.

So, long before many modern drugs such as antibiotics, tranquillisers, sleeping pills, antidepressants, painkillers and appetite suppressants came into being, wines were being prescribed by French doctors to their patients. This, it must be admitted, is a very much more pleasurable (and healthy) way of taking "medicine". The important point is that the wine should not be drunk in large quantities—no more than two glasses per meal for adults—but if the right wine is chosen it can help you digest your meal and relax after a hard day, and boost the vitamin and mineral content of your diet. Where the British sometimes go wrong is in drinking wine as an aperitif: without food, wine can have harmful effects, especially if you drink too much of it. But a good wine drunk with good food should have nothing but beneficial effects.

So, far from discouraging wine drinking, I can happily and confidently recommend a glass or two with your meal, for when you are feeling low, or if you are suffering from some minor ill.

- If you are anaemic or too pale, or are a vegetarian, I recommend the wines of Burgundy which are rich in iron and other minerals.
- If you have a weight problem, a dry white wine from Alsace (a Sylvaner, particularly) will act as a diuretic.
- If you are convalescing or suffering from fatigue, drink some champagne, some old Burgundy, or some Muscat.
- If you are suffering from nervous depression or merely a bit low, red Bordeaux wines, a Médoc or a Côte de Roussillon will help.
- For those undergoing the menopause, red Burgundies and St. Emilion wines are good.
- Banyuls and Monbazillac wines will help overcome the pains and traumas of PMT.
- To keep the circulatory system, especially the heart, in good order, many French doctors, phytotherapists recommend modest amounts of red wine.
- And, finally, if you want a stimulant, tonic or aphrodisiac wine, drink champagne, Chablis or white Bordeaux. *Salud!*

APPENDIX II
AROMATHERAPEUTIC MENUS

I HOPE that you have enjoyed reading this book and cooking some of the recipes in it. Here, in a selection of menus for specific occasions or ailments, I have put together ideas rather than specifics, but the principles of aromatherapeutic eating are there for you to see, appreciate and enjoy.

MENU 1: FOR THE KIDNEYS AND URINARY SYSTEM

If you have any sort of kidney or urinary problem you need aromatics that are stimulant, diuretic and cleansing, and which possess properties specific to this area. Vegetarian foods are very helpful.

Vegetable soup
=====

Braised celery and fennel
with
rice
=====

Strawberries in white wine

For the soup, gently fry some chopped onion, a few crushed juniper berries, some chopped fennel, sliced celery, asparagus tips and some parsley in a little olive oil until softened, then liquidise and add a dash of soya milk. All the vegetables are diuretic and good for kidney problems.

For the main course, braise celery and fennel in chunks

with some olive oil until tender. Sprinkle with finely chopped walnuts, parsley and a little extra virgin olive oil, and serve with whole rice. Celery and fennel fortify and protect against infections, as do walnuts.

Macerate some hulled raw strawberries in enough white wine to cover them for about 30 minutes. Drizzle a little honey on top to serve. To drink, try celery juice with lemon or lime juice or tomato juice.

MENU 2: APHRODISIAC

Before making love, you don't want to eat or drink too much. You need wonderful exhilarating foods, and aromatics that will enhance them and your own appetites. A little old-fashioned romance won't go amiss either: try dimmed lights, red candles, moody music and a sweet perfume—a few drops of ylang ylang, the essential oil of flowers of a tropical perfume tree, is very aphrodisiac.

Oysters with lemon and ginger
or
Ginseng soup with miso (see page 78)

A little red meat or pheasant
or other game bird
cooked with savory
or
Chicken cooked with
ginseng, angelica and cardamom
with
Braised celery hearts with
white soy flour sauce
spiked with a little Roquefort cheese

Millet, rye and wheat pancakes,
filled with rose jam (gul), walnuts or stem ginger
and black sesame seeds

Shellfish, particularly oysters, are always sexy, and the ginger will enhance their flavour and digestibility. You could put the oysters briefly under a hot grill, along with the aromatics. The soup hardly needs explanation, as ginseng has such a gentle and undeniable effect on libido.

A little red meat—beef steak or lamb cutlets—would be tasty, especially if grilled with peppercorns and savory. Savory would also bring its active aromatic constituents to bear on the assimilation of a briefly cooked game bird—pheasant or grouse, for instance. The chicken will be beautifully flavoured by the ginseng and angelica; cardamom is considered aphrodisiac in India, where it is widely used in poultry cooking.

The Turks swear by their rose jam, *gul,* as a sexual stimulant. Buy it in Turkish or Cypriot shops. Mix it with walnuts or ginger for vitality, and sprinkle with black sesame seeds, which are good for the reproductive system in general because of their calcium.

A Cloudy Bay sparkling wine from New Zealand is full of minerals and makes a wonderful aperitif. Dr. Maury recommended Médoc, Pouilly Fuissé or Champagne Brut. Also try the ginseng wine on page 77.

MENU 3: SEDATIVE

Instead of taking a tranquilliser or sleeping pill, you can eat yourself to sleep. You obviously won't want to eat too much, but you need foods that are rich in tranquillising bromine, as well as the famous lettuce and mandarin oranges. Try to eat earlier rather than later, and don't drink alcohol because it is too stimulant.

Lettuce hearts with basil and sesame seeds
or
Steamed asparagus

Monkfish (or chicken)
with
leeks and mandarin oranges

=====

Apple mousse
or
Compote of rhubarb

Cook the lettuce hearts very lightly in a little water, then add the shredded basil and the sesame seeds to serve in order to get the full calming benefit of all of the ingredients. Asparagus is good for the nervous system.

You need a little protein; this quantity would serve two people. Cut 300 g (10 oz) monkfish (or skinned chicken breast) into small cubes, brush with a little olive oil and grill, turning until done. Keep warm. Wash a couple of leeks, slice thinly, then cook in a very little water for a few minutes just to soften. Add a crushed garlic clove, the washed and grated skin of 2 large mandarin oranges, a chopped anchovy and 1 tablespoon chopped parsley. Cook for 10 minutes, stirring continually, then put on warmed plates and place the monkfish (or chicken) on top. Squeeze the mandarin orange juice over the fish (or chicken), and sprinkle with freshly ground black pepper.

Cook some washed apples, skin, core and all, until they "fall" (Bramleys do this well), then sieve. You want about 4 cups full (use a 150 ml/5 fl oz cup). Mix in 1 tablespoon blackcurrant, redcurrant or apple jelly, then fold in the very stiffly beaten white of a medium egg. Spoon into ramekins, and sprinkle with ground cinnamon and coarsely chopped hazelnuts. Apples are one of the richest sources of bromine. Rhubarb is another; simply stew in a little water or apple juice, adding honey to taste.

To drink, make a decoction of cereals. Boil 20 g (3/4 oz) each of barley, rye and oats in 1 litre (1 3/4 pints) water for 5–20 minutes. Leave to sit for 10 minutes, then strain. Mix the liquid with some apple juice and honey. It is very rich in minerals and vitamins.

MENU 4: ENERGISING

To energise yourself and others—perhaps a lunch before a

busy afternoon—you need foods that have a high content of glucose sugars and hydrocarbons, rich in solar energy. The chlorophyll of green leaves is the prime source, closely followed by fruit and then cereals. You also need all the vitamins, especially C.

Red pepper terrine
with
a green leaf salad

A little protein
(fish, meat, chicken or eggs, all optional)
with
whole rice, wild rice, soya beans
and fresh tomato sauce

Cantaloupe or Ogen melon
with
fresh orange juice

Red peppers are rich in vitamin C. Put 4 large peppers on a baking tray in the oven, preheated to 180°C/350°F/Gas 4, for about 30 minutes. Then remove and put in a sealed container such as a saucepan with a lid. Leave for about 10 minutes, then skin the peppers, seed them and cut into long strips. Layer in a terrine dish with olive oil, garlic to taste, and the herbs of your choice—I would use thyme or savory—until the dish is full. Refrigerate for about an hour before serving with rye bread and a salad of rocket, watercress, dandelion and raw spinach, plus a few bacon lardons and some garlic croûtons, perhaps.

You don't need to eat any protein, as the rice and beans by themselves are energising enough. Cook the well-soaked beans with some thyme and rosemary. Make a fresh tomato sauce, cooking flavourful tomatoes minimally with some chopped onion and garlic, or simply use the tomato dice "recipe" on page 186. Tomatoes too are very energising.

For their vitamin C content, serve a half melon, with a little redcurrant or raspberry jelly in the cavity that contained the seeds, with some fresh orange juice squeezed over. Many medical experts say that fruit is best eaten an hour after a meal, or even before the meal.

To drink I suggest orange juice, perhaps diluted with mineral water.

MENU 5: FOR THE LIVER

If you have liver problems you need decongestive foods, foods that are low in fat, and aromatics that dynamise bile secretion and ease digestion. You should avoid alcohol.

Carrot (or celery) soup
with
fresh rosemary

=========

Artichoke hearts with tapenade (see pages 123–124)
and herbs
with
Stir-fried soya beansprouts
and a watercress, rocket and dandelion salad

=========

Raspberries and strawberries
stewed in their own juice

First cook the artichoke hearts, keeping the water. Juice the carrots or celery and mix them with the artichoke water. Simmer together briefly with the rosemary. All are stimulant and benefit the liver.

Spread the artichoke hearts—whose cynarine content is very good for the liver—with some tapenade or black olive pâté, and sprinkle with lots of parsley and/or chervil. Stir-fry the soya sprouts in some olive oil (with a little rosemary if liked). Then, if in season, add a few thyme or rosemary flowers to the salad leaves.

Cook the berries very briefly in their own juices. Add a little apple juice if they are not very juicy. Both are good for hepatic imbalances. Drink chamomile tea or a hot lemon drink, decorated with a few mint leaves.

MENU 6: FOR THE SKIN

The skin needs cleansing and remineralising aromatics, together with a wealth of foods rich in vitamins A, C and E, as well as calcium and magnesium

Cucumber and tomato salad with
onion, parsley and almonds
or
Shredded cabbage salad
or
Pumpkin and red pepper soup (see page 142)

Fish pâté with rye bread
and a green salad
or
Chicken stir-fried with thyme
with
Pumpkin and carrot purée with cardamom

Bilberry sorbet
or
Apple or dried apricot compote

Cucumber and tomato together are detoxifying, and the chopped nuts sprinkled on top at the end are rich in magnesium. The cabbage is high in vitamin C; the soup ingredients are rich in A. Add a little fresh coriander to the soup, and perhaps a little cream which, in moderation, is good for the skin.

For the fish pâté, drain a tin of sardines and purée them in a food processor along with a little whisky, a few spring onions, a little wheatgerm oil and lots of fresh parsley. Serve on rye and sunflower seed bread, or brown toast, accompanied by a salad of aromatic green leaves—lettuce and nasturtium, for instance. The fish pâté is rich in calcium because of the little bones in the fish.

Stir-fry chicken breast, cut into small pieces, in a little sesame oil with some thyme leaves (these are antiseptic for the skin, and antioxidant). The vegetable purée is packed with vitamin A.

Bilberries are wonderful for the health of the skin, full of vitamin C and energising. Follow the sorbet instructions on page 146. Or cook chunks of apple or presoaked dried apricots in some fruit juice with added aromatics—a few bruised cardamom pods, say, or a cinnamon stick. Remove the spices before serving.

Drink celery and cucumber juice with a dash of fresh orange juice.

MENU 7: FOR THE LUNGS AND RESPIRATORY SYSTEM

The major requirement with most respiratory problems is opening up the chest and freeing the system of mucus. You also need foods that are rich in vitamin C, to counter the infections. Start the meal with a little whisky; I find this goes straight to where it is needed, helping me to breathe better. Or you could make an aromatic whisky: macerate pieces of quince or pomegranate in the whisky, along with some vanilla pod, cinnamon stick or a few cloves, and some crushed juniper berries.

Grated celeriac
with red cabbage and radishes
or
Sage and garlic soup (see page 75)
with seaweed

Baked white fish
with turnip and potato purée
or
A little red meat or smoked fish
with horseradish
with
Watercress and sorrel salad

Quince compote
or

Guava and apple compote
or
Pineapple sorbet (see page 146)

Celeriac, like celery, is good for the throat, the shredded cabbage is rich in vitamin C, and radishes—a few pink ones—make a pretty and therapeutic garnish. The sage and garlic soup is wonderful for colds and many respiratory infections, as is any seaweed.

Bake some white fish such as halibut or cod briefly in the oven, covered with some grated Gruyère cheese. Cook the puréed vegetables, which are very decongestant, with a couple of bay leaves. You could have a little cold roast beef or a small steak with the horseradish, or some smoked fish such as mackerel. Horseradish is very strongly expectorant.

Quinces are rich in vitamin C, as are guavas and apples. Peel the fruit and cook very gently with a very little water. Serve with some honey if you like. The pineapple sorbet is especially easy to eat if you have a sore throat.

Drink a mineral water flavoured and coloured with a little Cassis, the blackcurrant liqueur from France.

GLOSSARY

Acidulate To make acid. Acidulated water is water acidulated with an acid such as vinegar or lemon juice. This prevents oxidation—or browning—of fruit like apples.

Amino acids Organic molecules which form the building blocks of protein. Of the twenty amino acids in proteins, eight are nutritionally essential.

Antibacterial Ability to destroy bacteria.

Antioxidant A substance which prevents rancidity in food or, in the body, which prevents cell damage. Vitamins A, C and E are antioxidant in action, as is the trace mineral selenium.

Antirheumatic Preventing inflammation and aching of the joints.

Antiscorbutic Preventing scurvy.

Antiviral Preventing the passage and acceptance of a virus into the body.

Aperitive Awakening appetite.

Balsamic Soothing, restorative.

Betacarotene see **Vitamin A**

Bioflavonoids Nutrients known also as vitamin P. They are thought to be as effective in vitamin C deficiency diseases as vitamin C itself, and help in the action of vitamin C. Most fruit are rich in bioflavonoids such as citrin and rutin, especially citrus, and they are also found in green peppers, buckwheat, tea and red wine. They are vital in preserving health and strength of capillaries.

Biotin A water-soluble B vitamin, also known as vitamin H. It is essential for growth and maintenance of healthy nervous tissue. Food sources include offal (particularly liver), brewers' yeast, eggs, fish, meat and whole cereal grains.

Calcium This is an essential mineral required for bones and teeth, and for proper nerve and muscle function. Vitamin D is needed to help in its absorption. Deficiency can lead to rickets in children, osteomalacia and osteoporosis in adults. Food sources include dairy products, eggs, tinned sardines and watercress.

Carminative Having the property of expelling wind.

Cholesterol This is a fatty substance manufactured in the human body and carried in the bloodstream. Too high an intake of cholesterol in the diet (in egg yolks, meat and so on) can lead to a deposition of cholesterol, a "furring up", on the walls of arteries. This can cause heart disease. There are different types of cholesterol: HDL (high density lipoproteins) is "good" as it is cholesterol taken *from* the tissue to be excreted; LDL (low density lipoproteins) is "bad" as it is cholesterol being taken *to* the tissues and deposited. Cholesterol and other fats are processed by the liver.

Choline This is a B complex factor, associated with the B vitamins in food. It is manufactured in the body, so it is not a vitamin for man. It prevents a build up of fat in the liver.

Chologogic Benefiting the liver.

Citrin see **Bioflavonoids**

Cobalamine A water-soluble B vitamin, also known as vitamin B12. It contains the mineral cobalt. It is essential for a healthy nervous system, for nerve sheaths, and for the formation of red blood cells. Deficiency can cause a form of anaemia. As B12 is not found in plants, deficiency is a risk factor for vegans who eat no food of animal origin at all, and may have to take B12 supplements. Food sources include offal, fish, most dairy products and eggs.

Cobalt see **Cobalamine**

Copper An essential mineral, required for red blood cell formation. Food sources include oysters, liver, parsley, walnuts, peanuts, and a variety of other common foods.

Demineralisation Loss of vital nutrients (as after illness).

Diaphoretic Having the property of promoting perspiration.

Diuretic Increasing the flow of urine.

Emmenogogic Having the power to promote the menstrual discharge.

Emollient Having the power to soften and smoothe.

Endocrine glands Glands that produce secretions or hormones that pass directly into the bloodstream (ie insulin from the pancreas).

Expectorant That which clears the chest and lungs.

Fatty acids, essential (EFAs) Fatty acids vital for the body, and which cannot be manufactured in the body. Vegetable oils like linseed and safflower seed oil are rich in EFAs.

Fatty acids, monounsaturated Fats which, in chemical terms, contain one unsaturated or double bond. Olive oil is one such, and it is healthier in the diet than saturated fat. It can lower "bad" cholesterol levels, raise "good" cholesterol levels.

Fatty acids, polyunsaturated Fats which, in chemical terms, contain two or more unsaturated or double bonds. Plant oils (those from seeds, for instance) have high proportions of polyunsaturates—which *lower* blood cholesterol levels—although fish oils too are high.

Fatty acids, saturated Fats of animal origin which, in chemical terms, contain no unsaturated bonds. High intakes of dairy products and meat raise blood cholesterol levels.

Folic acid A water-soluble B vitamin which works with B12 in the division of cells, and in the growth and maintenance of healthy nervous and digestive systems. Deficiency can cause a form of anaemia. If deficiency occurs at conception and within the first few weeks of pregnancy, babies can be born with neural tube defect or spina bifida. All women planning pregnancy should eat foods rich in folic acid and take supplements preconceptually. Food sources include brewers' yeast, yeast extract, wheatgerm, offal, dark green vegetables, nuts and wholemeal bread.

Gluten Proteins which are present in wheat and, to a much lesser extent, in rye, oats and barley.

Hepatic Relating to the liver.

Inositol This is a B complex factor, associated with the B vitamins in food. It can be manufactured in the body, so it is not a vitamin for humans. It prevents the accumulation of fat in the liver.

Iodine An essential trace mineral, required for the normal functioning of the thyroid gland. Deficiency leads to goitre and cretinism. Seafoods are rich sources, and there is iodine in iodised salt, in dairy products, in some nuts and green vegetables.

Iron An essential trace mineral required by the blood, and involved in transporting oxygen in the body. A deficiency causes anaemia. Iron is not easily absorbed, especially from plant sources, but it can be helped by vitamin C. Liver and kidney are good sources of iron, as are dried apricots, dark green vegetables, eggs, meat and pulses.

Lactase An enzyme present in the intestinal digestive juices which splits lactose (milk sugar) into its constituents for absorption. The lack of this enzyme is known as lactase deficiency which thus leads to lactose malabsorption or intolerance.

Lactose The sugars in milk. See also **Lactase**.

Lecithin A liquid composed of vegetable oils, fatty acids and sugars. When purified, it becomes a granular substance used as a health-food supplement, a good source of choline and inositol.

Lignin A component of plant cell walls, therefore of dietary fibre.

Lysine One of the eight essential amino acids.

Magnesium An essential mineral required for the synthesis of protein, and muscle contraction. It is a component of chlorophyll, the green pigment in plants and vegetables. Other food sources include Brazil nuts, soya and wholemeal flours, and pulses.

Manganese An essential trace mineral required in the use of enzymes. Food sources include wheatgerm, whole grains, tea, nuts, legumes and leafy vegetables.

Minerals Nutrients essential in the diet in amounts of over 100 mg daily. Principal among these are calcium, copper, magnesium, phosphorus, and potassium. See also **Trace minerals.**

Nephritis A general term for inflammation of the kidneys.

Niacin A water-soluble B vitamin which includes nicotinic acid and nicotinamide. It is required for healthy nervous and digestive systems, and for the skin and tongue. A deficiency leads to pellagra. Food sources include brewers' yeast, yeast extract, meat, offal, oily fish, cheese, lentils, mushrooms and eggs.

Oestrogen A female sex hormone produced mainly by the ovaries. A fall in oestrogen levels heralds the menopause.

Pantothenic acid A water-soluble B vitamin which is needed by the adrenal glands, and by the whole body in times of stress. Food sources include brewers' yeast, offal, wheat, bran, wheatgerm, egg, mushrooms, peanuts and wholemeal bread.

Pectoral Good for diseases of the chest and lungs.

Phosphorus An essential mineral required for bones, teeth and the release of energy. Food sources include dairy products, liver, lentils, wholemeal bread, eggs, meat, fish, green vegetables and garlic.

Phytate A salt of phytic acid, an acid of inositol. Phytates are found in cereal grains and pulses, and they can prevent minerals being absorbed by the body.

Phytotherapy A therapy popular in France which treats illness through the use of plants. Prescribed plants are eaten for individual ailments, but aromatherapeutic principles are sometimes utilised as well.

Potassium An essential mineral required in nerve and muscle function, in enzyme activation and water/acid balance. Sodium or salt causes potassium depletion. Food sources include brewers' yeast, dried fruit, mushrooms, green vegetables, dates, lean meats, many fruit, pulses and grains.

Pyridoxine This is a water-soluble B vitamin, also known as vitamin B6. It is necessary for protein metabolism and for the blood, for growth, health of the nervous system and the skin. Food sources include brewers' yeast, liver, oily fish, wheatgerm, meat, nuts, wholemeal bread, avocados, bananas, pulses and green vegetables.

Riboflavin   A water-soluble B vitamin also known as vitamin B2. It is essential for the growth and maintenance of healthy skin and eyes.

Rutin   see **Bioflavonoids**

Salmonella   A bacterium which causes the food poisoning, salmonellosis. It is found mostly in cooked meat and meat pies, raw chicken and raw eggs, in ice cream and shellfish.

Selenium   An essential trace mineral required in a protective antioxidant role in much the same way as is vitamin E. Deficiency has caused heart and joint disease in areas where soil selenium is low. Food sources include wholemeal flours, meat, oily fish, dairy produce and garlic.

Stomachic   Good for the stomach.

Sudorific   Promoting or causing perspiration.

Thiamin   A water-soluble B vitamin, also known as vitamin B1. It is essential for the release of energy from carbohydrates, for growth, appetite, digestion and the nervous system. Food sources include brewers' yeast, yeast extract, wheatgerm, meat, rice, pulses and offal.

Trace minerals   Also known as trace elements or micronutrients. These are essential minerals, which are required in less than 100 mg amounts daily. They include cobalt, copper, iodine, iron, manganese, selenium and zinc.

Tryptophan   One of the eight essential amino acids.

Vitamins   Nutrients required for good health which must be present in the diet because they cannot be synthesised adequately within the body.

Vitamin A   This is obtained from animal sources (fish oils, liver, oily fish, dairy foods) primarily as retinol. Betacarotene is the precursor of A found in plant sources (green, orange and yellow fruit and vegetables), and is converted to retinol in the body. A is required for vision, the mucous membranes of the body, skin and teeth. A is also believed to protect against cancer. Retinol can be toxic in overdose; betacarotene is not toxic.

B complex vitamins   A group of water-soluble vitamins needed for growth, general health and digestion. See individual entries: **Biotin, Cobalamine, Folic acid, Niacin, Pantothenic acid, Pyridoxine, Riboflavin** and **Thiamin.**

Vitamin C A water-soluble vitamin, required for the absorption of iron, which acts as an antioxidant, helping wound-healing, and maintaining integrity of skin, bones, teeth, gums and many tissues of the body. Food sources include many fruit and vegetables. There is some C in liver.

Vitamin D A fat-soluble vitamin which occurs in a very few foods: cod liver oil, liver, egg yolk, fortified margarine and dairy products. The skin manufactures D when exposed to sunlight. It is required for the absorption and use of calcium, in bones and teeth.

Vitamin E A fat-soluble vitamin, known as the fertility vitamin, this is required for the health of blood cells and skin. It is antioxidant in action, working with selenium. Food sources include wheatgerm, vegetable and seed oils, eggs, nuts, avocados, dairy products, and cereal grains.

Vitamin K A fat-soluble vitamin required for the prevention of bloodclotting. Food sources include fresh green leafy vegetables and liver.

Vitamin P see **Bioflavonoids**

Zinc An essential trace mineral, required for the synthesis of protein, and for the health of bones, skin, eyes and male reproductive glands. Food sources include oysters, liver, meat, dairy products, pulses, wholemeal bread and eggs.

BIBLIOGRAPHY

AUBERT, Emmanuelle, *Les 9 Grains d'Or dans la Cuisine,* Editions le Courier du Livre, 1983

AUCKLAND HERB SOCIETY, *The Fragrant Kitchen,* 1983

ANDROUET, *Guide du Fromage,* Larousse, 1973

BARRIER CHAUCHART, Christian, *Pour Guérir, Menus et Recettes,* Editions Encre, 1985

COHEN, Prof. Gaston, Conference à la Radio Suisse, 1960

DEXTRAIT, Raymond, *La Cure Végétale,* Editions Vivre en Harmonie, 1960

Pourquoi? Comment? Manger des Ceréales, Editions Vivre en Harmonic, 1975

Le Foie se Méconnu, Collection La Santé dans Ma Poche, 1985

DUBOS, René and Pines, Maya, *Health and Disease,* Time-Life Books, 1965

EMMAUS, *The Encyclopedia of Common Diseases,* Rodale Books Inc., 1962

FLEMING, Susan, *The Little Exotic Fruit Book,* Piatkus, 1987

The Little Potato Book, Piatkus, 1987

Herbs: A Connoisseur's Guide, W. H. Smith, 1990

GRIGSON, Jane, *Jane Grigson's Vegetable Book,* Penguin, 1979

Jane Grigson's Fruit Book, Penguin, 1982

HIPPOCRATES, *History of Health and Medicine,* Pelican, 1978

HALVORSEN, Brian, *The Natural Dentist,* Century Arrow, 1986

LAGRIFFE, Louis, *Le Livre des Epices,* Marabout Service, 1968

LALANNE, Raymond, *L'Alimentation Humaine,* Editions Presses Universitaires

LAMBERT ORTIZ, Elizabeth, *The Encyclopedia of Herbs, Spices and Flavourings,* Dorling Kindersley, 1992

LAVER, Mary and SMITH, Margaret, *Diet for Life, A Cookbook for Arthritics,* Editions Dan, 1981

LECLERC, Dr. H., *Précis de Phytothérapie,* Editions Masson, 1976

LONGUE, Dr. René-Etienne, *Yoga de la Table,* 1964

LUST, John B., *Raw Juice Therapy,* Benedict Lust Publications, 1958

MABEY, Richard, *Food for Free,* Collins, 1972

MACMILLAN, H. F., *Tropical Planting and Gardening,* Macmillian, 1935

MARGARIÑOS, Hélène, *Cuisine pour une Vie Nouvelle,* Editions Debard, 1980

MAURY, Dr. E., *La Médécine par le Vin,* Editions Avtulen, 1988

MAURY, Marguerite, *The Secret of Life and Youth,* Macdonald, 1962

MAYES, Dr. Adrienne, *The A-Z of Nutritional Health,* Thorsons, 1991

MCCANCE & WIDDOWSON, *The Composition of Foods,* MAFF, 1987

MCGEE, Harold, *On Food and Cooking,* Unwin Hyman, 1984

MESSEGUE, Didier, *Les Plantes de Mon Père,* Robert Laffont, 1973

MESSEGUE, Maurice, *C'est la Nature qui a Raison,* Robert Laffont, 1972

MOORE, Mary Courtney, *Nutrition and Diet Therapy,* The CV Mosby Co., 1988

The Natural Foods Primer, Simon & Schuster, 1972

Nutrition, Your Key to Good Health, North Hollywood London Press, 1964

PASSMORE, Jacki, *The Letts Companion to Asian Food and Cooking,* Charles Letts, 1991

PENNINGTON, C. R., *Therapeutic Nutrition,* Chapman and Hall, 1988

PRICE, Dr. Weston, *Nutrition and Physical Degeneration,* Price-Pottenger Foundation, 1970

RAFAEL, Marcia, *The Natural Foods and Nutrition Handbook,* Harper and Row, 1972

RINZLER, Carol Ann, *Food Facts,* Bloomsbury, 1987

ROOT, Waverley, *Food,* Simon & Schuster, 1980

RYMAN, Danièle, *The Aromatherapy Handbook,* Century, 1984
Aromatherapy, Piatkus, 1991

SINCLAIR, Eleanor, *A Garden of Herbs,* Editions Rohde, 1926

STOBART, Tom, *Herbs, Spices and Flavourings,* Penguin, 1977
The Cook's Encyclopedia, Batsford, 1980

STORKOWSKI, Joseph, *Les Diastases, Collection 'Que Sais Je?'* Editions Presses Universitaires

SUZUKI, Daisetz Teitaro, *Essaies sur le Bouddhisme Zen,* Albin Michel

TREMOLIERES, Dr., *L'Alimentation Familiale,* Editions Institut National d'Hygiène, 1958

TRIMMER, Dr. Eric, *The Good Health Food Guide,* Piatkus, 1994

WAYLER, Thelma and KLEIN, Moses, *Applied Nutrition,* Macmillan, 1965

WINTER, Ruth, *Beware of the Food You Eat,* Signet Books, 1971
The Yellow Emperor's Classic of Internal Medicine, Williams and Wilkins, 1949

YUDKIN, John, *Sweet and Dangerous,* Peter Wyden Inc., 1972
The Penguin Encyclopedia of Nutrition, Viking, 1985

ZOTTOLA, Georges, *La Faim, La Soif et les Hommes,* Hachette, 1960

INDEX

TO KILL A MOCKINGBIRD

By HARPER LEE

WARNER BOOKS

A Time Warner Company

WARNER BOOKS EDITION

Published by arrangement with J. B. Lippincott Company, Subsidiary of Harper & Row Publishers, Inc., East Washington Square, Philadelphia, Pennsylvania 19105.

Warner Books, Inc.
1271 Avenue of the Americas
New York, N.Y. 10020

Visit our Web site at
www.warnerbooks.com

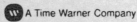 A Time Warner Company

Printed in the United States of America

First Warner Books Printing: December, 1982

60 59

Lawyers, I suppose, were children once.

CHARLES LAMB

Part One

Part One

When he was nearly thirteen, my brother Jem got his arm badly broken at the elbow. When it healed, and Jem's fears of never being able to play football were assuaged, he was seldom self-conscious about his injury. His left arm was somewhat shorter than his right; when he stood or walked, the back of his hand was at right angles to his body, his thumb parallel to his thigh. He couldn't have cared less, so long as he could pass and punt.

When enough years had gone by to enable us to look back on them, we sometimes discussed the events leading to his accident. I maintain that the Ewells started it all, but Jem, who was four years my senior, said it started long before that. He said it began the summer Dill came to us, when Dill first gave us the idea of making Boo Radley come out.

I said if he wanted to take a broad view of the thing, it really began with Andrew Jackson. If General Jackson hadn't run the Creeks up the creek, Simon Finch would never have paddled up the Alabama, and where would we be if he hadn't? We were far too old to settle an argument with a fist-fight, so we consulted Atticus. Our father said we were both right.

Being Southerners, it was a source of shame to some members of the family that we had no recorded ancestors on either side of the Battle of Hastings. All we had was Simon Finch, a fur-trapping apothecary from Cornwall whose piety was exceeded only by his stinginess. In England, Simon was irritated by the persecution of those who called themselves Methodists at the hands of their more liberal brethren, and as Simon called himself a Methodist, he worked his way across the Atlantic to Philadelphia, thence to Jamaica, thence to Mobile, and up the Saint Stephens. Mindful of John Wesley's strictures on the use of many words in buying and selling, Simon made a pile practicing medicine, but in this pursuit he was unhappy lest he be tempted into doing what he knew was not for the glory of God, as the putting on of gold and costly apparel. So Simon, having forgotten his teacher's dictum on the possession of human chattels, bought three slaves and with their aid established a homestead on the banks of the Alabama River some forty miles above Saint Stephens. He returned to Saint Stephens only once, to find a wife, and with her established a line that ran high to daughters. Simon lived to an impressive age and died rich.

It was customary for the men in the family to remain on Simon's homestead, Finch's Landing, and make their living from cotton. The place was self-sufficient: modest in comparison with the empires around it, the Landing nevertheless produced everything required to sustain life except ice, wheat flour, and articles of clothing, supplied by river-boats from Mobile.

Simon would have regarded with impotent fury the disturbance between the North and the South, as it left his descendants stripped of everything but their land, yet the tradition of living on the land remained unbroken until well into the twentieth century, when my father, Atticus Finch, went to Montgomery to read law, and his younger brother went to Boston to study medicine. Their sister Alexandra was the Finch who remained at the Landing: she married a taciturn man who spent most of his time lying in a hammock by the river wondering if his trot-lines were full.

When my father was admitted to the bar, he returned to Maycomb and began his practice. Maycomb, some twenty miles east of Finch's Landing, was the county seat of Maycomb County. Atticus's office in the courthouse contained little more than a hat rack, a spittoon, a checkerboard and an unsullied Code of Alabama. His first two clients were the last two persons hanged in the Maycomb County jail. Atticus had urged them to accept the state's generosity in allowing them to plead Guilty to second-degree murder and escape with their lives, but they were Haverfords, in Maycomb County a name synonymous with jackass. The Haverfords had dispatched Maycomb's leading blacksmith in a misunderstanding arising from the alleged wrongful detention of a mare, were imprudent enough to do it in the presence of three witnesses, and insisted that the-son-of-a-bitch-had-it-coming-to-him was a good enough defense for anybody. They persisted in pleading Not Guilty to first-degree murder, so there was nothing much Atticus could do for his clients except be present at their departure, an occasion that was probably the beginning of my father's profound distaste for the practice of criminal law.

During his first five years in Maycomb, Atticus practiced economy more than anything; for several years thereafter he invested his earnings in his brother's education. John Hale Finch was ten years younger than my father, and chose to study medicine at a time when cotton was not worth growing; but after getting Uncle Jack started, Atticus derived a reasonable income from the law. He liked Maycomb, he was Maycomb County born and bred; he knew his people, they knew him, and because of Simon Finch's industry, Atticus was related by blood or marriage to nearly every family in the town.

Maycomb was an old town, but it was a tired old town when I first knew it. In rainy weather the streets turned to red slop; grass grew on the sidewalks, the courthouse sagged in the square. Somehow, it was hotter then: a black dog suffered on a summer's day; bony mules hitched to Hoover carts flicked flies in the sweltering shade of the live oaks on the square. Men's stiff collars wilted by nine in the morning. Ladies bathed before noon, after their three-o'clock naps, and by nightfall were like soft teacakes with frostings of sweat and sweet talcum.

People moved slowly then. They ambled across the square, shuffled in and out of the stores around it, took their time about everything. A day was twenty-four hours long but seemed longer. There was no hurry, for there was nowhere to go, nothing to buy and no money to buy it with, nothing to see outside the boundaries of Maycomb County. But it was a time of vague optimism for some of the people: Maycomb County had recently been told that it had nothing to fear but fear itself.

We lived on the main residential street in town—Atticus, Jem and I, plus Calpurnia our cook. Jem and I found our father satisfactory: he played with us, read to us, and treated us with courteous detachment.

Calpurnia was something else again. She was all angles and bones; she was nearsighted; she squinted; her hand was wide as a bed slat and twice as hard. She was always ordering me out of the kitchen, asking me why I couldn't behave as well as Jem when she knew he was older, and calling me home when I wasn't ready to come. Our battles were epic and one-sided. Calpurnia always won, mainly because Atticus always took her side. She had been with us ever since Jem was born, and I had felt her tyrannical presence as long as I could remember.

Our mother died when I was two, so I never felt her absence. She was a Graham from Montgomery; Atticus met her when he was first elected to the state legislature. He was middle-aged then, she was fifteen years his junior. Jem was the product of their first year of marriage; four years later I was born, and two years later our mother died from a sudden heart attack. They said it ran in her family. I did not miss her, but I think Jem did. He remembered her clearly, and sometimes in the middle of a game he would sigh at length, then go off and play by himself behind the car-house. When he was like that, I knew better than to bother him.

When I was almost six and Jem was nearly ten, our summertime boundaries (within calling distance of Calpurnia) were Mrs. Henry Lafayette Dubose's house two doors to the north of us, and the Radley Place three doors to the south. We were never tempted to break them. The Radley Place was inhabited by an unknown entity the mere description of whom was enough to make us behave for days on end; Mrs. Dubose was plain hell.

That was the summer Dill came to us.

Early one morning as we were beginning our day's play in the back yard, Jem and I heard something next door in Miss Rachel Haverford's collard patch. We went to the wire fence to see if there was a puppy—Miss Rachel's rat terrier was expecting—instead we found someone sitting looking at us. Sitting down, he wasn't much higher than the collards. We stared at him until he spoke:

"Hey."

"Hey yourself," said Jem pleasantly.

"I'm Charles Baker Harris," he said. "I can read."

"So what?" I said.

"I just thought you'd like to know I can read. You got anything needs readin' I can do it. . . ."

"How old are you," asked Jem, "four-and-a-half?"

"Goin' on seven."

"Shoot no wonder, then," said Jem, jerking his thumb at me. "Scout yonder's been readin' ever since she was born, and she ain't even started to school yet. You look right puny for goin' on seven."

"I'm little but I'm old," he said.

Jem brushed his hair back to get a better look. "Why don't you come over, Charles Baker Harris?" he said. "Lord, what a name."

" 's not any funnier'n yours. Aunt Rachel says your name's Jeremy Atticus Finch."

Jem scowled. "I'm big enough to fit mine," he said. "Your name's longer'n you are. Bet it's a foot longer."

"Folks call me Dill," said Dill, struggling under the fence.

"Do better if you go over it instead of under it," I said. "Where'd you come from?"

Dill was from Meridian, Mississippi, was spending the summer with his aunt, Miss Rachel, and would be spending every summer in Maycomb from now on. His family was from Maycomb County originally, his mother worked for a photographer in Meridian, had entered his picture in a Beautiful Child contest and won five dollars. She gave the money to Dill, who went to the picture show twenty times on it.

"Don't have any picture shows here, except Jesus ones in the courthouse sometimes," said Jem. "Ever see anything good?"

Dill had seen *Dracula*, a revelation that moved Jem to eye him with the beginning of respect. "Tell it to us," he said.

Dill was a curiosity. He wore blue linen shorts that buttoned to his shirt, his hair was snow white and stuck to his head like duckfluff; he was a year my senior but I towered over him. As he told us the old tale his blue eyes would lighten and darken; his laugh was sudden and happy; he habitually pulled at a cowlick in the center of his forehead.

When Dill reduced Dracula to dust, and Jem said the show sounded better than the book, I asked Dill where his father was: "You ain't said anything about him."

"I haven't got one."

"Is he dead?"

"No . . ."

"Then if he's not dead you've got one, haven't you?"

Dill blushed and Jem told me to hush, a sure sign that Dill had been studied and found acceptable. Thereafter the summer passed in routine contentment. Routine contentment was: improving our treehouse that rested between giant twin chinaberry trees in the back yard, fussing, running through our list of dramas based on the works of Oliver Optic, Victor Appleton, and Edgar Rice Burroughs. In this matter we were lucky to have Dill. He played the character parts formerly thrust upon me—the ape in *Tarzan*, Mr. Crabtree in *The Rover Boys*, Mr. Damon in *Tom Swift*. Thus we came to know Dill as a pocket Merlin, whose head teemed with eccentric plans, strange longings, and quaint fancies.

But by the end of August our repertoire was vapid from countless reproductions, and it was then that Dill gave us the idea of making Boo Radley come out.

The Radley Place fascinated Dill. In spite of our warnings and explanations it drew him as the moon draws water, but drew him no nearer than the light-pole on the corner, a safe distance from the Radley gate. There he would stand, his arm around the fat pole, staring and wondering.

The Radley Place jutted into a sharp curve beyond our house. Walking south, one faced its porch; the sidewalk turned and ran beside the lot. The house was low, was once white with a deep front porch and green shutters, but had long ago darkened to the color of the slate-gray yard around it. Rain-rotted shingles drooped over the eaves of the veranda; oak trees kept the sun away. The remains of a picket drunkenly guarded the front yard—a "swept" yard that was never swept—where johnson grass and rabbit-tobacco grew in abundance.

Inside the house lived a malevolent phantom. People said

he existed, but Jem and I had never seen him. People said he went out at night when the moon was down, and peeped in windows. When people's azaleas froze in a cold snap, it was because he had breathed on them. Any stealthy small crimes committed in Maycomb were his work. Once the town was terrorized by a series of morbid nocturnal events: people's chickens and household pets were found mutilated; although the culprit was Crazy Addie, who eventually drowned himself in Barker's Eddy, people still looked at the Radley Place, unwilling to discard their initial suspicions. A Negro would not pass the Radley Place at night, he would cut across to the sidewalk opposite and whistle as he walked. The Maycomb school grounds adjoined the back of the Radley lot; from the Radley chickenyard tall pecan trees shook their fruit into the schoolyard, but the nuts lay untouched by the children: Radley pecans would kill you. A baseball hit into the Radley yard was a lost ball and no questions asked.

The misery of that house began many years before Jem and I were born. The Radleys, welcome anywhere in town, kept to themselves, a predilection unforgivable in Maycomb. They did not go to church, Maycomb's principal recreation, but worshiped at home; Mrs. Radley seldom if ever crossed the street for a mid-morning coffee break with her neighbors, and certainly never joined a missionary circle. Mr. Radley walked to town at eleven-thirty every morning and came back promptly at twelve, sometimes carrying a brown paper bag that the neighborhood assumed contained the family groceries. I never knew how old Mr. Radley made his living—Jem said he "bought cotton," a polite term for doing nothing—but Mr. Radley and his wife had lived there with their two sons as long as anybody could remember.

The shutters and doors of the Radley house were closed on Sundays, another thing alien to Maycomb's ways: closed doors meant illness and cold weather only. Of all days Sunday was the day for formal afternoon visiting: ladies wore corsets, men wore coats, children wore shoes. But to climb the Radley front steps and call, "He-y," of a Sunday afternoon was something their neighbors never did. The Radley house had no screen doors. I once asked Atticus if it ever had any; Atticus said yes, but before I was born.

According to neighborhood legend, when the younger Radley boy was in his teens he became acquainted with some of the Cunninghams from Old Sarum, an enormous and confusing tribe domiciled in the northern part of the county, and they formed the nearest thing to a gang ever seen in Maycomb. They did little, but enough to be discussed by the town and publicly warned from three pulpits: they hung around the barbershop; they rode the bus to Abbottsville on Sundays and went to the picture show; they attended dances at the county's riverside gambling hell, the Dew-Drop Inn & Fishing Camp; they experimented with stumphole whiskey. Nobody in Maycomb had nerve enough to tell Mr. Radley that his boy was in with the wrong crowd.

One night, in an excessive spurt of high spirits, the boys backed around the square in a borrowed flivver, resisted arrest by Maycomb's ancient beadle, Mr. Conner, and locked him in the courthouse outhouse. The town decided something had to be done; Mr. Conner said he knew who each and every one of them was, and he was bound and determined they wouldn't get away with it, so the boys came before the probate judge on charges of disorderly conduct, disturbing the peace, assault and battery, and using abusive and profane language in the presence and hearing of a female. The judge asked Mr. Conner why he included the last charge; Mr. Conner said they cussed so loud he was sure every lady in Maycomb heard them. The judge decided to send the boys to the state industrial school, where boys were sometimes sent for no other reason than to provide them with food and decent shelter: it was no prison and it was no disgrace. Mr. Radley thought it was. If the judge released Arthur, Mr. Radley would see to it that Arthur gave no further trouble. Knowing that Mr. Radley's word was his bond, the judge was glad to do so.

The other boys attended the industrial school and received the best secondary education to be had in the state; one of them eventually worked his way through engineering school at Auburn. The doors of the Radley house were closed on weekdays as well as Sundays, and Mr. Radley's boy was not seen again for fifteen years.

But there came a day, barely within Jem's memory, when Boo Radley was heard from and was seen by several people, but not by Jem. He said Atticus never talked much about the

Radleys: when Jem would question him Atticus's only answer was for him to mind his own business and let the Radleys mind theirs, they had a right to; but when it happened Jem said Atticus shook his head and said, "Mm, mm, mm."

So Jem received most of his information from Miss Stephanie Crawford, a neighborhood scold, who said she knew the whole thing. According to Miss Stephanie, Boo was sitting in the livingroom cutting some items from *The Maycomb Tribune* to paste in his scrapbook. His father entered the room. As Mr. Radley passed by, Boo drove the scissors into his parent's leg, pulled them out, wiped them on his pants, and resumed his activities.

Mrs. Radley ran screaming into the street that Arthur was killing them all, but when the sheriff arrived he found Boo still sitting in the livingroom, cutting up the *Tribune*. He was thirty-three years old then.

Miss Stephanie said old Mr. Radley said no Radley was going to any asylum, when it was suggested that a season in Tuscaloosa might be helpful to Boo. Boo wasn't crazy, he was high-strung at times. It was all right to shut him up, Mr. Radley conceded, but insisted that Boo not be charged with anything: he was not a criminal. The sheriff hadn't the heart to put him in jail alongside Negroes, so Boo was locked in the courthouse basement.

Boo's transition from the basement to back home was nebulous in Jem's memory. Miss Stephanie Crawford said some of the town council told Mr. Radley that if he didn't take Boo back, Boo would die of mold from the damp. Besides, Boo could not live forever on the bounty of the county.

Nobody knew what form of intimidation Mr. Radley employed to keep Boo out of sight, but Jem figured that Mr. Radley kept him chained to the bed most of the time. Atticus said no, it wasn't that sort of thing, that there were other ways of making people into ghosts.

My memory came alive to see Mrs. Radley occasionally open the front door, walk to the edge of the porch, and pour water on her cannas. But every day Jem and I would see Mr. Radley walking to and from town. He was a thin leathery man with colorless eyes, so colorless they did not reflect light. His cheekbones were sharp and his mouth was wide, with a thin upper lip and a full lower lip. Miss Stephanie Crawford said he was so upright he took the word of God as his only law, and we believed her, because Mr. Radley's posture was ramrod straight.

He never spoke to us. When he passed we would look at the ground and say, "Good morning, sir," and he would cough in reply. Mr. Radley's elder son lived in Pensacola; he came home at Christmas, and he was one of the few persons we ever saw enter or leave the place. From the day Mr. Radley took Arthur home, people said the house died.

But there came a day when Atticus told us he'd wear us out if we made any noise in the yard and commissioned Calpurnia to serve in his absence if she heard a sound out of us. Mr. Radley was dying.

He took his time about it. Wooden sawhorses blocked the road at each end of the Radley lot, straw was put down on the sidewalk, traffic was diverted to the back street. Dr. Reynolds parked his car in front of our house and walked to the Radley's every time he called. Jem and I crept around the yard for days. At last the sawhorses were taken away, and we stood watching from the front porch when Mr. Radley made his final journey past our house.

"There goes the meanest man ever God blew breath into," murmured Calpurnia, and she spat meditatively into the yard. We looked at her in surprise, for Calpurnia rarely commented on the ways of white people.

The neighborhood thought when Mr. Radley went under Boo would come out, but it had another think coming: Boo's elder brother returned from Pensacola and took Mr. Radley's place. The only difference between him and his father was their ages. Jem said Mr. Nathan Radley "bought cotton," too. Mr. Nathan would speak to us, however, when we said good morning, and sometimes we saw him coming from town with a magazine in his hand.

The more we told Dill about the Radleys, the more he wanted to know, the longer he would stand hugging the light-pole on the corner, the more he would wonder.

"Wonder what he does in there," he would murmur. "Looks like he'd just stick his head out the door."

Jem said, "He goes out, all right, when it's pitch dark. Miss Stephanie Crawford said she woke up in the middle of the night one time and saw him looking straight through the window at her . . . said his head was like a skull lookin' at her. Ain't you ever waked up at night and heard him, Dill? He walks like this—'' Jem slid his feet through the gravel. "Why do you think Miss Rachel locks up so tight at night? I've seen his tracks in our back yard many a mornin', and one night I heard him scratching on the back screen, but he was gone time Atticus got there.''

"Wonder what he looks like?'' said Dill.

Jem gave a reasonable description of Boo: Boo was about six-and-a-half feet tall, judging from his tracks; he dined on raw squirrels and any cats he could catch, that's why his hands were bloodstained—if you ate an animal raw, you could never wash the blood off. There was a long jagged scar that ran across his face; what teeth he had were yellow and rotten; his eyes popped, and he drooled most of the time.

"Let's try to make him come out,'' said Dill. "I'd like to see what he looks like.''

Jem said if Dill wanted to get himself killed, all he had to do was go up and knock on the front door.

Our first raid came to pass only because Dill bet Jem *The Gray Ghost* against two Tom Swifts that Jem wouldn't get any farther than the Radley gate. In all his life, Jem had never declined a dare.

Jem thought about it for three days. I suppose he loved honor more than his head, for Dill wore him down easily: "You're scared," Dill said, the first day. "Ain't scared, just respectful," Jem said. The next day Dill said, "You're too scared even to put your big toe in the front yard." Jem said he reckoned he wasn't, he'd passed the Radley Place every school day of his life.

"Always runnin'," I said.

But Dill got him the third day, when he told Jem that folks in Meridian certainly weren't as afraid as the folks in Maycomb, that he'd never seen such scary folks as the ones in Maycomb.

This was enough to make Jem march to the corner, where he stopped and leaned against the light-pole, watching the gate hanging crazily on its homemade hinge.

"I hope you've got it through your head that he'll kill us

each and every one, Dill Harris,'' said Jem, when we joined him. "Don't blame me when he gouges your eyes out. You started it, remember.''

"You're still scared,'' murmured Dill patiently.

Jem wanted Dill to know once and for all that he wasn't scared of anything "It's just that I can't think of a way to make him come out without him gettin' us.'' Besides, Jem had his little sister to think of.

When he said that, I knew he was afraid. Jem had his little sister to think of the time I dared him to jump off the top of the house: "If I got killed, what'd become of you?'' he asked. Then he jumped, landed unhurt, and his sense of responsibility left him until confronted by the Radley Place.

"You gonna run out on a dare?'' asked Dill. "If you are, then—''

"Dill, you have to think about these things,'' Jem said. "Lemme think a minute . . . it's sort of like making a turtle come out . . .''

"How's that?'' asked Dill.

"Strike a match under him.''

I told Jem if he set fire to the Radley house I was going to tell Atticus on him.

Dill said striking a match under a turtle was hateful.

"Ain't hateful, just persuades him—'s not like you'd chunk him in the fire,'' Jem growled.

"How do you know a match don't hurt him?''

"Turtles can't feel, stupid,'' said Jem.

"Were you ever a turtle, huh?''

"My stars, Dill! Now lemme think . . . reckon we can rock him. . . .''

Jem stood in thought so long that Dill made a mild concession: "I won't say you ran out on a dare an' I'll swap you *The Gray Ghost* if you just go up and touch the house.''

Jem brightened. "Touch the house, that all?''

Dill nodded.

"Sure that's all, now? I don't want you hollerin' something different the minute I get back.''

"Yeah, that's all,'' said Dill. "He'll probably come out after you when he sees you in the yard, then Scout 'n' me 'll jump on him and hold him down till we can tell him we ain't gonna hurt him.''

We left the corner, crossed the side street that ran in front of the Radley house, and stopped at the gate.

"Well go on," said Dill, "Scout and me's right behind you."

"I'm going," said Jem, "don't hurry me."

He walked to the corner of the lot, then back again, studying the simple terrain as if deciding how best to effect an entry, frowning and scratching his head.

Then I sneered at him.

Jem threw open the gate and sped to the side of the house, slapped it with his palm and ran back past us, not waiting to see if his foray was successful. Dill and I followed on his heels. Safely on our porch, panting and out of breath, we looked back.

The old house was the same, droopy and sick, but as we stared down the street we thought we saw an inside shutter move. Flick. A tiny, almost invisible movement, and the house was still.

2

Dill left us early in September, to return to Meridian. We saw him off on the five o'clock bus and I was miserable without him until it occurred to me that I would be starting to school in a week. I never looked forward more to anything in my life. Hours of wintertime had found me in the treehouse, looking over at the schoolyard, spying on multitudes of children through a two-power telescope Jem had given me, learning their games, following Jem's red jacket through wriggling circles of blind man's buff, secretly sharing their misfortunes and minor victories. I longed to join them.

Jem condescended to take me to school the first day, a job usually done by one's parents, but Atticus had said Jem would be delighted to show me where my room was. I think some money changed hands in this transaction, for as we trotted around the corner past the Radley Place I heard an unfamiliar jingle in Jem's pockets. When we slowed to a walk at the edge of the schoolyard, Jem was careful to explain that during school hours I was not to bother him, I was not to approach him with requests to enact a chapter of *Tarzan and the Ant Men*, to embarrass him with references to his private life, or tag along behind him at recess and noon. I was to stick with the first grade and he would stick with the fifth. In short, I was to leave him alone.

"You mean we can't play any more?" I asked.

"We'll do like we always do at home," he said, "but you'll see—school's different."

It certainly was. Before the first morning was over, Miss Caroline Fisher, our teacher, hauled me up to the front of the room and patted the palm of my hand with a ruler, then made me stand in the corner until noon.

Miss Caroline was no more than twenty-one. She had bright auburn hair, pink cheeks, and wore crimson fingernail polish. She also wore high-heeled pumps and a red-and-white-striped dress. She looked and smelled like a peppermint drop. She boarded across the street one door down from us in Miss Maudie Atkinson's upstairs front room, and when Miss Maudie introduced us to her, Jem was in a haze for days.

Miss Caroline printed her name on the blackboard and said, "This says I am Miss Caroline Fisher. I am from North Alabama, from Winston County." The class murmured apprehensively, should she prove to harbor her share of the peculiarities indigenous to that region. (When Alabama seceded from the Union on January 11, 1861, Winston County seceded from Alabama, and every child in Maycomb County knew it.) North Alabama was full of Liquor Interests, Big Mules, steel companies, Republicans, professors, and other persons of no background.

Miss Caroline began the day by reading us a story about cats. The cats had long conversations with one another, they wore cunning little clothes and lived in a warm house beneath a kitchen stove. By the time Mrs. Cat called the drugstore for an order of chocolate malted mice the class was wriggling like a bucketful of catawba worms. Miss Caroline seemed unaware that the ragged, denim-shirted and floursack-skirted first grade, most of whom had chopped cotton and fed hogs from the time they were able to walk, were immune to imaginative literature. Miss Caroline came to the end of the story and said, "*Oh*, my, wasn't that nice?"

Then she went to the blackboard and printed the alphabet in enormous square capitals, turned to the class and asked, "Does anybody know what these are?"

Everybody did; most of the first grade had failed it last year.

I suppose she chose me because she knew my name; as I read the alphabet a faint line appeared between her eyebrows, and after making me read most of *My First Reader* and the stock-market quotations from *The Mobile Register* aloud, she discovered that I was literate and looked at me with more than faint distaste. Miss Caroline told me to tell my father not to teach me any more, it would interfere with my reading.

"Teach me?" I said in surprise. "He hasn't taught me anything, Miss Caroline. Atticus ain't got time to teach me anything," I added, when Miss Caroline smiled and shook her head. "Why, he's so tired at night he just sits in the livingroom and reads."

"If he didn't teach you, who did?" Miss Caroline asked good-naturedly. "Somebody did. You weren't born reading *The Mobile Register*."

"Jem says I was. He read in a book where I was a Bullfinch instead of a Finch. Jem says my name's really Jean Louise Bullfinch, that I got swapped when I was born and I'm really a—"

Miss Caroline apparently thought I was lying. "Let's not let our imaginations run away with us, dear," she said. "Now you tell your father not to teach you any more. It's best to begin reading with a fresh mind. You tell him I'll take over from here and try to undo the damage—"

"Ma'am?"

"Your father does not know how to teach. You can have a seat now."

I mumbled that I was sorry and retired meditating upon my crime. I never deliberately learned to read, but somehow I had been wallowing illicitly in the daily papers. In the long hours of church—was it then I learned? I could not remember not being able to read hymns. Now that I was compelled to think about it, reading was something that just came to me, as learning to fasten the seat of my union suit without looking around, or achieving two bows from a snarl of shoelaces. I could not remember when the lines above Atticus's moving finger separated into words, but I had stared at them all the evenings in my memory, listening to the news of the day, Bills to Be Enacted into Laws, the diaries of Lorenzo Dow —anything Atticus happened to be reading when I crawled into his lap every night. Until I feared I would lose it, I never loved to read. One does not love breathing.

I knew I had annoyed Miss Caroline, so I let well enough alone and stared out the window until recess when Jem cut me from the covey of first-graders in the schoolyard. He asked how I was getting along. I told him.

"If I didn't have to stay I'd leave. Jem, that damn lady says Atticus's been teaching me to read and for him to stop it—"

"Don't worry, Scout," Jem comforted me. "Our teacher says Miss Caroline's introducing a new way of teaching. She learned about it in college. It'll be in all the grades soon. You don't have to learn much out of books that way—it's like if you wanta learn about cows, you go milk one, see?"

"Yeah Jem, but I don't wanta study cows, I—"

"Sure you do. You hafta know about cows, they're a big part of life in Maycomb County."

I contented myself with asking Jem if he'd lost his mind.

"I'm just trying to tell you the new way they're teachin' the first grade, stubborn. It's the Dewey Decimal System."

Having never questioned Jem's pronouncements, I saw no reason to begin now. The Dewey Decimal System consisted, in part, of Miss Caroline waving cards at us on which were printed "the," "cat," "rat," "man," and "you." No comment seemed to be expected of us, and the class received these impressionistic revelations in silence. I was bored, so I began a letter to Dill. Miss Caroline caught me writing and told me to tell my father to stop teaching me. "Besides," she said. "We don't write in the first grade, we print. You won't learn to write until you're in the third grade."

Calpurnia was to blame for this. It kept me from driving her crazy on rainy days, I guess. She would set me a writing task by scrawling the alphabet firmly across the top of a tablet, then copying out a chapter of the Bible beneath. If I reproduced her penmanship satisfactorily, she rewarded me with an open-faced sandwich of bread and butter and sugar. In Calpurnia's teaching, there was no sentimentality: I seldom pleased her and she seldom rewarded me.

"Everybody who goes home to lunch hold up your hands," said Miss Caroline, breaking into my new grudge against Calpurnia.

The town children did so, and she looked us over.

"Everybody who brings his lunch put it on top of his desk."

Molasses buckets appeared from nowhere, and the ceiling danced with metallic light. Miss Caroline walked up and down the rows peering and poking into lunch containers, nodding if the contents pleased her, frowning a little at others. She stopped at Walter Cunningham's desk. "Where's yours?" she asked.

Walter Cunningham's face told everybody in the first grade he had hookworms. His absence of shoes told us how he got them. People caught hookworms going barefooted in barnyards and hog wallows. If Walter had owned any shoes he would have worn them the first day of school and then discarded them until mid-winter. He did have on a clean shirt and neatly mended overalls.

"Did you forget your lunch this morning?" asked Miss Caroline.

Walter looked straight ahead. I saw a muscle jump in his skinny jaw.

"Did you forget it this morning?" asked Miss Caroline. Walter's jaw twitched again.

"Yeb'm," he finally mumbled.

Miss Caroline went to her desk and opened her purse. "Here's a quarter," she said to Walter. "Go and eat downtown today. You can pay me back tomorrow."

Walter shook his head. "Nome thank you ma'am," he drawled softly.

Impatience crept into Miss Caroline's voice: "Here Walter, come get it."

Walter shook his head again.

When Walter shook his head a third time someone whispered, "Go on and tell her, Scout."

I turned around and saw most of the town people and the entire bus delegation looking at me. Miss Caroline and I had conferred twice already, and they were looking at me in the innocent assurance that familiarity breeds understanding.

I rose graciously on Walter's behalf: "Ah—Miss Caroline?"

"What is it, Jean Louise?"

"Miss Caroline, he's a Cunningham."

I sat back down.

"What, Jean Louise?"

I thought I had made things sufficiently clear. It was clear enough to the rest of us: Walter Cunningham was sitting there lying his head off. He didn't forget his lunch, he didn't have any. He had none today nor would he have any tomorrow or the next day. He had probably never seen three quarters together at the same time in his life.

I tried again: "Walter's one of the Cunninghams, Miss Caroline."

"I beg your pardon, Jean Louise?"

"That's okay, ma'am, you'll get to know all the county folks after a while. The Cunninghams never took anything they can't pay back—no church baskets and no scrip stamps. They never took anything off of anybody, they get along on what they have. They don't have much, but they get along on it."

My special knowledge of the Cunningham tribe—one branch, that is—was gained from events of last winter. Walter's father was one of Atticus's clients. After a dreary conversation in our livingroom one night about his entailment, before Mr. Cunningham left he said, "Mr. Finch, I don't know when I'll ever be able to pay you."

"Let that be the least of your worries, Walter," Atticus said.

When I asked Jem what entailment was, and Jem described it as a condition of having your tail in a crack, I asked Atticus if Mr. Cunningham would ever pay us.

"Not in money," Atticus said, "but before the year's out I'll have been paid. You watch."

We watched. One morning Jem and I found a load of stovewood in the back yard. Later, a sack of hickory nuts appeared on the back steps. With Christmas came a crate of smilax and holly. That spring when we found a crokersack full of turnip greens, Atticus said Mr. Cunningham had more than paid him.

"Why does he pay you like that?" I asked.

"Because that's the only way he can pay me. He has no money."

"Are we poor, Atticus?"

Atticus nodded. "We are indeed."

Jem's nose wrinkled. "Are we as poor as the Cunninghams?"

"Not exactly. The Cunninghams are country folks, farmers, and the crash hit them hardest."

Atticus said professional people were poor because the farmers were poor. As Maycomb County was farm country, nickels and dimes were hard to come by for doctors and dentists and lawyers. Entailment was only a part of Mr. Cunningham's vexations. The acres not entailed were mortgaged to the hilt, and the little cash he made went to interest. If he held his mouth right, Mr. Cunningham could get a WPA job, but his land would go to ruin if he left it, and he was willing to go hungry to keep his land and vote as he pleased. Mr. Cunningham, said Atticus, came from a set breed of men.

As the Cunninghams had no money to pay a lawyer, they simply paid us with what they had. "Did you know," said Atticus, "that Dr. Reynolds works the same way? He charges some folks a bushel of potatoes for delivery of a baby. Miss Scout, if you give me your attention I'll tell you what entailment is. Jem's definitions are very nearly accurate sometimes."

If I could have explained these things to Miss Caroline, I would have saved myself some inconvenience and Miss Caroline subsequent mortification, but it was beyond my ability to explain things as well as Atticus, so I said, "You're shamin' him, Miss Caroline. Walter hasn't got a quarter at home to bring you, and you can't use any stovewood."

Miss Caroline stood stock still, then grabbed me by the collar and hauled me back to her desk. "Jean Louise, I've had about enough of you this morning," she said. "You're starting off on the wrong foot in every way, my dear. Hold out your hand."

I thought she was going to spit in it, which was the only

reason anybody in Maycomb held out his hand: it was a time-honored method of sealing oral contracts. Wondering what bargain we had made, I turned to the class for an answer, but the class looked back at me in puzzlement. Miss Caroline picked up her ruler, gave me half a dozen quick little pats, then told me to stand in the corner. A storm of laughter broke loose when it finally occurred to the class that Miss Caroline had whipped me.

When Miss Caroline threatened it with a similar fate the first grade exploded again, becoming cold sober only when the shadow of Miss Blount fell over them. Miss Blount, a native Maycombian as yet uninitiated in the mysteries of the Decimal System, appeared at the door hands on hips and announced: "If I hear another sound from this room I'll burn up everybody in it. Miss Caroline, the sixth grade cannot concentrate on the pyramids for all this racket!"

My sojourn in the corner was a short one. Saved by the bell, Miss Caroline watched the class file out for lunch. As I was the last to leave, I saw her sink down into her chair and bury her head in her arms. Had her conduct been more friendly toward me, I would have felt sorry for her. She was a pretty little thing.

3

Catching Walter Cunningham in the schoolyard gave me some pleasure, but when I was rubbing his nose in the dirt Jem came by and told me to stop. "You're bigger'n he is," he said.

"He's as old as you, nearly," I said. "He made me start off on the wrong foot."

"Let him go, Scout. Why?"

"He didn't have any lunch," I said, and explained my involvement in Walter's dietary affairs.

Walter had picked himself up and was standing quietly

listening to Jem and me. His fists were half cocked, as if expecting an onslaught from both of us. I stomped at him to chase him away, but Jem put out his hand and stopped me. He examined Walter with an air of speculation. "Your daddy Mr. Walter Cunningham from Old Sarum?" he asked, and Walter nodded.

Walter looked as if he had been raised on fish food: his eyes, as blue as Dill Harris's, were red-rimmed and watery. There was no color in his face except at the tip of his nose, which was moistly pink. He fingered the straps of his overalls, nervously picking at the metal hooks.

Jem suddenly grinned at him. "Come on home to dinner with us, Walter," he said. "We'd be glad to have you."

Walter's face brightened, then darkened.

Jem said, "Our daddy's a friend of your daddy's. Scout here, she's crazy—she won't fight you any more."

"I wouldn't be too certain of that," I said. Jem's free dispensation of my pledge irked me, but precious noontime minutes were ticking away. "Yeah Walter, I won't jump on you again. Don't you like butterbeans? Our Cal's a real good cook."

Walter stood where he was, biting his lip. Jem and I gave up, and we were nearly to the Radley Place when Walter called, "Hey, I'm comin'!"

When Walter caught up with us, Jem made pleasant conversation with him. "A hain't lives there," he said cordially, pointing to the Radley house. "Ever hear about him, Walter?"

"Reckon I have," said Walter. "Almost died first year I come to school and et them pecans—folks say he pizened 'em and put 'em over on the school side of the fence."

Jem seemed to have little fear of Boo Radley now that Walter and I walked beside him. Indeed, Jem grew boastful: "I went all the way up to the house once," he said to Walter.

"Anybody who went up to the house once oughta not to still run every time he passes it," I said to the clouds above.

"And who's runnin', Miss Priss?"

"You are, when ain't anybody with you."

By the time we reached our front steps Walter had forgotten he was a Cunningham. Jem ran to the kitchen and asked

Calpurnia to set an extra plate, we had company. Atticus greeted Walter and began a discussion about crops neither Jem nor I could follow.

"Reason I can't pass the first grade, Mr. Finch, is I've had to stay out ever' spring an' help Papa with the choppin', but there's another'n at the house now that's field size."

"Did you pay a bushel of potatoes for him?" I asked, but Atticus shook his head at me.

While Walter piled food on his plate, he and Atticus talked together like two men, to the wonderment of Jem and me. Atticus was expounding upon farm problems when Walter interrupted to ask if there was any molasses in the house. Atticus summoned Calpurnia, who returned bearing the syrup pitcher. She stood waiting for Walter to help himself. Walter poured syrup on his vegetables and meat with a generous hand. He would probably have poured it into his milk glass had I not asked what the sam hill he was doing.

The silver saucer clattered when he replaced the pitcher, and he quickly put his hands in his lap. Then he ducked his head.

Atticus shook his head at me again. "But he's gone and drowned his dinner in syrup," I protested. "He's poured it all over—"

It was then that Calpurnia requested my presence in the kitchen.

She was furious, and when she was furious Calpurnia's grammar became erratic. When in tranquility, her grammar was as good as anybody's in Maycomb. Atticus said Calpurnia had more education than most colored folks.

When she squinted down at me the tiny lines around her eyes deepened. "There's some folks who don't eat like us," she whispered fiercely, "but you ain't called on to contradict 'em at the table when they don't. That boy's yo' comp'ny and if he wants to eat up the table cloth you let him, you hear?"

"He ain't company, Cal, he's just a Cunningham—"

"Hush your mouth! Don't matter who they are, anybody sets foot in this house's yo' comp'ny, and don't you let me catch you remarkin' on their ways like you was so high and mighty! Yo' folks might be better'n the Cunninghams but it don't count for nothin' the way you're disgracin' 'em—if you can't act fit to eat at the table you can just set here and eat in the kitchen!''

Calpurnia sent me through the swinging door to the diningroom with a stinging smack. I retrieved my plate and finished dinner in the kitchen, thankful, though, that I was spared the humiliation of facing them again. I told Calpurnia to just wait, I'd fix her: one of these days when she wasn't looking I'd go off and drown myself in Barker's Eddy and then she'd be sorry. Besides, I added, she'd already gotten me in trouble once today: she had taught me to write and it was all her fault. "Hush your fussin'," she said.

Jem and Walter returned to school ahead of me: staying behind to advise Atticus of Calpurnia's iniquities was worth a solitary sprint past the Radley Place. "She likes Jem better'n she likes me, anyway," I concluded, and suggested that Atticus lose no time in packing her off.

"Have you ever considered that Jem doesn't worry her half as much?" Atticus's voice was flinty. "I've no intention of getting rid of her, now or ever. We couldn't operate a single day without Cal, have you ever thought of that? You think about how much Cal does for you, and you mind her, you hear?"

I returned to school and hated Calpurnia steadily until a sudden shriek shattered my resentments. I looked up to see Miss Caroline standing in the middle of the room, sheer horror flooding her face. Apparently she had revived enough to persevere in her profession.

"It's alive!" she screamed.

The male population of the class rushed as one to her assistance. Lord, I thought, she's scared of a mouse. Little Chuck Little, whose patience with all living things was phenomenal, said, "Which way did he go, Miss Caroline? Tell us where he went, quick! D.C.—" he turned to a boy behind him—"D.C., shut the door and we'll catch him. Quick, ma'am, where'd he go?"

Miss Caroline pointed a shaking finger not at the floor nor at a desk, but to a hulking individual unknown to me. Little Chuck's face contracted and he said gently, "You mean him, ma'am? Yessum, he's alive. Did he scare you some way?"

Miss Caroline said desperately, "I was just walking by when it crawled out of his hair . . . just crawled out of his hair—"

Little Chuck grinned broadly. "There ain't no need to fear a cootie, ma'am. Ain't you ever seen one? Now don't you be afraid, you just go back to your desk and teach us some more."

Little Chuck Little was another member of the population who didn't know where his next meal was coming from, but he was a born gentleman. He put his hand under her elbow and led Miss Caroline to the front of the room. "Now don't you fret, ma'am," he said. "There ain't no need to fear a cootie. I'll just fetch you some cool water."

The cootie's host showed not the faintest interest in the furor he had wrought. He searched the scalp above his forehead, located his guest and pinched it between his thumb and forefinger.

Miss Caroline watched the process in horrid fascination. Little Chuck brought water in a paper cup, and she drank it gratefully. Finally she found her voice. "What is your name, son?" she asked softly.

The boy blinked. "Who, me?" Miss Caroline nodded.

"Burris Ewell."

Miss Caroline inspected her roll-book. "I have a Ewell here, but I don't have a first name . . . would you spell your first name for me?"

"Don't know how. They call me Burris't home."

"Well, Burris," said Miss Caroline, "I think we'd better excuse you for the rest of the afternoon. I want you to go home and wash your hair."

From her desk she produced a thick volume, leafed through its pages and read for a moment. "A good home remedy for—Burris, I want you to go home and wash your hair with lye soap. When you've done that, treat your scalp with kerosene."

"What fer, missus?"

"To get rid of the—er, cooties. You see, Burris, the other children might catch them, and you wouldn't want that, would you?"

The boy stood up. He was the filthiest human I had ever

seen. His neck was dark gray, the backs of his hands were rusty, and his fingernails were black deep into the quick. He peered at Miss Caroline from a fist-sized clean space on his face. No one had noticed him, probably, because Miss Caroline and I had entertained the class most of the morning.

"And Burris," said Miss Caroline, "please bathe yourself before you come back tomorrow."

The boy laughed rudely. "You ain't sendin' me home, missus. I was on the verge of leavin'—I done done my time for this year."

Miss Caroline looked puzzled. "What do you mean by that?"

The boy did not answer. He gave a short contemptuous snort.

One of the elderly members of the class answered her: "He's one of the Ewells, ma'am," and I wondered if this explanation would be as unsuccessful as my attempt. But Miss Caroline seemed willing to listen. "Whole school's full of 'em. They come first day every year and then leave. The truant lady gets 'em here 'cause she threatens 'em with the sheriff, but she's give up tryin' to hold 'em. She reckons she's carried out the law just gettin' their names on the roll and runnin' 'em here the first day. You're supposed to mark 'em absent the rest of the year . . ."

"But what about their parents?" asked Miss Caroline, in genuine concern.

"Ain't got no mother," was the answer, "and their paw's right contentious."

Burris Ewell was flattered by the recital. "Been comin' to the first day o' the first grade fer three year now," he said expansively. "Reckon if I'm smart this year they'll promote me to the second. . . ."

Miss Caroline said, "Sit back down, please, Burris," and the moment she said it I knew she had made a serious mistake. The boy's condescension flashed to anger.

"You try and make me, missus."

Little Chuck Little got to his feet. "Let him go, ma'am," he said. "He's a mean one, a hard-down mean one. He's liable to start somethin', and there's some little folks here."

He was among the most diminutive of men, but when

Burris Ewell turned toward him, Little Chuck's right hand went to his pocket. "Watch your step, Burris," he said. "I'd soon's kill you as look at you. Now go home."

Burris seemed to be afraid of a child half his height, and Miss Caroline took advantage of his indecision: "Burris, go home. If you don't I'll call the principal," she said. "I'll have to report this, anyway."

The boy snorted and slouched leisurely to the door.

Safely out of range, he turned and shouted: "Report and be damned to ye! Ain't no snot-nosed slut of a schoolteacher ever born c'n make me do nothin'! You ain't makin' me go nowhere, missus. You just remember that, you ain't makin' me go nowhere!"

He waited until he was sure she was crying, then he shuffled out of the building.

Soon we were clustered around her desk, trying in our various ways to comfort her. He was a real mean one . . . below the belt . . . you ain't called on to teach folks like that . . . them ain't Maycomb's ways, Miss Caroline, not really . . . now don't you fret, ma'am. Miss Caroline, why don't you read us a story? That cat thing was real fine this mornin'. . . .

Miss Caroline smiled, blew her nose, said, "Thank you, darlings," dispersed us, opened a book and mystified the first grade with a long narrative about a toadfrog that lived in a hall.

When I passed the Radley Place for the fourth time that day—twice at a full gallop—my gloom had deepened to match the house. If the remainder of the school year were as fraught with drama as the first day, perhaps it would be mildly entertaining, but the prospect of spending nine months refraining from reading and writing made me think of running away.

By late afternoon most of my traveling plans were complete; when Jem and I raced each other up the sidewalk to meet Atticus coming home from work, I didn't give him much of a race. It was our habit to run meet Atticus the moment we saw him round the post office corner in the distance. Atticus seemed to have forgotten my noontime fall from grace; he was full of questions about school. My replies were monosyllabic and he did not press me.

Perhaps Calpurnia sensed that my day had been a grim one: she let me watch her fix supper. "Shut your eyes and open your mouth and I'll give you a surprise," she said.

It was not often that she made crackling bread, she said she never had time, but with both of us at school today had been an easy one for her. She knew I loved crackling bread.

"I missed you today," she said. "The house got so lonesome 'long about two o'clock I had to turn on the radio."

"Why? Jem 'n me ain't ever in the house unless it's rainin'."

"I know," she said, "But one of you's always in callin' distance. I wonder how much of the day I spend just callin' after you. Well," she said, getting up from the kitchen chair, "it's enough time to make a pan of cracklin' bread, I reckon. You run along now and let me get supper on the table."

Calpurnia bent down and kissed me. I ran along, wondering what had come over her. She had wanted to make up with me, that was it. She had always been too hard on me, she had at last seen the error of her fractious ways, she was sorry and too stubborn to say so. I was weary from the day's crimes.

After supper, Atticus sat down with the paper and called, "Scout, ready to read?" The Lord sent me more than I could bear, and I went to the front porch. Atticus followed me.

"Something wrong, Scout?"

I told Atticus I didn't feel very well and didn't think I'd go to school any more if it was all right with him.

Atticus sat down in the swing and crossed his legs. His fingers wandered to his watchpocket; he said that was the only way he could think. He waited in amiable silence, and I sought to reinforce my position: "You never went to school and you do all right, so I'll just stay home too. You can teach me like Granddaddy taught you 'n' Uncle Jack."

"No I can't," said Atticus. "I have to make a living. Besides, they'd put me in jail if I kept you at home—dose of magnesia for you tonight and school tomorrow."

"I'm feeling all right, really."

"Thought so. Now what's the matter?"

Bit by bit, I told him the day's misfortunes. "—and she said you taught me all wrong, so we can't ever read any more, ever. Please don't send me back, please sir."

Atticus stood up and walked to the end of the porch. When

he completed his examination of the wisteria vine he strolled back to me.

"First of all," he said, "if you can learn a simple trick, Scout, you'll get along a lot better with all kinds of folks. You never really understand a person until you consider things from his point of view—"

"Sir?"

"—until you climb into his skin and walk around in it."

Atticus said I had learned many things today, and Miss Caroline had learned several things herself. She had learned not to hand something to a Cunningham, for one thing, but if Walter and I had put ourselves in her shoes we'd have seen it was an honest mistake on her part. We could not expect her to learn all Maycomb's ways in one day, and we could not hold her responsible when she knew no better.

"I'll be dogged," I said. "I didn't know no better than not to read to her, and she held me responsible—listen Atticus, I don't have to go to school!" I was bursting with a sudden thought. "Burris Ewell, remember? He just goes to school the first day. The truant lady reckons she's carried out the law when she gets his name on the roll—"

"You can't do that, Scout," Atticus said. "Sometimes it's better to bend the law a little in special cases. In your case, the law remains rigid. So to school you must go."

"I don't see why I have to when he doesn't."

"Then listen."

Atticus said the Ewells had been the disgrace of Maycomb for three generations. None of them had done an honest day's work in his recollection. He said that some Christmas, when he was getting rid of the tree, he would take me with him and show me where and how they lived. They were people, but they lived like animals. "They can go to school any time they want to, when they show the faintest symptom of wanting an education," said Atticus. "There are ways of keeping them in school by force, but it's silly to force people like the Ewells into a new environment—"

"If I didn't go to school tomorrow, you'd force me to."

"Let us leave it at this," said Atticus dryly. "You, Miss Scout Finch, are of the common folk. You must obey the law." He said that the Ewells were members of an exclusive society made up of Ewells. In certain circumstances the common folk judiciously allowed them certain privileges by the simple method of becoming blind to some of the Ewells' activities. They didn't have to go to school, for one thing. Another thing, Mr. Bob Ewell, Burris's father, was permitted to hunt and trap out of season.

"Atticus, that's bad," I said. In Maycomb County, hunting out of season was a misdemeanor at law, a capital felony in the eyes of the populace.

"It's against the law, all right," said my father, "and it's certainly bad, but when a man spends his relief checks on green whiskey his children have a way of crying from hunger pains. I don't know of any landowner around here who begrudges those children any game their father can hit."

"Mr. Ewell shouldn't do that—"

"Of course he shouldn't, but he'll never change his ways. Are you going to take out your disapproval on his children?"

"No sir," I murmured, and made a final stand: "But if I keep on goin' to school, we can't ever read any more. . . ."

"That's really bothering you, isn't it?"

"Yes sir."

When Atticus looked down at me I saw the expression on his face that always made me expect something. "Do you know what a compromise is?" he asked.

"Bending the law?"

"No, an agreement reached by mutual concessions. It works this way," he said. "If you'll concede the necessity of going to school, we'll go on reading every night just as we always have. Is it a bargain?"

"Yes sir!"

"We'll consider it sealed without the usual formality," Atticus said, when he saw me preparing to spit.

As I opened the front screen door Atticus said, "By the way, Scout, you'd better not say anything at school about our agreement."

"Why not?"

"I'm afraid our activities would be received with considerable disapprobation by the more learned authorities."

Jem and I were accustomed to our father's last-will-and-testament diction, and we were at all times free to interrupt Atticus for a translation when it was beyond our understanding.

"Huh, sir?"

"I never went to school," he said, "but I have a feeling that if you tell Miss Caroline we read every night she'll get after me, and I wouldn't want her after *me*."

Atticus kept us in fits that evening, gravely reading columns of print about a man who sat on a flagpole for no discernible reason, which was reason enough for Jem to spend the following Saturday aloft in the treehouse. Jem sat from after breakfast until sunset and would have remained overnight had not Atticus severed his supply lines. I had spent most of the day climbing up and down, running errands for him, providing him with literature, nourishment and water, and was carrying him blankets for the night when Atticus said if I paid no attention to him, Jem would come down. Atticus was right.

4

The remainder of my schooldays were no more auspicious than the first. Indeed, they were an endless Project that slowly evolved into a Unit, in which miles of construction paper and wax crayon were expended by the State of Alabama in its well-meaning but fruitless efforts to teach me Group Dynamics. What Jem called the Dewey Decimal System was school-wide by the end of my first year, so I had no chance to compare it with other teaching techniques. I could only look around me: Atticus and my uncle, who went to school at home, knew everything—at least, what one didn't know the other did. Furthermore, I couldn't help noticing that my father had served for years in the state legislature, elected each time without opposition, innocent of the adjustments my teachers thought essential to the development of Good Citizenship. Jem, educated on a half-Decimal half-Duncecap basis, seemed to function effectively alone or in a group, but Jem was a poor example: no tutorial system devised by man could have stopped him from getting at books. As for me, I knew nothing except what I gathered from *Time* magazine and reading everything I could lay hands on at home, but as I inched sluggishly along the treadmill of the Maycomb County school system, I could not help receiving the impression that I was being cheated out of something. Out of what I knew not, yet I did not believe that twelve years of unrelieved boredom was exactly what the state had in mind for me.

As the year passed, released from school thirty minutes before Jem, who had to stay until three o'clock, I ran by the Radley Place as fast as I could, not stopping until I reached the safety of our front porch. One afternoon as I raced by, something caught my eye and caught it in such a way that I took a deep breath, a long look around, and went back.

Two live oaks stood at the edge of the Radley lot; their roots reached out into the side-road and made it bumpy. Something about one of the trees attracted my attention.

Some tinfoil was sticking in a knot-hole just above my eye level, winking at me in the afternoon sun. I stood on tiptoe, hastily looked around once more, reached into the hole, and withdrew two pieces of chewing gum minus their outer wrappers.

My first impulse was to get it into my mouth as quickly as possible, but I remembered where I was. I ran home, and on our front porch I examined my loot. The gum looked fresh. I sniffed it and it smelled all right. I licked it and waited for a while. When I did not die I crammed it into my mouth: Wrigley's Double-Mint.

When Jem came home he asked me where I got such a wad. I told him I found it.

"Don't eat things you find, Scout."

"This wasn't on the ground, it was in a tree."

Jem growled.

"Well it was," I said. "It was sticking in that tree yonder, the one comin' from school."

"Spit it out right now!"

I spat it out. The tang was fading, anyway. "I've been chewin' it all afternoon and I ain't dead yet, not even sick."

Jem stamped his foot. "Don't you know you're not supposed to even touch the trees over there? You'll get killed if you do!"

"You touched the house once!"

"That was different! You go gargle—right now, you hear me?"

"Ain't neither, it'll take the taste outa my mouth."

"You don't 'n' I'll tell Calpurnia on you!"

Rather than risk a tangle with Calpurnia, I did as Jem told me. For some reason, my first year of school had wrought a great change in our relationship: Calpurnia's tyranny, unfairness, and meddling in my business had faded to gentle grumblings of general disapproval. On my part, I went to much trouble, sometimes, not to provoke her.

Summer was on the way; Jem and I awaited it with impatience. Summer was our best season: it was sleeping on the back screened porch in cots, or trying to sleep in the treehouse; summer was everything good to eat; it was a thousand colors in a parched landscape; but most of all, summer was Dill.

The authorities released us early the last day of school, and Jem and I walked home together. "Reckon old Dill'll be coming home tomorrow," I said.

"Probably day after," said Jem. "Mis'sippi turns 'em loose a day later."

As we came to the live oaks at the Radley Place I raised my finger to point for the hundredth time to the knot-hole where I had found the chewing gum, trying to make Jem believe I had found it there, and found myself pointing at another piece of tinfoil.

"I see it, Scout! I see it—"

Jem looked around, reached up, and gingerly pocketed a tiny shiny package. We ran home, and on the front porch we looked at a small box patchworked with bits of tinfoil collected from chewing-gum wrappers. It was the kind of box wedding rings came in, purple velvet with a minute catch. Jem flicked open the tiny catch. Inside were two scrubbed and polished pennies, one on top of the other. Jem examined them.

"Indian-heads," he said. "Nineteen-six and Scout, one of 'em's nineteen-hundred. These are real old."

"Nineteen-hundred," I echoed. "Say—"

"Hush a minute, I'm thinkin'."

"Jem, you reckon that's somebody's hidin' place?"

"Naw, don't anybody much but us pass by there, unless it's some grown person's—"

"Grown folks don't have hidin' places. You reckon we ought to keep 'em, Jem?"

"I don't know what we could do, Scout. Who'd we give 'em back to? I know for a fact don't anybody go by there—Cecil goes by the back street an' all the way around by town to get home."

Cecil Jacobs, who lived at the far end of our street next door to the post office, walked a total of one mile per school day to avoid the Radley Place and old Mrs. Henry Lafayette Dubose. Mrs. Dubose lived two doors up the street from us; neighborhood opinion was unanimous that Mrs. Dubose was the meanest old woman who ever lived. Jem wouldn't go by her place without Atticus beside him.

"What you reckon we oughta do, Jem?"

Finders were keepers unless title was proven. Plucking an occasional camellia, getting a squirt of hot milk from Miss Maudie Atkinson's cow on a summer day, helping ourselves to someone's scuppernongs was part of our ethical culture, but money was different.

"Tell you what," said Jem. "We'll keep 'em till school starts, then go around and ask everybody if they're theirs. They're some bus child's, maybe—he was too taken up with gettin' outa school today an' forgot 'em. These are somebody's, I know that. See how they've been slicked up? They've been saved."

"Yeah, but why should somebody wanta put away chewing gum like that? You know it doesn't last."

"I don't know, Scout. But these are important to somebody. . . ."

"How's that, Jem . . . ?"

"Well, Indian-heads—well, they come from the Indians. They're real strong magic, they make you have good luck. Not like fried chicken when you're not lookin' for it, but things like long life 'n' good health, 'n' passin' six-weeks tests . . . these are real valuable to somebody. I'm gonna put 'em in my trunk."

Before Jem went to his room, he looked for a long time at the Radley Place. He seemed to be thinking again.

Two days later Dill arrived in a blaze of glory: he had
ridden the train by himself from Meridian to Maycomb Junction (a courtesy title—Maycomb Junction was in Abbott
County) where he had been met by Miss Rachel in Maycomb's one taxi; he had eaten dinner in the diner, he had
seen two twins hitched together get off the train in Bay St.
Louis and stuck to his story regardless of threats. He had
discarded the abominable blue shorts that were buttoned to
his shirts and wore real short pants with a belt; he was somewhat heavier, no taller, and said he had seen his father. Dill's
father was taller than ours, he had a black beard (pointed),
and was president of the L & N Railroad.

"I helped the engineer for a while," said Dill, yawning.

"In a pig's ear you did, Dill. Hush," said Jem. "What'll
we play today?"

"Tom and Sam and Dick," said Dill. "Let's go in the
front yard." Dill wanted the Rover Boys because there were
three respectable parts. He was clearly tired of being our
character man.

"I'm tired of those," I said. I was tired of playing Tom
Rover, who suddenly lost his memory in the middle of a
picture show and was out of the script until the end, when
he was found in Alaska.

"Make us up one, Jem," I said.

"I'm tired of makin' 'em up."

Our first days of freedom, and we were tired. I wondered
what the summer would bring.

We had strolled to the front yard, where Dill stood looking
down the street at the dreary face of the Radley Place. "I—
smell—death," he said. "I do, I mean it," he said, when I
told him to shut up.

"You mean when somebody's dyin' you can smell it?"

"No, I mean I can smell somebody an' tell if they're gonna
die. An old lady taught me how." Dill leaned over and sniffed
me. "Jean—Louise—Finch, you are going to die in three
days."

"Dill if you don't hush I'll knock you bowlegged. I mean
it, now—"

"Yawl hush," growled Jem, "you act like you believe in
Hot Steams."

"You act like you don't," I said.

"What's a Hot Steam?" asked Dill.

"Haven't you ever walked along a lonesome road at night and passed by a hot place?" Jem asked Dill. "A Hot Steam's somebody who can't get to heaven, just wallows around on lonesome roads an' if you walk through him, when you die you'll be one too, an' you'll go around at night suckin' people's breath—"

"How can you keep from passing through one?"

"You can't," said Jem. "Sometimes they stretch all the way across the road, but if you hafta go through one you say, 'Angel-bright, life-in-death; get off the road, don't suck my breath.' That keeps 'em from wrapping around you—"

"Don't you believe a word he says, Dill," I said. "Calpurnia says that's nigger-talk."

Jem scowled darkly at me, but said, "Well, are we gonna play anything or not?"

"Let's roll in the tire," I suggested.

Jem sighed. "You know I'm too big."

"You c'n push."

I ran to the back yard and pulled an old car tire from under the house. I slapped it up to the front yard. "I'm first," I said.

Dill said he ought to be first, he just got here.

Jem arbitrated, awarded me first push with an extra time for Dill, and I folded myself inside the tire.

Until it happened I did not realize that Jem was offended by my contradicting him on Hot Steams, and that he was patiently awaiting an opportunity to reward me. He did, by pushing the tire down the sidewalk with all the force in his body. Ground, sky and houses melted into a mad palette, my ears throbbed, I was suffocating. I could not put out my hands to stop, they were wedged between my chest and knees. I could only hope that Jem would outrun the tire and me, or that I would be stopped by a bump in the sidewalk. I heard him behind me, chasing and shouting.

The tire bumped on gravel, skeetered across the road, crashed into a barrier and popped me like a cork onto pavement. Dizzy and nauseated, I lay on the cement and shook my head still, pounded my ears to silence, and heard Jem's voice: "Scout, get away from there, come on!"

I raised my head and stared at the Radley Place steps in front of me. I froze.

"Come on, Scout, don't just lie there!" Jem was screaming. "Get up, can'tcha?"

I got to my feet, trembling as I thawed.

"Get the tire!" Jem hollered. "Bring it with you! Ain't you got any sense at all?"

When I was able to navigate, I ran back to them as fast as my shaking knees would carry me.

"Why didn't you bring it?" Jem yelled.

"Why don't *you* get it?" I screamed.

Jem was silent.

"Go on, it ain't far inside the gate. Why, you even touched the house once, remember?"

Jem looked at me furiously, could not decline, ran down the sidewalk, treaded water at the gate, then dashed in and retrieved the tire.

"See there?" Jem was scowling triumphantly. "Nothin' to it. I swear, Scout, sometimes you act so much like a girl it's mortifyin'."

There was more to it than he knew, but I decided not to tell him.

Calpurnia appeared in the front door and yelled, "Lemonade time! You all get in outa that hot sun 'fore you fry alive!" Lemonade in the middle of the morning was a summertime ritual. Calpurnia set a pitcher and three glasses on the porch, then went about her business. Being out of Jem's good graces did not worry me especially. Lemonade would restore his good humor.

Jem gulped down his second glassful and slapped his chest. "I know what we are going to play," he announced. "Something new, something different."

"What?" asked Dill.

"Boo Radley."

Jem's head at times was transparent: he had thought that up to make me understand he wasn't afraid of Radleys in any shape or form, to contrast his own fearless heroism with my cowardice.

"Boo Radley? How?" asked Dill.

Jem said, "Scout, you can be Mrs. Radley——"

"I declare if I will. I don't think——"

" 'Smatter?" said Dill. "Still scared?"

"He can get out at night when we're all asleep. . . ." I said.

Jem hissed. "Scout, how's he gonna know what we're doin'? Besides, I don't think he's still there. He died years ago and they stuffed him up the chimney."

Dill said, "Jem, you and me can play and Scout can watch if she's scared."

I was fairly sure Boo Radley was inside that house, but I couldn't prove it, and felt it best to keep my mouth shut or I would be accused of believing in Hot Steams, phenomena I was immune to in the daytime.

Jem parceled out our roles: I was Mrs. Radley, and all I had to do was come out and sweep the porch. Dill was old Mr. Radley: he walked up and down the sidewalk and coughed when Jem spoke to him. Jem, naturally, was Boo: he went under the front steps and shrieked and howled from time to time.

As the summer progressed, so did our game. We polished and perfected it, added dialogue and plot until we had manufactured a small play upon which we rang changes every day.

Dill was a villain's villain: he could get into any character part assigned him, and appear tall if height was part of the devilry required. He was as good as his worst performance; his worst performance was Gothic. I reluctantly played assorted ladies who entered the script. I never thought it as much fun as Tarzan, and I played that summer with more than vague anxiety despite Jem's assurances that Boo Radley was dead and nothing would get me, with him and Calpurnia there in the daytime and Atticus home at night.

Jem was a born hero.

It was a melancholy little drama, woven from bits and scraps of gossip and neighborhood legend: Mrs. Radley had been beautiful until she married Mr. Radley and lost all her money. She also lost most of her teeth, her hair, and her right forefinger (Dill's contribution. Boo bit it off one night when he couldn't find any cats and squirrels to eat.); she sat in the livingroom and cried most of the time, while Boo slowly whittled away all the furniture in the house.

The three of us were the boys who got into trouble; I was

the probate judge, for a change; Dill led Jem away and crammed him beneath the steps, poking him with the brush-broom. Jem would reappear as needed in the shapes of the sheriff, assorted townsfolk, and Miss Stephanie Crawford, who had more to say about the Radleys than anybody in Maycomb.

When it was time to play Boo's big scene, Jem would sneak into the house, steal the scissors from the sewing-machine drawer when Calpurnia's back was turned, then sit in the swing and cut up newspapers. Dill would walk by, cough at Jem, and Jem would fake a plunge into Dill's thigh. From where I stood it looked real.

When Mr. Nathan Radley passed us on his daily trip to town, we would stand still and silent until he was out of sight, then wonder what he would do to us if he suspected. Our activities halted when any of the neighbors appeared, and once I saw Miss Maudie Atkinson staring across the street at us, her hedge clippers poised in midair.

One day we were so busily playing Chapter XXV, Book II of One Man's Family, we did not see Atticus standing on the sidewalk looking at us, slapping a rolled magazine against his knee. The sun said twelve noon.

"What are you all playing?" he asked.

"Nothing," said Jem.

Jem's evasion told me our game was a secret, so I kept quiet.

"What are you doing with those scissors, then? Why are you tearing up that newspaper? If it's today's I'll tan you."

"Nothing."

"Nothing what?" said Atticus.

"Nothing, sir."

"Give me those scissors," Atticus said. "They're no things to play with. Does this by any chance have anything to do with the Radleys?"

"No sir," said Jem, reddening.

"I hope it doesn't," he said shortly, and went inside the house.

"Je-m . . ."

"Shut up! He's gone in the livingroom, he can hear us in there."

Safely in the yard, Dill asked Jem if we could play any more.

"I don't know. Atticus didn't say we couldn't—"

"Jem," I said, "I think Atticus knows it anyway."

"No he don't. If he did he'd say he did."

I was not so sure, but Jem told me I was being a girl, that girls always imagined things, that's why other people hated them so, and if I started behaving like one I could just go off and find some to play with.

"All right, you just keep it up then," I said. "You'll find out."

Atticus's arrival was the second reason I wanted to quit the game. The first reason happened the day I rolled into the Radley front yard. Through all the head-shaking, quelling of nausea and Jem-yelling, I had heard another sound, so low I could not have heard it from the sidewalk. Someone inside the house was laughing.

5

My nagging got the better of Jem eventually, as I knew it would, and to my relief we slowed down the game for a while. He still maintained, however, that Atticus hadn't said we couldn't, therefore we could; and if Atticus ever said we couldn't, Jem had thought of a way around it: he would simply change the names of the characters and then we couldn't be accused of playing anything.

Dill was in hearty agreement with this plan of action. Dill was becoming something of a trial anyway, following Jem about. He had asked me earlier in the summer to marry him, then he promptly forgot about it. He staked me out, marked as his property, said I was the only girl he would ever love, then he neglected me. I beat him up twice but it did no good, he only grew closer to Jem. They spent days together in the treehouse plotting and planning, calling me only when they needed a third party. But I kept aloof from their more fool-hardy schemes for a while, and on pain of being called a girl, I spent most of the remaining twilights that summer sitting with Miss Maudie Atkinson on her front porch.

Jem and I had always enjoyed the free run of Miss Maudie's yard if we kept out of her azaleas, but our contact with her was not clearly defined. Until Jem and Dill excluded me from their plans, she was only another lady in the neighborhood, but a relatively benign presence.

Our tacit treaty with Miss Maudie was that we could play on her lawn, eat her scuppernongs if we didn't jump on the arbor, and explore her vast back lot, terms so generous we seldom spoke to her, so careful were we to preserve the delicate balance of our relationship, but Jem and Dill drove me closer to her with their behavior.

Miss Maudie hated her house: time spent indoors was time wasted. She was a widow, a chameleon lady who worked in her flower beds in an old straw hat and men's coveralls, but after her five o'clock bath she would appear on the porch and reign over the street in magisterial beauty.

She loved everything that grew in God's earth, even the weeds. With one exception. If she found a blade of nut grass in her yard it was like the Second Battle of the Marne: she swooped down upon it with a tin tub and subjected it to blasts from beneath with a poisonous substance she said was so powerful it'd kill us all if we didn't stand out of the way.

"Why can't you just pull it up?" I asked, after witnessing a prolonged campaign against a blade not three inches high.

"Pull it up, child, pull it up?" She picked up the limp sprout and squeezed her thumb up its tiny stalk. Microscopic grains oozed out. "Why, one sprig of nut grass can ruin a whole yard. Look here. When it comes fall this dries up and the wind blows it all over Maycomb County!" Miss Maudie's face likened such an occurrence unto an Old Testament pestilence.

Her speech was crisp for a Maycomb County inhabitant. She called us by all our names, and when she grinned she revealed two minute gold prongs clipped to her eyeteeth. When I admired them and hoped I would have some even-tually, she said, "Look here." With a click of her tongue she thrust out her bridgework, a gesture of cordiality that cemented our friendship.

Miss Maudie's benevolence extended to Jem and Dill, whenever they paused in their pursuits: we reaped the benefits of a talent Miss Maudie had hitherto kept hidden from us. She made the best cakes in the neighborhood. When she was admitted into our confidence, every time she baked she made a big cake and three little ones, and she would call across the street: "Jem Finch, Scout Finch, Charles Baker Harris, come here!" Our promptness was always rewarded.

In summertime, twilights are long and peaceful. Often as not, Miss Maudie and I would sit silently on her porch, watching the sky go from yellow to pink as the sun went down, watching flights of martins sweep low over the neighborhood and disappear behind the schoolhouse rooftops.

"Miss Maudie," I said one evening, "do you think Boo Radley's still alive?"

"His name's Arthur and he's alive," she said. She was rocking slowly in her big oak chair. "Do you smell my mimosa? It's like angels' breath this evening."

"Yessum. How do you know?"

"Know what, child?"

"That B——Mr. Arthur's still alive?"

"What a morbid question. But I suppose it's a morbid subject. I know he's alive, Jean Louise, because I haven't seen him carried out yet."

"Maybe he died and they stuffed him up the chimney."

"Where did you get such a notion?"

"That's what Jem said he thought they did."

"S-ss-ss. He gets more like Jack Finch every day."

Miss Maudie had known Uncle Jack Finch, Atticus's brother, since they were children. Nearly the same age, they had grown up together at Finch's Landing. Miss Maudie was the daughter of a neighboring landowner, Dr. Frank Buford. Dr. Buford's profession was medicine and his obsession was anything that grew in the ground, so he stayed poor. Uncle Jack Finch confined his passion for digging to his window boxes in Nashville and stayed rich. We saw Uncle Jack every Christmas, and every Christmas he yelled across the street for Miss Maudie to come marry him. Miss Maudie would yell back, "Call a little louder, Jack Finch, and they'll hear you at the post office, I haven't heard you yet!" Jem and I thought this a strange way to ask for a lady's hand in marriage, but then Uncle Jack was rather strange. He said he was trying to get Miss Maudie's goat, that he had been trying unsuccessfully for forty years, that he was the last person in the world Miss Maudie would think about marrying but the first person she thought about teasing, and the best defense to her was spirited offense, all of which we understood clearly.

"Arthur Radley just stays in the house, that's all," said Miss Maudie. "Wouldn't you stay in the house if you didn't want to come out?"

"Yessum, but I'd wanta come out. Why doesn't he?"

Miss Maudie's eyes narrowed. "You know that story as well as I do."

"I never heard why, though. Nobody ever told me why."

Miss Maudie settled her bridgework. "You know old Mr. Radley was a foot-washing Baptist—"

"That's what you are, ain't it?"

"My shell's not that hard, child. I'm just a Baptist."

"Don't you all believe in foot-washing?"

"We do. At home in the bathtub."

"But we can't have communion with you all—"

Apparently deciding that it was easier to define primitive baptistry than closed communion, Miss Maudie said: "Foot-washers believe anything that's pleasure is a sin. Did you know some of 'em came out of the woods one Saturday and passed by this place and told me me and my flowers were going to hell?"

"Your flowers, too?"

"Yes ma'am. They'd burn right with me. They thought I spent too much time in God's outdoors and not enough time inside the house reading the Bible."

My confidence in pulpit Gospel lessened at the vision of Miss Maudie stewing forever in various Protestant hells. True enough, she had an acid tongue in her head, and she did not go about the neighborhood doing good, as did Miss Stephanie Crawford. But while no one with a grain of sense trusted Miss Stephanie, Jem and I had considerable faith in Miss Maudie. She had never told on us, had never played cat-and-mouse with us, she was not at all interested in our private lives. She was our friend. How so reasonable a creature could live in peril of everlasting torment was incomprehensible.

"That ain't right, Miss Maudie. You're the best lady I know."

Miss Maudie grinned. "Thank you ma'am. Thing is, foot-washers think women are a sin by definition. They take the Bible literally, you know."

"Is that why Mr. Arthur stays in the house, to keep away from women?"

"I've no idea."

"It doesn't make sense to me. Looks like if Mr. Arthur was hankerin' after heaven he'd come out on the porch at least. Atticus says God's loving folks like you love yourself—"

Miss Maudie stopped rocking, and her voice hardened. "You are too young to understand it," she said, "but sometimes the Bible in the hand of one man is worse than a whiskey bottle in the hand of—oh, of your father."

I was shocked. "Atticus doesn't drink whiskey," I said. "He never drunk a drop in his life—nome, yes he did. He said he drank some one time and didn't like it."

Miss Maudie laughed. "Wasn't talking about your father," she said. "What I meant was, if Atticus Finch drank until he was drunk he wouldn't be as hard as some men are at their best. There are just some kind of men who—who're so busy worrying about the next world they've never learned to live in this one, and you can look down the street and see the results."

"Do you think they're true, all those things they say about B—Mr. Arthur?"

"What things?"

I told her.

"That is three-fourths colored folks and one-fourth Stephanie Crawford," said Miss Maudie grimly. "Stephanie Crawford even told me once she woke up in the middle of the night and found him looking in the window at her. I said what did you do, Stephanie, move over in the bed and make room for him? That shut her up a while."

I was sure it did. Miss Maudie's voice was enough to shut anybody up.

"No, child," she said, "that is a sad house. I remember

Arthur Radley when he was a boy. He always spoke nicely to me, no matter what folks said he did. Spoke as nicely as he knew how."

"You reckon he's crazy?"

Miss Maudie shook her head. "If he's not he should be by now. The things that happen to people we never really know. What happens in houses behind closed doors, what secrets—"

"Atticus don't ever do anything to Jem and me in the house that he don't do in the yard," I said, feeling it my duty to defend my parent.

"Gracious child, I was raveling a thread, wasn't even thinking about your father, but now that I am I'll say this: Atticus Finch is the same in his house as he is on the public streets. How'd you like some fresh poundcake to take home?"

I liked it very much.

Next morning when I awakened I found Jem and Dill in the back yard deep in conversation. When I joined them, as usual they said go away.

"Will not. This yard's as much mine as it is yours, Jem Finch. I got just as much right to play in it as you have."

Dill and Jem emerged from a brief huddle: "If you stay you've got to do what we tell you," Dill warned.

"We-ll," I said, "who's so high and mighty all of a sudden?"

"If you don't say you'll do what we tell you, we ain't gonna tell you anything," Dill continued.

"You act like you grew ten inches in the night! All right, what is it?"

Jem said placidly, "We are going to give a note to Boo Radley."

"Just how?" I was trying to fight down the automatic terror rising in me. It was all right for Miss Maudie to talk—she was old and snug on her porch. It was different for us.

Jem was merely going to put the note on the end of a fishing pole and stick it through the shutters. If anyone came along, Dill would ring the bell.

Dill raised his right hand. In it was my mother's silver dinner-bell.

"I'm goin' around to the side of the house," said Jem.

"We looked yesterday from across the street, and there's a shutter loose. Think maybe I can make it stick on the window sill, at least."

"Jem—"

"Now you're in it and you can't get out of it, you'll just stay in it, Miss Priss!"

"Okay, okay, but I don't wanta watch. Jem, somebody was—"

"Yes you will, you'll watch the back end of the lot and Dill's gonna watch the front of the house an' up the street, an' if anybody comes he'll ring the bell. That clear?"

"All right then. What'd you write him?"

Dill said, "We're askin' him real politely to come out sometimes, and tell us what he does in there—we said we wouldn't hurt him and we'd buy him an ice cream."

"You all've gone crazy, he'll kill us!"

Dill said, "It's my idea. I figure if he'd come out and sit a spell with us he might feel better."

"How do you know he don't feel good?"

"Well how'd you feel if you'd been shut up for a hundred years with nothin' but cats to eat? I bet he's got a beard down to here—"

"Like your daddy's?"

"He ain't got a beard, he—" Dill stopped, as if trying to remember.

"Uh huh, caughtcha," I said. "You said 'fore you were off the train good your daddy had a black beard—"

"If it's all the same to you he shaved it off last summer! Yeah, an' I've got the letter to prove it—he sent me two dollars, too!"

"Keep on—I reckon he even sent you a mounted police uniform! That'n never showed up, did it? You just keep on tellin' 'em, son—"

Dill Harris could tell the biggest ones I ever heard. Among other things, he had been up in a mail plane seventeen times, he had been to Nova Scotia, he had seen an elephant, and his granddaddy was Brigadier General Joe Wheeler and left him his sword.

"You all hush," said Jem. He scuttled beneath the house and came out with a yellow bamboo pole. "Reckon this is long enough to reach from the sidewalk?"

"Anybody who's brave enough to go up and touch the house hadn't oughta use a fishin' pole," I said. "Why don't you just knock the front door down?"

"This—is—different," said Jem, "how many times do I have to tell you that?"

Dill took a piece of paper from his pocket and gave it to Jem. The three of us walked cautiously toward the old house. Dill remained at the light-pole on the front corner of the lot, and Jem and I edged down the sidewalk parallel to the side of the house. I walked beyond Jem and stood where I could see around the curve.

"All clear," I said. "Not a soul in sight."

Jem looked up the sidewalk to Dill, who nodded.

Jem attached the note to the end of the fishing pole, let the pole out across the yard and pushed it toward the window he had selected. The pole lacked several inches of being long enough, and Jem leaned over as far as he could. I watched him making jabbing motions for so long, I abandoned my post and went to him.

"Can't get it off the pole," he muttered, "or if I got it off I can't make it stay. G'on back down the street, Scout."

I returned and gazed around the curve at the empty road. Occasionally I looked back at Jem, who was patiently trying to place the note on the window sill. It would flutter to the ground and Jem would jab it up, until I thought if Boo Radley ever received it he wouldn't be able to read it. I was looking down the street when the dinner-bell rang.

Shoulder up, I reeled around to face Boo Radley and his bloody fangs; instead, I saw Dill ringing the bell with all his might in Atticus's face.

Jem looked so awful I didn't have the heart to tell him I told him so. He trudged along, dragging the pole behind him on the sidewalk.

Atticus said, "Stop ringing that bell."

Dill grabbed the clapper; in the silence that followed, I wished he'd start ringing it again. Atticus pushed his hat to the back of his head and put his hands on his hips. "Jem," he said, "what were you doing?"

"Nothin', sir."

"I don't want any of that. Tell me."

"I was—we were just tryin' to give somethin' to Mr. Radley."

"What were you trying to give him?"

"Just a letter."

"Let me see it."

Jem held out a filthy piece of paper. Atticus took it and tried to read it. "Why do you want Mr. Radley to come out?"

Dill said, "We thought he might enjoy us . . ." and dried up when Atticus looked at him.

"Son," he said to Jem, "I'm going to tell you something and tell you one time: stop tormenting that man. That goes for the other two of you."

What Mr. Radley did was his own business. If he wanted to come out, he would. If he wanted to stay inside his own house he had the right to stay inside free from the attentions of inquisitive children, which was a mild term for the likes of us. How would we like it if Atticus barged in on us without knocking, when we were in our rooms at night? We were, in effect, doing the same thing to Mr. Radley. What Mr. Radley did might seem peculiar to us, but it did not seem peculiar to him. Furthermore, had it never occurred to us that the civil way to communicate with another being was by the front door instead of a side window? Lastly, we were to stay away from that house until we were invited there, we were not to play an asinine game he had seen us playing or make fun of anybody on this street or in this town—

"We weren't makin' fun of him, we weren't laughin' at him," said Jem, "we were just—"

"So that was what you were doing, wasn't it?"

"Makin' fun of him?"

"No," said Atticus, "putting his life's history on display for the edification of the neighborhood."

Jem seemed to swell a little. "I didn't say we were doin' that, I didn't say it!"

Atticus grinned dryly. "You just told me," he said. "You stop this nonsense right now, every one of you."

Jem gaped at him.

"You want to be a lawyer, don't you?" Our father's mouth was suspiciously firm, as if he were trying to hold it in line.

Jem decided there was no point in quibbling, and was

silent. When Atticus went inside the house to retrieve a file he had forgotten to take to work that morning, Jem finally realized that he had been done in by the oldest lawyer's trick on record. He waited a respectful distance from the front steps, watched Atticus leave the house and walk toward town. When Atticus was out of earshot Jem yelled after him: "I thought I wanted to be a lawyer but I ain't so sure now!"

6

"Yes," said our father, when Jem asked him if we could go over and sit by Miss Rachel's fishpool with Dill, as this was his last night in Maycomb. "Tell him so long for me, and we'll see him next summer."

We leaped over the low wall that separated Miss Rachel's yard from our driveway. Jem whistled bob-white and Dill answered in the darkness.

"Not a breath blowing," said Jem. "Looka yonder."

He pointed to the east. A gigantic moon was rising behind Miss Maudie's pecan trees. "That makes it seem hotter," he said.

"Cross in it tonight?" asked Dill, not looking up. He was constructing a cigarette from newspaper and string.

"No, just the lady. Don't light that thing, Dill, you'll stink up this whole end of town."

There was a lady in the moon in Maycomb. She sat at a dresser combing her hair.

"We're gonna miss you, boy," I said. "Reckon we better watch for Mr. Avery?"

Mr. Avery boarded across the street from Mrs. Henry Lafayette Dubose's house. Besides making change in the collection plate every Sunday, Mr. Avery sat on the porch every night until nine o'clock and sneezed. One evening we were privileged to witness a performance by him which seemed to have been his positively last, for he never did it again so long as we watched. Jem and I were leaving Miss Rachel's front

steps one night when Dill stopped us: "Golly, looka yonder."
He pointed across the street. At first we saw nothing but a
kudzu-covered front porch, but a closer inspection revealed
an arc of water descending from the leaves and splashing in
the yellow circle of the street light, some ten feet from source
to earth, it seemed to us. Jem said Mr. Avery misfigured,
Dill said he must drink a gallon a day, and the ensuing contest
to determine relative distances and respective prowess only
made me feel left out again, as I was untalented in this area.

Dill stretched, yawned, and said altogether too casually,
"I know what, let's go for a walk."

He sounded fishy to me. Nobody in Maycomb just went
for a walk. "Where to, Dill?"

Dill jerked his head in a southerly direction.

Jem said, "Okay." When I protested, he said sweetly,
"You don't have to come along, Angel May."

"You don't have to go. Remember—"

Jem was not one to dwell on past defeats: it seemed the
only message he got from Atticus was insight into the art of
cross examination. "Scout, we ain't gonna do anything,
we're just goin' to the street light and back."

We strolled silently down the sidewalk, listening to porch
swings creaking with the weight of the neighborhood, listening to the soft night-murmurs of the grown people on our
street. Occasionally we heard Miss Stephanie Crawford
laugh.

"Well?" said Dill.

"Okay," said Jem. "Why don't you go on home, Scout?"

"What are you gonna do?"

Dill and Jem were simply going to peep in the window with
the loose shutter to see if they could get a look at Boo Radley,
and if I didn't want to go with them I could go straight home
and keep my fat flopping mouth shut, that was all.

"But what in the sam holy hill did you wait till tonight?"

Because nobody could see them at night, because Atticus
would be so deep in a book he wouldn't hear the Kingdom
coming, because if Boo Radley killed them they'd miss school
instead of vacation, and because it was easier to see inside
a dark house in the dark than in the daytime, did I understand?

"Jem, *please*—"

"Scout, I'm tellin' you for the last time, shut your trap or go home—I declare to the Lord you're gettin' more like a girl every day!''

With that, I had no option but to join them. We thought it was better to go under the high wire fence at the rear of the Radley lot, we stood less chance of being seen. The fence enclosed a large garden and a narrow wooden outhouse.

Jem held up the bottom wire and motioned Dill under it. I followed, and held up the wire for Jem. It was a tight squeeze for him. ''Don't make a sound,'' he whispered. ''Don't get in a row of collards whatever you do, they'll wake the dead.''

With this thought in mind, I made perhaps one step per minute. I moved faster when I saw Jem far ahead beckoning in the moonlight. We came to the gate that divided the garden from the back yard. Jem touched it. The gate squeaked.

''Spit on it,'' whispered Dill.

''You've got us in a box, Jem,'' I muttered. ''We can't get out of here so easy.''

''Sh-h. Spit on it, Scout.''

We spat ourselves dry, and Jem opened the gate slowly, lifting it aside and resting it on the fence. We were in the back yard.

The back of the Radley house was less inviting than the front: a ramshackle porch ran the width of the house; there were two doors and two dark windows between the doors. Instead of a column, a rough two-by-four supported one end of the roof. An old Franklin stove sat in a corner of the porch; above it a hat-rack mirror caught the moon and shone eerily.

''Ar-r,'' said Jem softly, lifting his foot.

'' 'Smatter?''

''Chickens,'' he breathed.

That we would be obliged to dodge the unseen from all directions was confirmed when Dill ahead of us spelled G-o-d in a whisper. We crept to the side of the house, around to the window with the hanging shutter. The sill was several inches taller than Jem.

''Give you a hand up,'' he muttered to Dill. ''Wait, though.'' Jem grabbed his left wrist and my right wrist, I grabbed my left wrist and Jem's right wrist, we crouched, and Dill sat on our saddle. We raised him and he caught the window sill.

"Hurry," Jem whispered, "we can't last much longer."

Dill punched my shoulder, and we lowered him to the ground.

"What'd you see?"

"Nothing. Curtains. There's a little teeny light way off somewhere, though."

"Let's get away from here," breathed Jem. "Let's go 'round in back again. Sh-h," he warned me, as I was about to protest.

"Let's try the back window."

"Dill, *no*," I said.

Dill stopped and let Jem go ahead. When Jem put his foot on the bottom step, the step squeaked. He stood still, then tried his weight by degrees. The step was silent. Jem skipped two steps, put his foot on the porch, heaved himself to it, and teetered a long moment. He regained his balance and dropped to his knees. He crawled to the window, raised his head and looked in.

Then I saw the shadow. It was the shadow of a man with a hat on. At first I thought it was a tree, but there was no wind blowing, and tree-trunks never walked. The back porch was bathed in moonlight, and the shadow, crisp as toast, moved across the porch toward Jem.

Dill saw it next. He put his hands to his face.

When it crossed Jem, Jem saw it. He put his arms over his head and went rigid.

The shadow stopped about a foot beyond Jem. Its arm came out from its side, dropped, and was still. Then it turned and moved back across Jem, walked along the porch and off the side of the house, returning as it had come.

Jem leaped off the porch and galloped toward us. He flung open the gate, danced Dill and me through, and shooed us between two rows of swishing collards. Halfway through the collards I tripped; as I tripped the roar of a shotgun shattered the neighborhood.

Dill and Jem dived beside me. Jem's breath came in sobs: "Fence by the schoolyard!—hurry, Scout!"

Jem held the bottom wire; Dill and I rolled through and were halfway to the shelter of the schoolyard's solitary oak when we sensed that Jem was not with us. We ran back and found him struggling in the fence, kicking his pants off to get loose. He ran to the oak tree in his shorts.

Safely behind it, we gave way to numbness, but Jem's mind was racing: "We gotta get home, they'll miss us."

We ran across the schoolyard, crawled under the fence to Deer's Pasture behind our house, climbed our back fence and were at the back steps before Jem would let us pause to rest.

Respiration normal, the three of us strolled as casually as we could to the front yard. We looked down the street and saw a circle of neighbors at the Radley front gate.

"We better go down there," said Jem. "They'll think it's funny if we don't show up."

Mr. Nathan Radley was standing inside his gate, a shotgun broken across his arm. Atticus was standing beside Miss Maudie and Miss Stephanie Crawford. Miss Rachel and Mr. Avery were near by. None of them saw us come up.

We eased in beside Miss Maudie, who looked around. "Where were you all, didn't you hear the commotion?"

"What happened?" asked Jem.

"Mr. Radley shot at a Negro in his collard patch."

"Oh. Did he hit him?"

"No," said Miss Stephanie. "Shot in the air. Scared him pale, though. Says if anybody sees a white nigger around, that's the one. Says he's got the other barrel waitin' for the next sound he hears in that patch, an' next time he won't aim high, be it dog, nigger, or—Jem *Finch*!"

"Ma'am?" asked Jem.

Atticus spoke. "Where're your pants, son?"

"Pants, sir?"

"Pants."

It was no use. In his shorts before God and everybody. I sighed.

"Ah—Mr. Finch?"

In the glare from the streetlight, I could see Dill hatching one: his eyes widened, his fat cherub face grew rounder.

"What is it, Dill?" asked Atticus.

"Ah—I won 'em from him," he said vaguely.

"Won them? How?"

Dill's hand sought the back of his head. He brought it forward and across his forehead. "We were playin' strip poker up yonder by the fishpool," he said.

Jem and I relaxed. The neighbors seemed satisfied: they all stiffened. But what was strip poker?

We had no chance to find out: Miss Rachel went off like the town fire siren: "Do-o-o Jee-sus, Dill Harris! Gamblin' by my fishpool? I'll strip-poker you, sir!"

Atticus saved Dill from immediate dismemberment. "Just a minute, Miss Rachel," he said. "I've never heard of 'em doing that before. Were you all playing cards?"

Jem fielded Dill's fly with his eyes shut: "No sir, just with matches."

I admired my brother. Matches were dangerous, but cards were fatal.

"Jem, Scout," said Atticus, "I don't want to hear of poker in any form again. Go by Dill's and get your pants, Jem. Settle it yourselves."

"Don't worry, Dill," said Jem, as we trotted up the side-walk, "she ain't gonna get you. He'll talk her out of it. That was fast thinkin', son. Listen . . . you hear?"

We stopped, and heard Atticus's voice: ". . . not serious . . . they all go through it, Miss Rachel. . . ."

Dill was comforted, but Jem and I weren't. There was the problem of Jem showing up some pants in the morning.

" 'd give you some of mine," said Dill, as we came to Miss Rachel's steps. Jem said he couldn't get in them, but thanks anyway. We said good-bye, and Dill went inside the house. He evidently remembered he was engaged to me, for he ran back out and kissed me swiftly in front of Jem. "Yawl write, hear?" he bawled after us.

Had Jem's pants been safely on him, we would not have slept much anyway. Every night-sound I heard from my cot on the back porch was magnified three-fold; every scratch of feet on gravel was Boo Radley seeking revenge, every passing Negro laughing in the night was Boo Radley loose and after us; insects splashing against the screen were Boo Radley's insane fingers picking the wire to pieces; the chinaberry trees were malignant, hovering, alive. I lingered between sleep and wakefulness until I heard Jem murmur.

"Sleep, Little Three-Eyes?"

"Are you crazy?"

"Sh-h. Atticus's light's out."

In the waning moonlight I saw Jem swing his feet to the floor.

"I'm goin' after 'em," he said.

I sat upright. "You can't. I won't let you."

He was struggling into his shirt. "I've got to."

"You do an' I'll wake up Atticus."

"You do and I'll kill you."

I pulled him down beside me on the cot. I tried to reason with him. "Mr. Nathan's gonna find 'em in the morning, Jem. He knows you lost 'em. When he shows 'em to Atticus it'll be pretty bad, that's all there is to it. Go'n back to bed."

"That's what I know," said Jem. "That's why I'm goin' after 'em."

I began to feel sick. Going back to that place by himself —I remembered Miss Stephanie: Mr. Nathan had the other barrel waiting for the next sound he heard, be it nigger, dog . . . Jem knew that better than I.

I was desperate: "Look, it ain't worth it, Jem. A lickin' hurts but it doesn't last. You'll get your head shot off, Jem. Please . . ."

He blew out his breath patiently. "I—it's like this, Scout," he muttered. "Atticus ain't ever whipped me since I can remember. I wanta keep it that way."

This was a thought. It seemed that Atticus threatened us every other day. "You mean he's never caught you at anything."

"Maybe so, but—I just wanta keep it that way, Scout. We shouldn'a done that tonight, Scout."

It was then, I suppose, that Jem and I first began to part company. Sometimes I did not understand him, but my periods of bewilderment were short-lived. This was beyond me. "Please," I pleaded, "can'tcha just think about it for a minute—by yourself on that place—"

"Shut up!"

"It's not like he'd never speak to you again or somethin' . . . I'm gonna wake him up, Jem, I swear I am—"

Jem grabbed my pajama collar and wrenched it tight. "Then I'm goin' with you—" I choked.

"No you ain't, you'll just make noise."

It was no use. I unlatched the back door and held it while he crept down the steps. It must have been two o'clock. The moon was setting and the lattice-work shadows were fading into fuzzy nothingness. Jem's white shirt-tail dipped and bobbed like a small ghost dancing away to escape the coming morning. A faint breeze stirred and cooled the sweat running down my sides.

He went the back way, through Deer's Pasture, across the schoolyard and around to the fence, I thought—at least that was the way he was headed. It would take longer, so it was not time to worry yet. I waited until it was time to worry and listened for Mr. Radley's shotgun. Then I thought I heard the back fence squeak. It was wishful thinking.

Then I heard Atticus cough. I held my breath. Sometimes when we made a midnight pilgrimage to the bathroom we would find him reading. He said he often woke up during the night, checked on us, and read himself back to sleep. I waited for his light to go on, straining my eyes to see it flood the hall. It stayed off, and I breathed again.

The night-crawlers had retired, but ripe chinaberries drummed on the roof when the wind stirred, and the darkness was desolate with the barking of distant dogs.

There he was, returning to me. His white shirt bobbed over the back fence and slowly grew larger. He came up the back steps, latched the door behind him, and sat on his cot. Wordlessly, he held up his pants. He lay down, and for a while I heard his cot trembling. Soon he was still. I did not hear him stir again.

7

Jem stayed moody and silent for a week. As Atticus had once advised me to do, I tried to climb into Jem's skin and walk around in it: if I had gone alone to the Radley Place at two in the morning, my funeral would have been held the next afternoon. So I left Jem alone and tried not to bother him.

School started. The second grade was as bad as the first,

only worse—they still flashed cards at you and wouldn't let you read or write. Miss Caroline's progress next door could be estimated by the frequency of laughter; however, the usual crew had flunked the first grade again, and were helpful in keeping order. The only thing good about the second grade was that this year I had to stay as late as Jem, and we usually walked home together at three o'clock.

One afternoon when we were crossing the schoolyard toward home, Jem suddenly said: "There's something I didn't tell you."

As this was his first complete sentence in several days, I encouraged him: "About what?"

"About that night."

"You've never told me anything about that night," I said.

Jem waved my words away as if fanning gnats. He was silent for a while, then he said, "When I went back for my breeches—they were all in a tangle when I was gettin' out of 'em, I couldn't get 'em loose. When I went back—" Jem took a deep breath. "When I went back, they were folded across the fence . . . like they were expectin' me."

"Across—"

"And something else—" Jem's voice was flat. "Show you when we get home. They'd been sewed up. Not like a lady sewed 'em, like somethin' I'd try to do. All crooked. It's almost like—"

"—somebody knew you were comin' back for 'em."

Jem shuddered. "Like somebody was readin' my mind . . . like somebody could tell what I was gonna do. Can't anybody tell what I'm gonna do lest they know me, can they, Scout?"

Jem's question was an appeal. I reassured him: "Can't anybody tell what you're gonna do lest they live in the house with you, and even I can't tell sometimes."

We were walking past our tree. In its knot-hole rested a ball of gray twine.

"Don't take it, Jem," I said. "This is somebody's hidin' place."

"I don't think so, Scout."

"Yes it is. Somebody like Walter Cunningham comes down here every recess and hides his things—and we come along and take 'em away from him. Listen, let's leave it and wait a couple of days. If it ain't gone then, we'll take it, okay?"

"Okay, you might be right," said Jem. "It must be some little kid's place—hides his things from the bigger folks. You know it's only when school's in that we've found things."

"Yeah," I said, "but we never go by here in the summertime."

We went home. Next morning the twine was where we had left it. When it was still there on the third day, Jem pocketed it. From then on, we considered everything we found in the knot-hole our property.

The second grade was grim, but Jem assured me that the older I got the better school would be, that he started off the same way, and it was not until one reached the sixth grade that one learned anything of value. The sixth grade seemed to please him from the beginning: he went through a brief Egyptian Period that baffled me—he tried to walk flat a great deal, sticking one arm in front of him and one in back of him, putting one foot behind the other. He declared Egyptians walked that way; I said if they did I didn't see how they got anything done, but Jem said they accomplished more than the Americans ever did, they invented toilet paper and perpetual embalming, and asked where would we be today if they hadn't? Atticus told me to delete the adjectives and I'd have the facts.

There are no clearly defined seasons in South Alabama; summer drifts into autumn, and autumn is sometimes never followed by winter, but turns to a days-old spring that melts into summer again. That fall was a long one, hardly cool enough for a light jacket. Jem and I were trotting in our orbit one mild October afternoon when our knot-hole stopped us again. Something white was inside this time.

Jem let me do the honors: I pulled out two small images carved in soap. One was the figure of a boy, the other wore a crude dress.

Before I remembered that there was no such thing as hoodooing, I shrieked and threw them down.

Jem snatched them up. "What's the matter with you?" he yelled. He rubbed the figures free of red dust. "These are good," he said. "I've never seen any these good."

He held them down to me. They were almost perfect miniatures of two children. The boy had on shorts, and a shock of soapy hair fell to his eyebrows. I looked up at Jem. A point of straight brown hair kicked downwards from his part. I had never noticed it before.

Jem looked from the girl-doll to me. The girl-doll wore bangs. So did I.

"These are us," he said.

"Who did 'em, you reckon?"

"Who do we know around here who whittles?" he asked.

"Mr. Avery."

"Mr. Avery just does like this. I mean carves."

Mr. Avery averaged a stick of stovewood per week; he honed it down to a toothpick and chewed it.

"There's old Miss Stephanie Crawford's sweetheart," I said.

"He carves all right, but he lives down the country. When would he ever pay any attention to us?"

"Maybe he sits on the porch and looks at us instead of Miss Stephanie. If I was him, I would."

Jem stared at me so long I asked what was the matter, but got Nothing, Scout for an answer. When we went home, Jem put the dolls in his trunk.

Less than two weeks later we found a whole package of chewing gum, which we enjoyed, the fact that everything on the Radley Place was poison having slipped Jem's memory.

The following week the knot-hole yielded a tarnished medal. Jem showed it to Atticus, who said it was a spelling medal, that before we were born the Maycomb County schools had spelling contests and awarded medals to the winners. Atticus said someone must have lost it, and had we asked around? Jem camel-kicked me when I tried to say where we had found it. Jem asked Atticus if he remembered anybody who ever won one, and Atticus said no.

Our biggest prize appeared four days later. It was a pocket watch that wouldn't run, on a chain with an aluminum knife.

"You reckon it's white gold, Jem?"

"Don't know. I'll show it to Atticus."

Atticus said it would probably be worth ten dollars, knife, chain and all, if it were new. "Did you swap with somebody at school?" he asked.

"Oh, no sir!" Jem pulled out his grandfather's watch that Atticus let him carry once a week if Jem were careful with it. On the days he carried the watch, Jem walked on eggs. "Atticus, if it's all right with you, I'd rather have this one instead. Maybe I can fix it."

When the new wore off his grandfather's watch, and carrying it became a day's burdensome task, Jem no longer felt the necessity of ascertaining the hour every five minutes.

He did a fair job, only one spring and two tiny pieces left over, but the watch would not run. "Oh-h," he sighed, "it'll never go. Scout—?"

"Huh?"

"You reckon we oughta write a letter to whoever's leaving us these things?"

"That'd be right nice, Jem, we can thank 'em—what's wrong?"

Jem was holding his ears, shaking his head from side to side. "I don't get it, I just don't get it—I don't know why, Scout . . ." He looked toward the livingroom. "I've gotta good mind to tell Atticus—no, I reckon not."

"I'll tell him for you."

"No, don't do that, Scout. Scout?"

"Wha-t?"

He had been on the verge of telling me something all evening; his face would brighten and he would lean toward me, then he would change his mind. He changed it again. "Oh, nothin'."

"Here, let's write a letter." I pushed a tablet and pencil under his nose.

"Okay. Dear Mister . . ."

"How do you know it's a man? I bet it's Miss Maudie—been bettin' that for a long time."

"Ar-r, Miss Maudie can't chew gum—" Jem broke into a grin. "You know, she can talk real pretty sometimes. One time I asked her to have a chew and she said no thanks, that—chewing gum cleaved to her palate and rendered her speechless," said Jem carefully. "Doesn't that sound nice?"

"Yeah, she can say nice things sometimes. She wouldn't have a watch and chain anyway."

"Dear sir," said Jem. "We appreciate the—no, we appreciate everything which you have put into the tree for us. Yours very truly, Jeremy Atticus Finch."

"He won't know who you are if you sign it like that, Jem."

Jem erased his name and wrote, "Jem Finch." I signed, "Jean Louise Finch (Scout)," beneath it. Jem put the note in an envelope.

Next morning on the way to school he ran ahead of me and stopped at the tree. Jem was facing me when he looked up, and I saw him go stark white.

"Scout!"

I ran to him.

Someone had filled our knot-hole with cement.

"Don't you cry, now, Scout . . . don't cry now, don't you worry—" he muttered at me all the way to school.

When we went home for dinner Jem bolted his food, ran to the porch and stood on the steps. I followed him. "Hasn't passed by yet," he said.

Next day Jem repeated his vigil and was rewarded.

"Hidy do, Mr. Nathan," he said.

"Morning Jem, Scout," said Mr. Radley, as he went by.

"Mr. Radley," said Jem.

Mr. Radley turned around.

"Mr. Radley, ah—did you put cement in that hole in that tree down yonder?"

"Yes," he said. "I filled it up."

"Why'd you do it, sir?"

"Tree's dying. You plug 'em with cement when they're sick. You ought to know that, Jem."

Jem said nothing more about it until late afternoon. When we passed our tree he gave it a meditative pat on its cement, and remained deep in thought. He seemed to be working himself into a bad humor, so I kept my distance.

As usual, we met Atticus coming home from work that evening. When we were at our steps Jem said, "Atticus, look down yonder at that tree, please sir."

"What tree, son?"

"The one on the corner of the Radley lot comin' from school."

"Yes?"

"Is that tree dyin'?"

"Why no, son, I don't think so. Look at the leaves, they're all green and full, no brown patches anywhere—"

"It ain't even sick?"

"That tree's as healthy as you are, Jem. Why?"

"Mr. Nathan Radley said it was dyin'."

"Well maybe it is. I'm sure Mr. Radley knows more about his trees than we do."

Atticus left us on the porch. Jem leaned on a pillar, rubbing his shoulders against it.

"Do you itch, Jem?" I asked as politely as I could. He did not answer. "Come on in, Jem," I said.

"After while."

He stood there until nightfall, and I waited for him. When we went in the house I saw he had been crying; his face was dirty in the right places, but I thought it odd that I had not heard him.

8

For reasons unfathomable to the most experienced prophets in Maycomb County, autumn turned to winter that year. We had two weeks of the coldest weather since 1885, Atticus said. Mr. Avery said it was written on the Rosetta Stone that when children disobeyed their parents, smoked cigarettes and made war on each other, the seasons would change: Jem and I were burdened with the guilt of contributing to the aberrations of nature, thereby causing unhappiness to our neighbors and discomfort to ourselves.

Old Mrs. Radley died that winter, but her death caused hardly a ripple—the neighborhood seldom saw her, except when she watered her cannas. Jem and I decided that Boo had got her at last, but when Atticus returned from the Radley house he said she died of natural causes, to our disappointment.

"Ask him," Jem whispered.

"You ask him, you're the oldest."

"That's why you oughta ask him."

"Atticus," I said, "did you see Mr. Arthur?"

Atticus looked sternly around his newspaper at me: "I did not."

Jem restrained me from further questions. He said Atticus was still touchous about us and the Radleys and it wouldn't do to push him any. Jem had a notion that Atticus thought our activities that night last summer were not solely confined to strip poker. Jem had no firm basis for his ideas, he said it was merely a twitch.

Next morning I awoke, looked out the window and nearly died of fright. My screams brought Atticus from his bathroom half-shaven.

"The world's endin', Atticus! Please do something—!" I dragged him to the window and pointed.

"No it's not," he said. "It's snowing."

Jem asked Atticus would it keep up. Jem had never seen snow either, but he knew what it was. Atticus said he didn't know any more about snow than Jem did. "I think, though, if it's watery like that, it'll turn to rain."

The telephone rang and Atticus left the breakfast table to answer it. "That was Eula May," he said when he returned. "I quote—'As it has not snowed in Maycomb County since 1885, there will be no school today.' "

Eula May was Maycomb's leading telephone operator. She was entrusted with issuing public announcements, wedding invitations, setting off the fire siren, and giving first-aid instructions when Dr. Reynolds was away.

When Atticus finally called us to order and bade us look at our plates instead of out the windows, Jem asked, "How do you make a snowman?"

"I haven't the slightest idea," said Atticus. "I don't want you all to be disappointed, but I doubt if there'll be enough snow for a snowball, even."

Calpurnia came in and said she thought it was sticking.

When we ran to the back yard, it was covered with a feeble layer of soggy snow.

"We shouldn't walk about in it," said Jem. "Look, every step you take's wasting it."

I looked back at my mushy footprints. Jem said if we waited until it snowed some more we could scrape it all up for a snowman. I stuck out my tongue and caught a fat flake. It burned.

"Jem, it's hot!"

"No it ain't, it's so cold it burns. Now don't eat it, Scout, you're wasting it. Let it come down."

"But I want to walk in it."

"I know what, we can go walk over at Miss Maudie's."

Jem hopped across the front yard. I followed in his tracks. When we were on the sidewalk in front of Miss Maudie's, Mr. Avery accosted us. He had a pink face and a big stomach below his belt.

"See what you've done?" he said. "Hasn't snowed in Maycomb since Appomattox. It's bad children like you makes the seasons change."

I wondered if Mr. Avery knew how hopefully we had watched last summer for him to repeat his performance, and reflected that if this was our reward, there was something to say for sin. I did not wonder where Mr. Avery gathered his meteorological statistics: they came straight from the Rosetta Stone.

"Jem Finch, you Jem Finch!"

"Miss Maudie's callin' you, Jem."

"You all stay in the middle of the yard. There's some thrift buried under the snow near the porch. Don't step on it!"

"Yessum!" called Jem. "It's beautiful, ain't it, Miss Maudie?"

"Beautiful my hind foot! If it freezes tonight it'll carry off all my azaleas!"

Miss Maudie's old sunhat glistened with snow crystals. She was bending over some small bushes, wrapping them in burlap bags. Jem asked her what she was doing that for.

"Keep 'em warm," she said.

"How can flowers keep warm? They don't circulate."

"I cannot answer that question, Jem Finch. All I know is

if it freezes tonight these plants'll freeze, so you cover 'em up. Is that clear?''

"Yessum. Miss Maudie?"

"What, sir?"

"Could Scout and me borrow some of your snow?"

"Heavens alive, take it all! There's an old peach basket under the house, haul it off in that." Miss Maudie's eyes narrowed. "Jem Finch, what are you going to do with my snow?"

"You'll see," said Jem, and we transferred as much snow as we could from Miss Maudie's yard to ours, a slushy operation.

"What are we gonna do, Jem?" I asked.

"You'll see," he said. "Now get the basket and haul all the snow you can rake up from the back yard to the front. Walk back in your tracks, though," he cautioned.

"Are we gonna have a snow baby, Jem?"

"No, a real snowman. Gotta work hard, now."

Jem ran to the back yard, produced the garden hoe and began digging quickly behind the woodpile, placing any worms he found to one side. He went in the house, returned with the laundry hamper, filled it with earth and carried it to the front yard.

When we had five baskets of earth and two baskets of snow, Jem said we were ready to begin.

"Don't you think this is kind of a mess?" I asked.

"Looks messy now, but it won't later," he said.

Jem scooped up an armful of dirt, patted it into a mound on which he added another load, and another until he had constructed a torso.

"Jem, I ain't ever heard of a nigger snowman," I said.

"He won't be black long," he grunted.

Jem procured some peachtree switches from the back yard, plaited them, and bent them into bones to be covered with dirt.

"He looks like Stephanie Crawford with her hands on her hips," I said. "Fat in the middle and little-bitty arms."

"I'll make 'em bigger." Jem sloshed water over the mud man and added more dirt. He looked thoughtfully at it for a moment, then he molded a big stomach below the figure's waistline. Jem glanced at me, his eyes twinkling: "Mr. Avery's sort of shaped like a snowman, ain't he?"

Jem scooped up some snow and began plastering it on. He permitted me to cover only the back, saving the public parts for himself. Gradually Mr. Avery turned white.

Using bits of wood for eyes, nose, mouth, and buttons, Jem succeeded in making Mr. Avery look cross. A stick of stovewood completed the picture. Jem stepped back and viewed his creation.

"It's lovely, Jem," I said. "Looks almost like he'd talk to you."

"It is, ain't it?" he said shyly.

We could not wait for Atticus to come home for dinner, but called and said we had a big surprise for him. He seemed surprised when he saw most of the back yard in the front yard, but he said we had done a jim-dandy job. "I didn't know how you were going to do it," he said to Jem, "but from now on I'll never worry about what'll become of you, son, you'll always have an idea."

Jem's ears reddened from Atticus's compliment, but he looked up sharply when he saw Atticus stepping back. Atticus squinted at the snowman a while. He grinned, then laughed. "Son, I can't tell what you're going to be—an engineer, a lawyer, or a portrait painter. You've perpetrated a near libel here in the front yard. We've got to disguise this fellow."

Atticus suggested that Jem hone down his creation's front a little, swap a broom for the stovewood, and put an apron on him.

Jem explained that if he did, the snowman would become muddy and cease to be a snowman.

"I don't care what you do, so long as you do something," said Atticus. "You can't go around making caricatures of the neighbors."

"Ain't a characterture," said Jem. "It looks just like him."

"Mr. Avery might not think so."

"I know what!" said Jem. He raced across the street, disappeared into Miss Maudie's back yard and returned triumphant. He stuck her sunhat on the snowman's head and jammed her hedge-clippers into the crook of his arm. Atticus said that would be fine.

Miss Maudie opened her front door and came out on the porch. She looked across the street at us. Suddenly she grinned. "Jem Finch," she called. "You devil, bring me back my hat, sir!"

Jem looked up at Atticus, who shook his head. "She's just fussing," he said. "She's really impressed with your—accomplishments."

Atticus strolled over to Miss Maudie's sidewalk, where they engaged in an arm-waving conversation, the only phrase of which I caught was ". . . erected an absolute morphodite in that yard! Atticus, you'll never raise 'em!"

The snow stopped in the afternoon, the temperature dropped, and by nightfall Mr. Avery's direst predictions came true: Calpurnia kept every fireplace in the house blazing, but we were cold. When Atticus came home that evening he said we were in for it, and asked Calpurnia if she wanted to stay with us for the night. Calpurnia glanced up at the high ceilings and long windows and said she thought she'd be warmer at her house. Atticus drove her home in the car.

Before I went to sleep Atticus put more coal on the fire in my room. He said the thermometer registered sixteen, that it was the coldest night in his memory, and that our snowman outside was frozen solid.

Minutes later, it seemed, I was awakened by someone shaking me. Atticus's overcoat was spread across me. "Is it morning already?"

"Baby, get up."

Atticus was holding out my bathrobe and coat. "Put your robe on first," he said.

Jem was standing beside Atticus, groggy and tousled. He was holding his overcoat closed at the neck, his other hand was jammed into his pocket. He looked strangely overweight.

"Hurry, hon," said Atticus. "Here're your shoes and socks."

Stupidly, I put them on. "Is it morning?"

"No, it's a little after one. Hurry now."

That something was wrong finally got through to me. "What's the matter?"

By then he did not have to tell me. Just as the birds know

where to go when it rains, I knew when there was trouble in our street. Soft taffeta-like sounds and muffled scurrying sounds filled me with helpless dread.

"Whose is it?"

"Miss Maudie's, hon," said Atticus gently.

At the front door, we saw fire spewing from Miss Maudie's diningroom windows. As if to confirm what we saw, the town fire siren wailed up the scale to a treble pitch and remained there, screaming.

"It's gone, ain't it?" moaned Jem.

"I expect so," said Atticus. "Now listen, both of you. Go down and stand in front of the Radley Place. Keep out of the way, do you hear? See which way the wind's blowing?"

"Oh," said Jem. "Atticus, reckon we oughta start moving the furniture out?"

"Not yet, son. Do as I tell you. Run now. Take care of Scout, you hear? Don't let her out of your sight."

With a push, Atticus started us toward the Radley front gate. We stood watching the street fill with men and cars while fire silently devoured Miss Maudie's house. "Why don't they hurry, why don't they hurry . . ." muttered Jem.

We saw why. The old fire truck, killed by the cold, was being pushed from town by a crowd of men. When the men attached its hose to a hydrant, the hose burst and water shot up, tinkling down on the pavement.

"Oh-h Lord, Jem . . ."

Jem put his arm around me. "Hush, Scout," he said. "It ain't time to worry yet. I'll let you know when."

The men of Maycomb, in all degrees of dress and undress, took furniture from Miss Maudie's house to a yard across the street. I saw Atticus carrying Miss Maudie's heavy oak rocking chair, and thought it sensible of him to save what she valued most.

Sometimes we heard shouts. Then Mr. Avery's face appeared in an upstairs window. He pushed a mattress out the window into the street and threw down furniture until men shouted, "Come down from there, Dick! The stairs are going! Get outta there, Mr. Avery!"

Mr. Avery began climbing through the window.

"Scout, he's stuck . . ." breathed Jem. "Oh God . . ."

Mr. Avery was wedged tightly. I buried my head under Jem's arm and didn't look again until Jem cried, "He's got loose, Scout! He's all right!"

I looked up to see Mr. Avery cross the upstairs porch. He swung his legs over the railing and was sliding down a pillar when he slipped. He fell, yelled, and hit Miss Maudie's shrubbery.

Suddenly I noticed that the men were backing away from Miss Maudie's house, moving down the street toward us. They were no longer carrying furniture. The fire was well into the second floor and had eaten its way to the roof: window frames were black against a vivid orange center.

"Jem, it looks like a pumpkin—"

"Scout, look!"

Smoke was rolling off our house and Miss Rachel's house like fog off a riverbank, and men were pulling hoses toward them. Behind us, the fire truck from Abbottsville screamed around the curve and stopped in front of our house.

"That book . . ." I said.

"What?" said Jem.

"That Tom Swift book, it ain't mine, it's Dill's . . ."

"Don't worry, Scout, it ain't time to worry yet," said Jem. He pointed. "Looka yonder."

In a group of neighbors, Atticus was standing with his hands in his overcoat pockets. He might have been watching a football game. Miss Maudie was beside him.

"See there, he's not worried yet," said Jem.

"Why ain't he on top of one of the houses?"

"He's too old, he'd break his neck."

"You think we oughta make him get our stuff out?"

"Let's don't pester him, he'll know when it's time," said Jem.

The Abbottsville fire truck began pumping water on our house; a man on the roof pointed to places that needed it most. I watched our Absolute Morphodite go black and crumble; Miss Maudie's sunhat settled on top of the heap. I could not see her hedge-clippers. In the heat between our house, Miss Rachel's and Miss Maudie's, the men had long ago shed coats and bathrobes. They worked in pajama tops and nightshirts stuffed into their pants, but I became aware that I was slowly freezing where I stood. Jem tried to keep me warm, but his arm was not enough. I pulled free of it and clutched my shoulders. By dancing a little, I could feel my feet.

Another fire truck appeared and stopped in front of Miss Stephanie Crawford's. There was no hydrant for another hose, and the men tried to soak her house with hand extinguishers.

Miss Maudie's tin roof quelled the flames. Roaring, the house collapsed; fire gushed everywhere, followed by a flurry of blankets from men on top of the adjacent houses, beating out sparks and burning chunks of wood.

It was dawn before the men began to leave, first one by one, then in groups. They pushed the Maycomb fire truck back to town, the Abbottsville truck departed, the third one remained. We found out next day it had come from Clark's Ferry, sixty miles away.

Jem and I slid across the street. Miss Maudie was staring at the smoking black hole in her yard, and Atticus shook his head to tell us she did not want to talk. He led us home, holding onto our shoulders to cross the icy street. He said Miss Maudie would stay with Miss Stephanie for the time being.

"Anybody want some hot chocolate?" he asked. I shuddered when Atticus started a fire in the kitchen stove.

As we drank our cocoa I noticed Atticus looking at me, first with curiosity, then with sternness. "I thought I told you and Jem to stay put," he said.

"Why, we did. We stayed—"

"Then whose blanket is that?"

"Blanket?"

"Yes ma'am, blanket. It isn't ours."

I looked down and found myself clutching a brown woolen blanket I was wearing around my shoulders, squaw-fashion.

"Atticus, I don't know, sir . . . I—"

I turned to Jem for an answer, but Jem was even more bewildered than I. He said he didn't know how it got there, we did exactly as Atticus had told us, we stood down by the Radley gate away from everybody, we didn't move an inch —Jem stopped.

"Mr. Nathan was at the fire," he babbled, "I saw him, I saw him, he was tuggin' that mattress—Atticus, I swear . . ."

"That's all right, son." Atticus grinned slowly. "Looks

like all of Maycomb was out tonight, in one way or another. Jem, there's some wrapping paper in the pantry, I think. Go get it and we'll—"

"Atticus, no sir!"

Jem seemed to have lost his mind. He began pouring out our secrets right and left in total disregard for my safety if not for his own, omitting nothing, knot-hole, pants and all.

". . . Mr. Nathan put cement in that tree, Atticus, an' he did it to stop us findin' things—he's crazy, I reckon, like they say, but Atticus, I swear to God he ain't ever harmed us, he ain't ever hurt us, he coulda cut my throat from ear to ear that night but he tried to mend my pants instead . . . he ain't ever hurt us, Atticus—"

Atticus said, "Whoa, son," so gently that I was greatly heartened. It was obvious that he had not followed a word Jem said, for all Atticus said was, "You're right. We'd better keep this and the blanket to ourselves. Someday, maybe, Scout can thank him for covering her up."

"Thank who?" I asked.

"Boo Radley. You were so busy looking at the fire you didn't know it when he put the blanket around you."

My stomach turned to water and I nearly threw up when Jem held out the blanket and crept toward me. "He sneaked out of the house—turn 'round—sneaked up, an' went like this!"

Atticus said dryly, "Do not let this inspire you to further glory, Jeremy."

Jem scowled, "I ain't gonna do anything to him," but I watched the spark of fresh adventure leave his eyes. "Just think, Scout," he said, "if you'd just turned around, you'da seen him."

Calpurnia woke us at noon. Atticus had said we need not go to school that day, we'd learn nothing after no sleep. Calpurnia said for us to try and clean up the front yard.

Miss Maudie's sunhat was suspended in a thin layer of ice, like a fly in amber, and we had to dig under the dirt for her hedge-clippers. We found her in her back yard, gazing at her frozen charred azaleas.

"We're bringing back your things, Miss Maudie," said Jem. "We're awful sorry."

Miss Maudie looked around, and the shadow of her old

grin crossed her face. "Always wanted a smaller house, Jem Finch. Gives me more yard. Just think, I'll have more room for my azaleas now!"

"You ain't grievin', Miss Maudie?" I asked, surprised. Atticus said her house was nearly all she had.

"Grieving, child? Why, I hated that old cow barn. Thought of settin' fire to it a hundred times myself, except they'd lock me up."

"But—"

"Don't you worry about me, Jean Louise Finch. There are ways of doing things you don't know about. Why, I'll build me a little house and take me a couple of roomers and—gracious, I'll have the finest yard in Alabama. Those Bellingraths'll look plain puny when I get started!"

Jem and I looked at each other. "How'd it catch, Miss Maudie?" he asked.

"I don't know, Jem. Probably the flue in the kitchen. I kept a fire in there last night for my potted plants. Hear you had some unexpected company last night, Miss Jean Louise."

"How'd you know?"

"Atticus told me on his way to town this morning. Tell you the truth, I'd like to've been with you. And I'd've had sense enough to turn around, too."

Miss Maudie puzzled me. With most of her possessions gone and her beloved yard a shambles, she still took a lively and cordial interest in Jem's and my affairs.

She must have seen my perplexity. She said, "Only thing I worried about last night was all the danger and commotion it caused. This whole neighborhood could have gone up. Mr. Avery'll be in bed for a week—he's right stove up. He's too old to do things like that and I told him so. Soon as I can get my hands clean and when Stephanie Crawford's not looking, I'll make him a Lane cake. That Stephanie's been after my recipe for thirty years, and if she thinks I'll give it to her just because I'm staying with her she's got another think coming."

I reflected that if Miss Maudie broke down and gave it to her, Miss Stephanie couldn't follow it anyway. Miss Maudie had once let me see it: among other things, the recipe called for one large cup of sugar.

It was a still day. The air was so cold and clear we heard

the courthouse clock clank, rattle and strain before it struck the hour. Miss Maudie's nose was a color I had never seen before, and I inquired about it.

"I've been out here since six o'clock," she said. "Should be frozen by now." She held up her hands. A network of tiny lines crisscrossed her palms, brown with dirt and dried blood.

"You've ruined 'em," said Jem. "Why don't you get a colored man?" There was no note of sacrifice in his voice when he added, "Or Scout'n'me, we can help you."

Miss Maudie said, "Thank you sir, but you've got a job of your own over there." She pointed to our yard.

"You mean the Morphodite?" I asked. "Shoot, we can rake him up in a jiffy."

Miss Maudie stared down at me, her lips moving silently. Suddenly she put her hands to her head and whooped. When we left her, she was still chuckling.

Jem said he didn't know what was the matter with her—that was just Miss Maudie.

9

"You can just take that back, boy!"

This order, given by me to Cecil Jacobs, was the beginning of a rather thin time for Jem and me. My fists were clenched and I was ready to let fly. Atticus had promised me he would wear me out if he ever heard of me fighting any more; I was far too old and too big for such childish things, and the sooner I learned to hold in, the better off everybody would be. I soon forgot.

Cecil Jacobs made me forget. He had announced in the schoolyard the day before that Scout Finch's daddy defended niggers. I denied it, but told Jem.

"What'd he mean sayin' that?" I asked.

"Nothing," Jem said. "Ask Atticus, he'll tell you."

"Do you defend niggers, Atticus?" I asked him that evening.

"Of course I do. Don't say nigger, Scout. That's common."

" 's what everybody at school says."

"From now on it'll be everybody less one—"

"Well if you don't want me to grow up talkin' that way, why do you send me to school?"

My father looked at me mildly, amusement in his eyes. Despite our compromise, my campaign to avoid school had continued in one form or another since my first day's dose of it: the beginning of last September had brought on sinking spells, dizziness, and mild gastric complaints. I went so far as to pay a nickel for the privilege of rubbing my head against the head of Miss Rachel's cook's son, who was afflicted with a tremendous ringworm. It didn't take.

But I was worrying another bone. "Do all lawyers defend n-Negroes, Atticus?"

"Of course they do, Scout."

"Then why did Cecil say you defended niggers? He made it sound like you were runnin' a still."

Atticus sighed. "I'm simply defending a Negro—his name's Tom Robinson. He lives in that little settlement beyond the town dump. He's a member of Calpurnia's church, and Cal knows his family well. She says they're clean-living folks. Scout, you aren't old enough to understand some things yet, but there's been some high talk around town to the effect that I shouldn't do much about defending this man. It's a peculiar case—it won't come to trial until summer session. John Taylor was kind enough to give us a postponement . . ."

"If you shouldn't be defendin' him, then why are you doin' it?"

"For a number of reasons," said Atticus. "The main one is, if I didn't I couldn't hold up my head in town, I couldn't represent this county in the legislature, I couldn't even tell you or Jem not to do something again."

"You mean if you didn't defend that man, Jem and me wouldn't have to mind you any more?"

"That's about right."

"Why?"

"Because I could never ask you to mind me again. Scout, simply by the nature of the work, every lawyer gets at least one case in his lifetime that affects him personally. This one's mine, I guess. You might hear some ugly talk about it at school, but do one thing for me if you will: you just hold your head high and keep those fists down. No matter what anybody says to you, don't you let 'em get your goat. Try fighting with your head for a change . . . it's a good one, even if it does resist learning."

"Atticus, are we going to win it?"

"No, honey."

"Then why—"

"Simply because we were licked a hundred years before we started is no reason for us not to try to win," Atticus said.

"You sound like Cousin Ike Finch," I said. Cousin Ike Finch was Maycomb County's sole surviving Confederate veteran. He wore a General Hood type beard of which he was inordinately vain. At least once a year Atticus, Jem and I called on him, and I would have to kiss him. It was horrible. Jem and I would listen respectfully to Atticus and Cousin Ike rehash the war. "Tell you, Atticus," Cousin Ike would say, "the Missouri Compromise was what licked us, but if I had to go through it agin I'd walk every step of the way there an' every step back jist like I did before an' furthermore we'd whip 'em this time . . . now in 1864, when Stonewall Jackson came around by—I beg your pardon, young folks. Ol' Blue Light was in heaven then, God rest his saintly brow. . . ."

"Come here, Scout," said Atticus. I crawled into his lap and tucked my head under his chin. He put his arms around me and rocked me gently. "It's different this time," he said. "This time we aren't fighting the Yankees, we're fighting our friends. But remember this, no matter how bitter things get, they're still our friends and this is still our home."

With this in mind, I faced Cecil Jacobs in the schoolyard next day: "You gonna take that back, boy?"

"You gotta make me first!" he yelled. "My folks said your daddy was a disgrace an' that nigger oughta hang from the water-tank!"

I drew a bead on him, remembered what Atticus had said, then dropped my fists and walked away, "Scout's a cow—

ward!'' ringing in my ears. It was the first time I ever walked away from a fight.

Somehow, if I fought Cecil I would let Atticus down. Atticus so rarely asked Jem and me to do something for him, I could take being called a coward for him. I felt extremely noble for having remembered, and remained noble for three weeks. Then Christmas came and disaster struck.

Jem and I viewed Christmas with mixed feelings. The good side was the tree and Uncle Jack Finch. Every Christmas Eve day we met Uncle Jack at Maycomb Junction, and he would spend a week with us.

A flip of the coin revealed the uncompromising lineaments of Aunt Alexandra and Francis.

I suppose I should include Uncle Jimmy, Aunt Alexandra's husband, but as he never spoke a word to me in my life except to say, ''Get off the fence,'' once, I never saw any reason to take notice of him. Neither did Aunt Alexandra. Long ago, in a burst of friendliness, Aunty and Uncle Jimmy produced a son named Henry, who left home as soon as was humanly possible, married, and produced Francis. Henry and his wife deposited Francis at his grandparents' every Christmas, then pursued their own pleasures.

No amount of sighing could induce Atticus to let us spend Christmas day at home. We went to Finch's Landing every Christmas in my memory. The fact that Aunty was a good cook was some compensation for being forced to spend a religious holiday with Francis Hancock. He was a year older than I, and I avoided him on principle: he enjoyed everything I disapproved of, and disliked my ingenuous diversions.

Aunt Alexandra was Atticus's sister, but when Jem told me about changelings and siblings, I decided that she had been swapped at birth, that my grandparents had perhaps received a Crawford instead of a Finch. Had I ever harbored the mystical notions about mountains that seem to obsess lawyers and judges, Aunt Alexandra would have been analogous to Mount Everest: throughout my early life, she was cold and there.

When Uncle Jack jumped down from the train Christmas Eve day, we had to wait for the porter to hand him two long packages. Jem and I always thought it funny when Uncle

Jack pecked Atticus on the cheek; they were the only two men we ever saw kiss each other. Uncle Jack shook hands with Jem and swung me high, but not high enough: Uncle Jack was a head shorter than Atticus; the baby of the family, he was younger than Aunt Alexandra. He and Aunty looked alike, but Uncle Jack made better use of his face: we were never wary of his sharp nose and chin.

He was one of the few men of science who never terrified me, probably because he never behaved like a doctor. Whenever he performed a minor service for Jem and me, as removing a splinter from a foot, he would tell us exactly what he was going to do, give us an estimation of how much it would hurt, and explain the use of any tongs he employed. One Christmas I lurked in corners nursing a twisted splinter in my foot, permitting no one to come near me. When Uncle Jack caught me, he kept me laughing about a preacher who hated going to church so much that every day he stood at his gate in his dressing-gown, smoking a hookah and delivering five-minute sermons to any passers-by who desired spiritual comfort. I interrupted to make Uncle Jack let me know when he would pull it out, but he held up a bloody splinter in a pair of tweezers and said he yanked it while I was laughing, that was what was known as relativity.

"What's in those packages?" I asked him, pointing to the long thin parcels the porter had given him.

"None of your business," he said.

Jem said, "How's Rose Aylmer?"

Rose Aylmer was Uncle Jack's cat. She was a beautiful yellow female Uncle Jack said was one of the few women he could stand permanently. He reached into his coat pocket and brought out some snapshots. We admired them.

"She's gettin' fat," I said.

"I should think so. She eats all the leftover fingers and ears from the hospital."

"Aw, that's a damn story," I said.

"I beg your pardon?"

Atticus said, "Don't pay any attention to her, Jack. She's trying you out. Cal says she's been cussing fluently for a week, now."

Uncle Jack raised his eyebrows and said nothing. I was proceeding on the dim theory, aside from the innate attractiveness of such words, that if Atticus discovered I had picked them up at school he wouldn't make me go.

But at supper that evening when I asked him to pass the damn ham, please, Uncle Jack pointed at me. "See me afterwards, young lady," he said.

When supper was over, Uncle Jack went to the livingroom and sat down. He slapped his thighs for me to come sit on his lap. I liked to smell him: he was like a bottle of alcohol and something pleasantly sweet. He pushed back my bangs and looked at me. "You're more like Atticus than your mother," he said. "You're also growing out of your pants a little."

"I reckon they fit all right."

"You like words like damn and hell now, don't you?"

I said I reckoned so.

"Well I don't," said Uncle Jack, "not unless there's extreme provocation connected with 'em. I'll be here a week, and I don't want to hear any words like that while I'm here. Scout, you'll get in trouble if you go around saying things like that. You want to grow up to be a lady, don't you?"

I said not particularly.

"Of course you do. Now let's get to the tree."

We decorated the tree until bedtime, and that night I dreamed of the two long packages for Jem and me. Next morning Jem and I dived for them: they were from Atticus, who had written Uncle Jack to get them for us, and they were what we had asked for.

"Don't point them in the house," said Atticus, when Jem aimed at a picture on the wall.

"You'll have to teach 'em to shoot," said Uncle Jack.

"That's your job," said Atticus. "I merely bowed to the inevitable."

It took Atticus's courtroom voice to drag us away from the tree. He declined to let us take our air rifles to the Landing (I had already begun to think of shooting Francis) and said if we made one false move he'd take them away from us for good.

Finch's Landing consisted of three hundred and sixty-six steps down a high bluff and ending in a jetty. Farther down stream, beyond the bluff, were traces of an old cotton landing, where Finch Negroes had loaded bales and produce, unloaded blocks of ice, flour and sugar, farm equipment, and feminine apparel. A two-rut road ran from the riverside and vanished among dark trees. At the end of the road was a two-storied white house with porches circling it upstairs and downstairs. In his old age, our ancestor Simon Finch had built it to please his nagging wife; but with the porches all resemblance to ordinary houses of its era ended. The internal arrangements of the Finch house were indicative of Simon's guilelessness and the absolute trust with which he regarded his offspring.

There were six bedrooms upstairs, four for the eight female children, one for Welcome Finch, the sole son, and one for visiting relatives. Simple enough; but the daughters' rooms could be reached only by one staircase, Welcome's room and the guestroom only by another. The Daughters' Staircase was in the ground-floor bedroom of their parents, so Simon always knew the hours of his daughters' nocturnal comings and goings.

There was a kitchen separate from the rest of the house, tacked onto it by a wooden catwalk; in the back yard was a rusty bell on a pole, used to summon field hands or as a distress signal; a widow's walk was on the roof, but no widows walked there—from it, Simon oversaw his overseer, watched the river-boats, and gazed into the lives of surrounding landholders.

There went with the house the usual legend about the Yankees: one Finch female, recently engaged, donned her complete trousseau to save it from raiders in the neighborhood; she became stuck in the door to the Daughters' Staircase but was doused with water and finally pushed through. When we arrived at the Landing, Aunt Alexandra kissed Uncle Jack, Francis kissed Uncle Jack, Uncle Jimmy shook hands silently with Uncle Jack, Jem and I gave our presents to Francis, who gave us a present. Jem felt his age and gravitated to the adults, leaving me to entertain our cousin. Francis was eight and slicked back his hair.

"What'd you get for Christmas?" I asked politely.

"Just what I asked for," he said. Francis had requested a pair of knee-pants, a red leather booksack, five shirts and an untied bow tie.

"That's nice," I lied. "Jem and me got air rifles, and Jem got a chemistry set—"

"A toy one, I reckon."

"No, a real one. He's gonna make me some invisible ink, and I'm gonna write to Dill in it."

Francis asked what was the use of that.

"Well, can't you just see his face when he gets a letter from me with nothing in it? It'll drive him nuts."

Talking to Francis gave me the sensation of settling slowly to the bottom of the ocean. He was the most boring child I ever met. As he lived in Mobile, he could not inform on me to school authorities, but he managed to tell everything he knew to Aunt Alexandra, who in turn unburdened herself to Atticus, who either forgot it or gave me hell, whichever struck his fancy. But the only time I ever heard Atticus speak sharply to anyone was when I once heard him say, "Sister, I do the best I can with them!" It had something to do with my going around in overalls.

Aunt Alexandra was fanatical on the subject of my attire. I could not possibly hope to be a lady if I wore breeches; when I said I could do nothing in a dress, she said I wasn't supposed to be doing things that required pants. Aunt Alexandra's vision of my deportment involved playing with small stoves, tea sets, and wearing the Add-A-Pearl necklace she gave me when I was born; furthermore, I should be a ray of sunshine in my father's lonely life. I suggested that one could be a ray of sunshine in pants just as well, but Aunty said that one had to behave like a sunbeam, that I was born good but had grown progressively worse every year. She hurt my feelings and set my teeth permanently on edge, but when I asked Atticus about it, he said there were already enough sunbeams in the family and to go on about my business, he didn't mind me much the way I was.

At Christmas dinner, I sat at the little table in the dining-room; Jem and Francis sat with the adults at the dining table. Aunty had continued to isolate me long after Jem and Francis graduated to the big table. I often wondered what she thought I'd do, get up and throw something? I sometimes thought of asking her if she would let me sit at the big table with the rest of them just once, I would prove to her how civilized I could be; after all, I ate at home every day with no major mishaps. When I begged Atticus to use his influence, he said he had none—we were guests, and we sat where she told us to sit. He also said Aunt Alexandra didn't understand girls much, she'd never had one.

But her cooking made up for everything: three kinds of meat, summer vegetables from her pantry shelves; peach pickles, two kinds of cake and ambrosia constituted a modest Christmas dinner. Afterwards, the adults made for the livingroom and sat around in a dazed condition. Jem lay on the floor, and I went to the back yard. "Put on your coat," said Atticus dreamily, so I didn't hear him.

Francis sat beside me on the back steps. "That was the best yet," I said.

"Grandma's a wonderful cook," said Francis. "She's gonna teach me how."

"Boys don't cook." I giggled at the thought of Jem in an apron.

"Grandma says all men should learn to cook, that men oughta be careful with their wives and wait on 'em when they don't feel good," said my cousin.

"I don't want Dill waitin' on me," I said. "I'd rather wait on him."

"Dill?"

"Yeah. Don't say anything about it yet, but we're gonna get married as soon as we're big enough. He asked me last summer."

Francis hooted.

"What's the matter with him?" I asked. "Ain't anything the matter with him."

"You mean that little runt Grandma says stays with Miss Rachel every summer?"

"That's exactly who I mean."

"I know all about him," said Francis.

"What about him?"

"Grandma says he hasn't got a home—"

"Has too, he lives in Meridian."

"—he just gets passed around from relative to relative, and Miss Rachel keeps him every summer."

"Francis, that's not so!"

Francis grinned at me. "You're mighty dumb sometimes, Jean Louise. Guess you don't know any better, though."

"What do you mean?"

"If Uncle Atticus lets you run around with stray dogs, that's his own business, like Grandma says, so it ain't your fault. I guess it ain't your fault if Uncle Atticus is a nigger-lover besides, but I'm here to tell you it certainly does mortify the rest of the family—"

"Francis, what the hell do you mean?"

"Just what I said. Grandma says it's bad enough he lets you all run wild, but now he's turned out a nigger-lover we'll never be able to walk the streets of Maycomb agin. He's ruinin' the family, that's what he's doin'."

Francis rose and sprinted down the catwalk to the old kitchen. At a safe distance he called, "He's nothin' but a nigger-lover!"

"He is not!" I roared. "I don't know what you're talkin' about, but you better cut it out this red hot minute!"

I leaped off the steps and ran down the catwalk. It was easy to collar Francis. I said take it back quick.

Francis jerked loose and sped into the old kitchen. "Nigger-lover!" he yelled.

When stalking one's prey, it is best to take one's time. Say nothing, and as sure as eggs he will become curious and emerge. Francis appeared at the kitchen door. "You still mad, Jean Louise?" he asked tentatively.

"Nothing to speak of," I said.

Francis came out on the catwalk.

"You gonna take it back, Fra—ancis?" But I was too quick on the draw. Francis shot back into the kitchen, so I retired to the steps. I could wait patiently. I had sat there perhaps five minutes when I heard Aunt Alexandra speak: "Where's Francis?"

"He's out yonder in the kitchen."

"He knows he's not supposed to play in there."

Francis came to the door and yelled, "Grandma, she's got me in here and she won't let me out!"

"What is all this, Jean Louise?"

I looked up at Aunt Alexandra. "I haven't got him in there, Aunty, I ain't holdin' him."

"Yes she is," shouted Francis, "she won't let me out!"

"Have you all been fussing?"

"Jean Louise got mad at me, Grandma," called Francis.

"Francis, come out of there! Jean Louise, if I hear another word out of you I'll tell your father. Did I hear you say hell a while ago?"

"Nome."

"I thought I did. I'd better not hear it again."

Aunt Alexandra was a back-porch listener. The moment she was out of sight Francis came out head up and grinning. "Don't you fool with me," he said.

He jumped into the yard and kept his distance, kicking tufts of grass, turning around occasionally to smile at me. Jem appeared on the porch, looked at us, and went away. Francis climbed the mimosa tree, came down, put his hands in his pockets and strolled around the yard. "Hah!" he said. I asked him who he thought he was, Uncle Jack? Francis said he reckoned I got told, for me to just sit there and leave him alone.

"I ain't botherin' you," I said.

Francis looked at me carefully, concluded that I had been sufficiently subdued, and crooned softly, "Nigger-lover . . ."

This time, I split my knuckle to the bone on his front teeth. My left impaired, I sailed in with my right, but not for long. Uncle Jack pinned my arms to my sides and said, "Stand still!"

Aunt Alexandra ministered to Francis, wiping his tears away with her handkerchief, rubbing his hair, patting his cheek. Atticus, Jem, and Uncle Jimmy had come to the back porch when Francis started yelling.

"Who started this?" said Uncle Jack.

Francis and I pointed at each other. "Grandma," he bawled, "she called me a whore-lady and jumped on me!"

"Is that true, Scout?" said Uncle Jack.

"I reckon so."

When Uncle Jack looked down at me, his features were like Aunt Alexandra's. "You know I told you you'd get in trouble if you used words like that? I told you, didn't I?"

"Yes sir, but—"

"Well, you're in trouble now. Stay there."

I was debating whether to stand there or run, and tarried in indecision a moment too long: I turned to flee but Uncle

Jack was quicker. I found myself suddenly looking at a tiny ant struggling with a bread crumb in the grass.

"I'll never speak to you again as long as I live! I hate you an' despise you an' hope you die tomorrow!" A statement that seemed to encourage Uncle Jack, more than anything. I ran to Atticus for comfort, but he said I had it coming and it was high time we went home. I climbed into the back seat of the car without saying good-bye to anyone, and at home I ran to my room and slammed the door. Jem tried to say something nice, but I wouldn't let him.

When I surveyed the damage there were only seven or eight red marks, and I was reflecting upon relativity when someone knocked on the door. I asked who it was; Uncle Jack answered.

"Go away!"

Uncle Jack said if I talked like that he'd lick me again, so I was quiet. When he entered the room I retreated to a corner and turned my back on him. "Scout," he said, "do you still hate me?"

"Go on, please sir."

"Why, I didn't think you'd hold it against me," he said. "I'm disappointed in you—you had that coming and you know it."

"Didn't either."

"Honey, you can't go around calling people—"

"You ain't fair," I said, "you ain't fair."

Uncle Jack's eyebrows went up. "Not fair? How not?"

"You're real nice, Uncle Jack, an' I reckon I love you even after what you did, but you don't understand children much."

Uncle Jack put his hands on his hips and looked down at me. "And why do I not understand children, Miss Jean Louise? Such conduct as yours required little understanding. It was obstreperous, disorderly and abusive—"

"You gonna give me a chance to tell you? I don't mean to sass you, I'm just tryin' to tell you."

Uncle Jack sat down on the bed. His eyebrows came together, and he peered up at me from under them. "Proceed," he said.

I took a deep breath. "Well, in the first place you never

stopped to gimme a chance to tell you my side of it—you just lit right into me. When Jem an' I fuss Atticus doesn't ever just listen to Jem's side of it, he hears mine too, an' in the second place you told me never to use words like that except in ex-extreme provocation, and Francis provocated me enough to knock his block off—''

Uncle Jack scratched his head. "What was your side of it, Scout?''

"Francis called Atticus somethin', an' I wasn't about to take it off him.''

"What did Francis call him?''

"A nigger-lover. I ain't very sure what it means, but the way Francis said it—tell you one thing right now, Uncle Jack, I'll be—I swear before God if I'll sit there and let him say somethin' about Atticus.''

"He called Atticus that?''

"Yes sir, he did, an' a lot more. Said Atticus'd be the ruination of the family an' he let Jem an me run wild. . . .''

From the look on Uncle Jack's face, I thought I was in for it again. When he said, "We'll see about this," I knew Francis was in for it. "I've a good mind to go out there tonight.''

"Please sir, just let it go. Please.''

"I've no intention of letting it go," he said. "Alexandra should know about this. The idea of—wait'll I get my hands on that boy. . . .''

"Uncle Jack, please promise me somethin', please sir. Promise you won't tell Atticus about this. He—he asked me one time not to let anything I heard about him make me mad, an' I'd ruther him think we were fightin' about somethin' else instead. Please promise . . .''

"But I don't like Francis getting away with something like that—''

"He didn't. You reckon you could tie up my hand? It's still bleedin' some.''

"Of course I will, baby. I know of no hand I would be more delighted to tie up. Will you come this way?''

Uncle Jack gallantly bowed me to the bathroom. While he cleaned and bandaged my knuckles, he entertained me with a tale about a funny nearsighted old gentleman who had a cat named Hodge, and who counted all the cracks in the sidewalk when he went to town. "There now," he said. "You'll have a very unladylike scar on your wedding-ring finger."

"Thank you sir. Uncle Jack?"

"Ma'am?"

"What's a whore-lady?"

Uncle Jack plunged into another long tale about an old Prime Minister who sat in the House of Commons and blew feathers in the air and tried to keep them there when all about him men were losing their heads. I guess he was trying to answer my question, but he made no sense whatsoever.

Later, when I was supposed to be in bed, I went down the hall for a drink of water and heard Atticus and Uncle Jack in the livingroom:

"I shall never marry, Atticus."

"Why?"

"I might have children."

Atticus said, "You've a lot to learn, Jack."

"I know. Your daughter gave me my first lessons this afternoon. She said I didn't understand children much and told me why. She was quite right. Atticus, she told me how I should have treated her—oh dear, I'm so sorry I romped on her."

Atticus chuckled. "She earned it, so don't feel too remorseful."

I waited, on tenterhooks, for Uncle Jack to tell Atticus my side of it. But he didn't. He simply murmured, "Her use of bathroom invective leaves nothing to the imagination. But she doesn't know the meaning of half she says—she asked me what a whore-lady was . . ."

"Did you tell her?"

"No, I told her about Lord Melbourne."

"Jack! When a child asks you something, answer him, for goodness' sake. But don't make a production of it. Children are children, but they can spot an evasion quicker than adults, and evasion simply muddles 'em. No," my father mused, "you had the right answer this afternoon, but the wrong reasons. Bad language is a stage all children go through, and it dies with time when they learn they're not attracting attention with it. Hotheadedness isn't. Scout's got to learn to keep her head and learn soon, with what's in store for her these next few months. She's coming along, though. Jem's getting older and she follows his example a good bit now. All she needs is assistance sometimes.''

"Atticus, you've never laid a hand on her."

"I admit that. So far I've been able to get by with threats. Jack, she minds me as well as she can. Doesn't come up to scratch half the time, but she tries.''

"That's not the answer," said Uncle Jack.

"No, the answer is she knows I know she tries. That's what makes the difference. What bothers me is that she and Jem will have to absorb some ugly things pretty soon. I'm not worried about Jem keeping his head, but Scout'd just as soon jump on someone as look at him if her pride's at stake. . . .''

I waited for Uncle Jack to break his promise. He still didn't.

"Atticus, how bad is this going to be? You haven't had too much chance to discuss it.''

"It couldn't be worse, Jack. The only thing we've got is a black man's word against the Ewells'. The evidence boils down to you-did—I-didn't. The jury couldn't possibly be expected to take Tom Robinson's word against the Ewells' —are you acquainted with the Ewells?''

Uncle Jack said yes, he remembered them. He described them to Atticus, but Atticus said, "You're a generation off. The present ones are the same, though.''

"What are you going to do, then?"

"Before I'm through, I intend to jar the jury a bit—I think we'll have a reasonable chance on appeal, though. I really can't tell at this stage, Jack. You know, I'd hoped to get through life without a case of this kind, but John Taylor pointed at me and said, 'You're It.' ''

"Let this cup pass from you, eh?''

"Right. But do you think I could face my children otherwise? You know what's going to happen as well as I do, Jack, and I hope and pray I can get Jem and Scout through it without bitterness, and most of all, without catching Maycomb's usual disease. Why reasonable people go stark raving mad when anything involving a Negro comes up, is something I don't pretend to understand . . . I just hope that Jem and Scout come to me for their answers instead of listening to the town. I hope they trust me enough. . . . Jean Louise?''

My scalp jumped. I stuck my head around the corner. "Sir?"

"Go to bed."

I scurried to my room and went to bed. Uncle Jack was a prince of a fellow not to let me down. But I never figured out how Atticus knew I was listening, and it was not until many years later that I realized he wanted me to hear every word he said.

10

Atticus was feeble: he was nearly fifty. When Jem and I asked him why he was so old, he said he got started late, which we felt reflected upon his abilities and manliness. He was much older than the parents of our school contemporaries, and there was nothing Jem or I could say about him when our classmates said, "*My* father—"

Jem was football crazy. Atticus was never too tired to play keep-away, but when Jem wanted to tackle him Atticus would say, "I'm too old for that, son."

Our father didn't do anything. He worked in an office, not in a drugstore. Atticus did not drive a dump-truck for the county, he was not the sheriff, he did not farm, work in a garage, or do anything that could possibly arouse the admiration of anyone.

Besides that, he wore glasses. He was nearly blind in his left eye, and said left eyes were the tribal curse of the Finches. Whenever he wanted to see something well, he turned his head and looked from his right eye.

He did not do the things our schoolmates' fathers did: he never went hunting, he did not play poker or fish or drink or smoke. He sat in the livingroom and read.

With these attributes, however, he would not remain as inconspicuous as we wished him to: that year, the school buzzed with talk about him defending Tom Robinson, none of which was complimentary. After my bout with Cecil

Jacobs when I committed myself to a policy of cowardice, word got around that Scout Finch wouldn't fight any more, her daddy wouldn't let her. This was not entirely correct: I wouldn't fight publicly for Atticus, but the family was private ground. I would fight anyone from a third cousin upwards tooth and nail. Francis Hancock, for example, knew that.

When he gave us our air-rifles Atticus wouldn't teach us to shoot. Uncle Jack instructed us in the rudiments thereof; he said Atticus wasn't interested in guns. Atticus said to Jem one day, "I'd rather you shot at tin cans in the back yard, but I know you'll go after birds. Shoot all the bluejays you want, if you can hit 'em, but remember it's a sin to kill a mockingbird."

That was the only time I ever heard Atticus say it was a sin to do something, and I asked Miss Maudie about it.

"Your father's right," she said. "Mockingbirds don't do one thing but make music for us to enjoy. They don't eat up people's gardens, don't nest in corncribs, they don't do one thing but sing their hearts out for us. That's why it's a sin to kill a mockingbird."

"Miss Maudie, this is an old neighborhood, ain't it?"

"Been here longer than the town."

"Nome, I mean the folks on our street are all old. Jem and me's the only children around here. Mrs. Dubose is close on to a hundred and Miss Rachel's old and so are you and Atticus."

"I don't call fifty very old," said Miss Maudie tartly. "Not being wheeled around yet, am I? Neither's your father. But I must say Providence was kind enough to burn down that old mausoleum of mine, I'm too old to keep it up—maybe you're right, Jean Louise, this is a settled neighborhood. You've never been around young folks much, have you?"

"Yessum, at school."

"I mean young grown-ups. You're lucky, you know. You and Jem have the benefit of your father's age. If your father was thirty you'd find life quite different."

"I sure would. Atticus can't do anything. . . ."

"You'd be surprised," said Miss Maudie. "There's life in him yet."

"What can he do?"

"Well, he can make somebody's will so airtight can't anybody meddle with it."

"Shoot . . ."

"Well, did you know he's the best checker-player in this town? Why, down at the Landing when we were coming up, Atticus Finch could beat everybody on both sides of the river."

"Good Lord, Miss Maudie, Jem and me beat him all the time."

"It's about time you found out it's because he lets you. Did you know he can play a Jew's Harp?"

This modest accomplishment served to make me even more ashamed of him.

"*Well* . . ." she said.

"Well, what, Miss Maudie?"

"Well nothing. Nothing—it seems with all that you'd be proud of him. Can't everybody play a Jew's Harp. Now keep out of the way of the carpenters. You'd better go home, I'll be in my azaleas and can't watch you. Plank might hit you."

I went to the back yard and found Jem plugging away at a tin can, which seemed stupid with all the bluejays around. I returned to the front yard and busied myself for two hours erecting a complicated breastworks at the side of the porch, consisting of a tire, an orange crate, the laundry hamper, the porch chairs, and a small U.S. flag Jem gave me from a popcorn box.

When Atticus came home to dinner he found me crouched down aiming across the street. "What are you shooting at?"

"Miss Maudie's rear end."

Atticus turned and saw my generous target bending over her bushes. He pushed his hat to the back of his head and crossed the street. "Maudie," he called, "I thought I'd better warn you. You're in considerable peril."

Miss Maudie straightened up and looked toward me. She said, "Atticus, you are a devil from hell."

When Atticus returned he told me to break camp. "Don't you ever let me catch you pointing that gun at anybody again," he said.

I wished my father was a devil from hell. I sounded out Calpurnia on the subject. "Mr. Finch? Why, he can do lots of things "

"Like what?" I asked.

Calpurnia scratched her head. "Well, I don't rightly know," she said.

Jem underlined it when he asked Atticus if he was going out for the Methodists and Atticus said he'd break his neck if he did, he was just too old for that sort of thing. The Methodists were trying to pay off their church mortgage, and had challenged the Baptists to a game of touch football. Everybody in town's father was playing, it seemed, except Atticus. Jem said he didn't even want to go, but he was unable to resist football in any form, and he stood gloomily on the sidelines with Atticus and me watching Cecil Jacobs's father make touchdowns for the Baptists.

One Saturday Jem and I decided to go exploring with our air-rifles to see if we could find a rabbit or a squirrel. We had gone about five hundred yards beyond the Radley Place when I noticed Jem squinting at something down the street. He had turned his head to one side and was looking out of the corners of his eyes.

"Whatcha looking at?"

"That old dog down yonder," he said.

"That's old Tim Johnson, ain't it?"

"Yeah."

Tim Johnson was the property of Mr. Harry Johnson who drove the Mobile bus and lived on the southern edge of town. Tim was a liver-colored bird dog, the pet of Maycomb.

"What's he doing?"

"I don't know, Scout. We better go home."

"Aw Jem, it's February."

"I don't care, I'm gonna tell Cal."

We raced home and ran to the kitchen.

"Cal," said Jem, "can you come down the sidewalk a minute?"

"What for, Jem? I can't come down the sidewalk every time you want me."

"There's somethin' wrong with an old dog down yonder."

Calpurnia sighed. "I can't wrap up any dog's foot now. There's some gauze in the bathroom, go get it and do it yourself."

Jem shook his head. "He's sick, Cal. Something's wrong with him."

"What's he doin', trying to catch his tail?"

"No, he's doin' like this."

Jem gulped like a goldfish, hunched his shoulders and twitched his torso. "He's goin' like that, only not like he means to."

"Are you telling me a story, Jem Finch?" Calpurnia's voice hardened.

"No Cal, I swear I'm not."

"Was he runnin'?"

"No, he's just moseyin' along, so slow you can't hardly tell it. He's comin' this way."

Calpurnia rinsed her hands and followed Jem into the yard. "I don't see any dog," she said.

She followed us beyond the Radley Place and looked where Jem pointed. Tim Johnson was not much more than a speck in the distance, but he was closer to us. He walked erratically, as if his right legs were shorter than his left legs. He reminded me of a car stuck in a sandbed.

"He's gone lopsided," said Jem.

Calpurnia stared, then grabbed us by the shoulders and ran us home. She shut the wood door behind us, went to the telephone and shouted, "Gimme Mr. Finch's office!"

"Mr. Finch!" she shouted. "This is Cal. I swear to God there's a mad dog down the street a piece—he's comin' this way, yes sir, he's—Mr. Finch, I declare he is—old Tim Johnson, yes sir . . . yessir . . . yes—"

She hung up and shook her head when we tried to ask her what Atticus had said. She rattled the telephone hook and said, "Miss Eula May—now ma'am, I'm through talkin' to Mr. Finch, please don't connect me no more—listen, Miss Eula May, can you call Miss Rachel and Miss Stephanie Crawford and whoever's got a phone on this street and tell 'em a mad dog's comin'? Please ma'am!"

Calpurnia listened. "I know it's February, Miss Eula May, but I know a mad dog when I see one. Please ma'am hurry!"

Calpurnia asked Jem, "Radleys got a phone?"

Jem looked in the book and said no. "They won't come out anyway, Cal."

"I don't care, I'm gonna tell 'em."

She ran to the front porch, Jem and I at her heels. "You stay in that house!" she yelled.

Calpurnia's message had been received by the neighborhood. Every wood door within our range of vision was closed tight. We saw no trace of Tim Johnson. We watched Calpurnia running toward the Radley Place, holding her skirt and apron above her knees. She went up to the front steps and banged on the door. She got no answer, and she shouted, "Mr. Nathan, Mr. Arthur, mad dog's comin'! Mad dog's comin'!"

"She's supposed to go around in back," I said.

Jem shook his head. "Don't make any difference now," he said.

Calpurnia pounded on the door in vain. No one acknowledged her warning; no one seemed to have heard it.

As Calpurnia sprinted to the back porch a black Ford swung into the driveway. Atticus and Mr. Heck Tate got out.

Mr. Heck Tate was the sheriff of Maycomb County. He was as tall as Atticus, but thinner. He was long-nosed, wore boots with shiny metal eye-holes, boot pants and a lumber jacket. His belt had a row of bullets sticking in it. He carried a heavy rifle. When he and Atticus reached the porch, Jem opened the door.

"Stay inside, son," said Atticus. "Where is he, Cal?"

"He oughta be here by now," said Calpurnia, pointing down the street.

"Not runnin', is he?" asked Mr. Tate.

"Naw sir, he's in the twitchin' stage, Mr. Heck."

"Should we go after him, Heck?" asked Atticus.

"We better wait, Mr. Finch. They usually go in a straight line, but you never can tell. He might follow the curve—hope he does or he'll go straight in the Radley back yard. Let's wait a minute."

"Don't think he'll get in the Radley yard," said Atticus. "Fence'll stop him. He'll probably follow the road. . . ."

I thought mad dogs foamed at the mouth, galloped, leaped and lunged at throats, and I thought they did it in August. Had Tim Johnson behaved thus, I would have been less frightened.

Nothing is more deadly than a deserted, waiting street. The trees were still, the mockingbirds were silent, the carpenters at Miss Maudie's house had vanished. I heard Mr. Tate sniff, then blow his nose. I saw him shift his gun to the crook of his arm. I saw Miss Stephanie Crawford's face framed in the glass window of her front door. Miss Maudie appeared and stood beside her. Atticus put his foot on the rung of a chair and rubbed his hand slowly down the side of his thigh.

"There he is," he said softly.

Tim Johnson came into sight, walking dazedly in the inner rim of the curve parallel to the Radley house.

"Look at him," whispered Jem. "Mr. Heck said they walked in a straight line. He can't even stay in the road."

"He looks more sick than anything," I said.

"Let anything get in front of him and he'll come straight at it."

Mr. Tate put his hand to his forehead and leaned forward. "He's got it all right, Mr. Finch."

Tim Johnson was advancing at a snail's pace, but he was not playing or sniffing at foliage: he seemed dedicated to one course and motivated by an invisible force that was inching him toward us. We could see him shiver like a horse shedding flies; his jaw opened and shut; he was alist, but he was being pulled gradually toward us.

"He's lookin' for a place to die," said Jem.

Mr. Tate turned around. "He's far from dead, Jem, he hasn't got started yet."

Tim Johnson reached the side street that ran in front of the Radley Place, and what remained of his poor mind made him pause and seem to consider which road he would take. He made a few hesitant steps and stopped in front of the Radley gate; then he tried to turn around, but was having difficulty.

Atticus said, "He's within range, Heck. You better get him before he goes down the side street—Lord knows who's around the corner. Go inside, Cal."

Calpurnia opened the screen door, latched it behind her, then unlatched it and held onto the hook. She tried to block Jem and me with her body, but we looked out from beneath her arms.

"Take him, Mr. Finch." Mr. Tate handed the rifle to Atticus; Jem and I nearly fainted.

"Don't waste time, Heck," said Atticus. "Go on."

"Mr. Finch, this is a one-shot job."

Atticus shook his head vehemently: "Don't just stand there, Heck! He won't wait all day for you—"

"For God's sake, Mr. Finch, look where he is! Miss and you'll go straight into the Radley house! I can't shoot that well and you know it!"

"I haven't shot a gun in thirty years—"

Mr. Tate almost threw the rifle at Atticus. "I'd feel mighty comfortable if you did now," he said.

In a fog, Jem and I watched our father take the gun and walk out into the middle of the street. He walked quickly, but I thought he moved like an underwater swimmer: time had slowed to a nauseating crawl.

When Atticus raised his glasses Calpurnia murmured, "Sweet Jesus help him," and put her hands to her cheeks.

Atticus pushed his glasses to his forehead; they slipped down, and he dropped them in the street. In the silence, I heard them crack. Atticus rubbed his eyes and chin; we saw him blink hard.

In front of the Radley gate, Tim Johnson had made up what was left of his mind. He had finally turned himself around, to pursue his original course up our street. He made two steps forward, then stopped and raised his head. We saw his body go rigid.

With movements so swift they seemed simultaneous, Atticus's hand yanked a ball-tipped lever as he brought the gun to his shoulder.

The rifle cracked. Tim Johnson leaped, flopped over and crumpled on the sidewalk in a brown-and-white heap. He didn't know what hit him.

Mr. Tate jumped off the porch and ran to the Radley Place. He stopped in front of the dog, squatted, turned around and tapped his finger on his forehead above his left eye. "You were a little to the right, Mr. Finch," he called.

"Always was," answered Atticus. "If I had my 'druthers I'd take a shotgun."

He stooped and picked up his glasses, ground the broken lenses to powder under his heel, and went to Mr. Tate and stood looking down at Tim Johnson.

Doors opened one by one, and the neighborhood slowly came alive. Miss Maudie walked down the steps with Miss Stephanie Crawford.

Jem was paralyzed. I pinched him to get him moving, but

when Atticus saw us coming he called, "Stay where you are."

When Mr. Tate and Atticus returned to the yard, Mr. Tate was smiling. "I'll have Zeebo collect him," he said. "You haven't forgot much, Mr. Finch. They say it never leaves you."

Atticus was silent.

"Atticus?" said Jem.

"Yes?"

"Nothin'."

"I saw that, One-Shot Finch!"

Atticus wheeled around and faced Miss Maudie. They looked at one another without saying anything, and Atticus got into the sheriff's car. "Come here," he said to Jem. "Don't you go near that dog, you understand? Don't go near him, he's just as dangerous dead as alive."

"Yes sir," said Jem. "Atticus—"

"What, son?"

"Nothing."

"What's the matter with you, boy, can't you talk?" said Mr. Tate, grinning at Jem. "Didn't you know your daddy's—"

"Hush, Heck," said Atticus, "let's go back to town."

When they drove away, Jem and I went to Miss Stephanie's front steps. We sat waiting for Zeebo to arrive in the garbage truck.

Jem sat in numb confusion, and Miss Stephanie said, "Uh, uh, uh, who'da thought of a mad dog in February? Maybe he wadn't mad, maybe he was just crazy. I'd hate to see Harry Johnson's face when he gets in from the Mobile run and finds Atticus Finch's shot his dog. Bet he was just full of fleas from somewhere—"

Miss Maudie said Miss Stephanie'd be singing a different tune if Tim Johnson was still coming up the street, that they'd find out soon enough, they'd send his head to Montgomery.

Jem became vaguely articulate: " 'd you see him, Scout? 'd you see him just standin' there? . . . 'n' all of a sudden he just relaxed all over, an' it looked like that gun was a part of him . . . an' he did it so quick, like . . . I hafta aim for ten minutes 'fore I can hit somethin'. . . ."

Miss Maudie grinned wickedly. "Well now, Miss Jean Louise," she said, "still think your father can't do anything? Still ashamed of him?"

"Nome," I said meekly.

"Forgot to tell you the other day that besides playing the Jew's Harp, Atticus Finch was the deadest shot in Maycomb County in his time."

"Dead shot . . ." echoed Jem.

"That's what I said, Jem Finch. Guess you'll change *your* tune now. The very idea, didn't you know his nickname was Ol' One-Shot when he was a boy? Why, down at the Landing when he was coming up, if he shot fifteen times and hit fourteen doves he'd complain about wasting ammunition."

"He never said anything about that," Jem muttered.

"Never said anything about it, did he?"

"No ma'am."

"Wonder why he never goes huntin' now," I said.

"Maybe I can tell you," said Miss Maudie. "If your father's anything, he's civilized in his heart. Marksmanship's a gift of God, a talent—oh, you have to practice to make it perfect, but shootin's different from playing the piano or the like. I think maybe he put his gun down when he realized that God had given him an unfair advantage over most living things. I guess he decided he wouldn't shoot till he had to, and he had to today."

"Looks like he'd be proud of it," I said.

"People in their right minds never take pride in their talents," said Miss Maudie.

We saw Zeebo drive up. He took a pitchfork from the back of the garbage truck and gingerly lifted Tim Johnson. He pitched the dog onto the truck, then poured something from a gallon jug on and around the spot where Tim fell. "Don't yawl come over here for a while," he called.

When we went home I told Jem we'd really have something to talk about at school on Monday. Jem turned on me.

"Don't say anything about it, Scout," he said.

"What? I certainly am. Ain't everybody's daddy the deadest shot in Maycomb County."

Jem said, "I reckon if he'd wanted us to know it, he'da told us. If he was proud of it, he'da told us."

"Maybe it just slipped his mind," I said.

"Naw, Scout, it's something you wouldn't understand. Atticus is real old, but I wouldn't care if he couldn't do anything—I wouldn't care if he couldn't do a blessed thing."

Jem picked up a rock and threw it jubilantly at the carhouse. Running after it, he called back: "Atticus is a gentleman, just like me!"

11

When we were small, Jem and I confined our activities to the southern neighborhood, but when I was well into the second grade at school and tormenting Boo Radley became passé, the business section of Maycomb drew us frequently up the street past the real property of Mrs. Henry Lafayette Dubose. It was impossible to go to town without passing her house unless we wished to walk a mile out of the way. Previous minor encounters with her left me with no desire for more, but Jem said I had to grow up some time.

Mrs. Dubose lived alone except for a Negro girl in constant attendance, two doors up the street from us in a house with steep front steps and a dog-trot hall. She was very old; she spent most of each day in bed and the rest of it in a wheelchair. It was rumored that she kept a CSA pistol concealed among her numerous shawls and wraps.

Jem and I hated her. If she was on the porch when we passed, we would be raked by her wrathful gaze, subjected to ruthless interrogation regarding our behavior, and given a melancholy prediction on what we would amount to when we grew up, which was always nothing. We had long ago given up the idea of walking past her house on the opposite side of the street; that only made her raise her voice and let the whole neighborhood in on it.

We could do nothing to please her. If I said as sunnily as I could, "Hey, Mrs. Dubose," I would receive for an answer, "Don't you say hey to me, you ugly girl! You say good afternoon, Mrs. Dubose!"

She was vicious. Once she heard Jem refer to our father as "Atticus" and her reaction was apoplectic. Besides being the sassiest, most disrespectful mutts who ever passed her way, we were told that it was quite a pity our father had not remarried after our mother's death. A lovelier lady than our mother never lived, she said, and it was heartbreaking the way Atticus Finch let his children run wild. I did not remember our mother, but Jem did—he would tell me about her sometimes—and he went livid when Mrs. Dubose shot us this message.

Jem, having survived Boo Radley, a mad dog and other terrors, had concluded that it was cowardly to stop at Miss Rachel's front steps and wait, and had decreed that we must run as far as the post office corner each evening to meet Atticus coming from work. Countless evenings Atticus would find Jem furious at something Mrs. Dubose had said when we went by.

"Easy does it, son," Atticus would say. "She's an old lady and she's ill. You just hold your head high and be a gentleman. Whatever she says to you, it's your job not to let her make you mad."

Jem would say she must not be very sick, she hollered so. When the three of us came to her house, Atticus would sweep off his hat, wave gallantly to her and say, "Good evening, Mrs. Dubose! You look like a picture this evening."

I never heard Atticus say like a picture of what. He would tell her the courthouse news, and would say he hoped with all his heart she'd have a good day tomorrow. He would return his hat to his head, swing me to his shoulders in her very presence, and we would go home in the twilight. It was times like these when I thought my father, who hated guns and had never been to any wars, was the bravest man who ever lived.

The day after Jem's twelfth birthday his money was burning up his pockets, so we headed for town in the early afternoon. Jem thought he had enough to buy a miniature steam engine for himself and a twirling baton for me.

I had long had my eye on that baton: it was at V. J. Elmore's, it was bedecked with sequins and tinsel, it cost seventeen cents. It was then my burning ambition to grow up and twirl with the Maycomb County High School band.

Having developed my talent to where I could throw up a stick and almost catch it coming down, I had caused Calpurnia to deny me entrance to the house every time she saw me with a stick in my hand. I felt that I could overcome this defect with a real baton, and I thought it generous of Jem to buy one for me.

Mrs. Dubose was stationed on her porch when we went by.

"Where are you two going at this time of day?" she shouted. "Playing hooky, I suppose. I'll just call up the principal and tell him!" She put her hands on the wheels of her chair and executed a perfect right face.

"Aw, it's Saturday, Mrs. Dubose," said Jem.

"Makes no difference if it's Saturday," she said obscurely. "I wonder if your father knows where you are?"

"Mrs. Dubose, we've been goin' to town by ourselves since we were this high." Jem placed his hand palm down about two feet above the sidewalk.

"Don't you lie to me!" she yelled. "Jeremy Finch, Maudie Atkinson told me you broke down her scuppernong arbor this morning. She's going to tell your father and then you'll wish you never saw the light of day! If you aren't sent to the reform school before next week, my name's not Dubose!"

Jem, who hadn't been near Miss Maudie's scuppernong arbor since last summer, and who knew Miss Maudie wouldn't tell Atticus if he had, issued a general denial.

"Don't you contradict me!" Mrs. Dubose bawled. "And *you*—" she pointed an arthritic finger at me—"what are you doing in those overalls? You should be in a dress and camisole, young lady! You'll grow up waiting on tables if somebody doesn't change your ways—a Finch waiting on tables at the O.K. Café—hah!"

I was terrified. The O.K. Café was a dim organization on the north side of the square. I grabbed Jem's hand but he shook me loose.

"Come on, Scout," he whispered. "Don't pay any attention to her, just hold your head high and be a gentleman."

But Mrs. Dubose held us: "Not only a Finch waiting on tables but one in the courthouse lawing for niggers!"

Jem stiffened. Mrs. Dubose's shot had gone home and she knew it:

"Yes indeed, what has this world come to when a Finch goes against his raising? I'll tell you!" She put her hand to her mouth. When she drew it away, it trailed a long silver thread of saliva. "Your father's no better than the niggers and trash he works for!"

Jem was scarlet. I pulled at his sleeve, and we were followed up the sidewalk by a philippic on our family's moral degeneration, the major premise of which was that half the Finches were in the asylum anyway, but if our mother were living we would not have come to such a state.

I wasn't sure what Jem resented most, but I took umbrage at Mrs. Dubose's assessment of the family's mental hygiene. I had become almost accustomed to hearing insults aimed at Atticus. But this was the first one coming from an adult. Except for her remarks about Atticus, Mrs. Dubose's attack was only routine. There was a hint of summer in the air— in the shadows it was cool, but the sun was warm, which meant good times coming: no school and Dill.

Jem bought his steam engine and we went by Elmore's for my baton. Jem took no pleasure in his acquisition; he jammed it in his pocket and walked silently beside me toward home. On the way home I nearly hit Mr. Link Deas, who said, "Look out now, Scout!" when I missed a toss, and when we approached Mrs. Dubose's house my baton was grimy from having picked it up out of the dirt so many times.

She was not on the porch.

In later years, I sometimes wondered exactly what made Jem do it, what made him break the bonds of "You just be a gentleman, son," and the phase of self-conscious rectitude he had recently entered. Jem had probably stood as much guff about Atticus lawing for niggers as had I, and I took it for granted that he kept his temper—he had a naturally tranquil disposition and a slow fuse. At the time, however, I thought the only explanation for what he did was that for a few minutes he simply went mad.

What Jem did was something I'd do as a matter of course had I not been under Atticus's interdict, which I assumed included not fighting horrible old ladies. We had just come to her gate when Jem snatched my baton and ran flailing wildly up the steps into Mrs. Dubose's front yard, forgetting everything Atticus had said, forgetting that she packed a pistol under her shawls, forgetting that if Mrs. Dubose missed, her girl Jessie probably wouldn't.

He did not begin to calm down until he had cut the tops off every camellia bush Mrs. Dubose owned, until the ground was littered with green buds and leaves. He bent my baton against his knee, snapped it in two and threw it down.

By that time I was shrieking. Jem yanked my hair, said he didn't care, he'd do it again if he got a chance, and if I didn't shut up he'd pull every hair out of my head. I didn't shut up and he kicked me. I lost my balance and fell on my face. Jem picked me up roughly but looked like he was sorry. There was nothing to say.

We did not choose to meet Atticus coming home that evening. We skulked around the kitchen until Calpurnia threw us out. By some voo-doo system Calpurnia seemed to know all about it. She was a less than satisfactory source of palliation, but she did give Jem a hot biscuit-and-butter which he tore in half and shared with me. It tasted like cotton.

We went to the livingroom. I picked up a football magazine, found a picture of Dixie Howell, showed it to Jem and said, "This looks like you." That was the nicest thing I could think to say to him, but it was no help. He sat by the windows, hunched down in a rocking chair, scowling, waiting. Daylight faded.

Two geological ages later, we heard the soles of Atticus's shoes scrape the front steps. The screen door slammed, there was a pause—Atticus was at the hat rack in the hall—and we heard him call, "Jem!" His voice was like the winter wind.

Atticus switched on the ceiling light in the livingroom and found us there, frozen still. He carried my baton in one hand; its filthy yellow tassel trailed on the rug. He held out his other hand; it contained fat camellia buds.

"Jem," he said, "are you responsible for this?"

"Yes sir."

"Why'd you do it?"

Jem said softly, "She said you lawed for niggers and trash."

"You did this because she said that?"

Jem's lips moved, but his, "Yes sir," was inaudible.

"Son, I have no doubt that you've been annoyed by your

contemporaries about me lawing for niggers, as you say, but to do something like this to a sick old lady is inexcusable. I strongly advise you to go down and have a talk with Mrs. Dubose," said Atticus. "Come straight home afterward."

Jem did not move.

"Go on, I said."

I followed Jem out of the livingroom. "Come back here," Atticus said to me. I came back.

Atticus picked up the *Mobile Press* and sat down in the rocking chair Jem had vacated. For the life of me, I did not understand how he could sit there in cold blood and read a newspaper when his only son stood an excellent chance of being murdered with a Confederate Army relic. Of course Jem antagonized me sometimes until I could kill him, but when it came down to it he was all I had. Atticus did not seem to realize this, or if he did he didn't care.

I hated him for that, but when you are in trouble you become easily tired: soon I was hiding in his lap and his arms were around me.

"You're mighty big to be rocked," he said.

"You don't care what happens to him," I said. "You just send him on to get shot at when all he was doin' was standin' up for you."

Atticus pushed my head under his chin. "It's not time to worry yet," he said. "I never thought Jem'd be the one to lose his head over this—thought I'd have more trouble with you."

I said I didn't see why we had to keep our heads anyway, that nobody I knew at school had to keep his head about anything.

"Scout," said Atticus, "when summer comes you'll have to keep your head about far worse things . . . it's not fair for you and Jem, I know that, but sometimes we have to make the best of things, and the way we conduct ourselves when the chips are down—well, all I can say is, when you and Jem are grown, maybe you'll look back on this with some compassion and some feeling that I didn't let you down. This case, Tom Robinson's case, is something that goes to the essence of a man's conscience—Scout, I couldn't go to church and worship God if I didn't try to help that man."

"Atticus, you must be wrong. . . ."

"How's that?"

"Well, most folks seem to think they're right and you're wrong. . . ."

"They're certainly entitled to think that, and they're entitled to full respect for their opinions," said Atticus, "but before I can live with other folks I've got to live with myself. The one thing that doesn't abide by majority rule is a person's conscience."

When Jem returned, he found me still in Atticus's lap. "Well, son?" said Atticus. He set me on my feet, and I made a secret reconnaissance of Jem. He seemed to be all in one piece, but he had a queer look on his face. Perhaps she had given him a dose of calomel.

"I cleaned it up for her and said I was sorry, but I ain't, and that I'd work on 'em ever Saturday and try to make 'em grow back out."

"There was no point in saying you were sorry if you aren't," said Atticus. "Jem, she's old and ill. You can't hold her responsible for what she says and does. Of course, I'd rather she'd have said it to me than to either of you, but we can't always have our 'druthers."

Jem seemed fascinated by a rose in the carpet. "Atticus," he said, "she wants me to read to her."

"Read to her?"

"Yes sir. She wants me to come every afternoon after school and Saturdays and read to her out loud for two hours. Atticus, do I have to?"

"Certainly."

"But she wants me to do it for a month."

"Then you'll do it for a month."

Jem planted his big toe delicately in the center of the rose and pressed it in. Finally he said, "Atticus, it's all right on the sidewalk but inside it's—it's all dark and creepy. There's shadows and things on the ceiling. . . ."

Atticus smiled grimly. "That should appeal to your imagination. Just pretend you're inside the Radley house."

The following Monday afternoon Jem and I climbed the steep front steps to Mrs. Dubose's house and padded down the open hallway. Jem, armed with *Ivanhoe* and full of superior knowledge, knocked at the second door on the left.

"Mrs. Dubose?" he called.

Jessie opened the wood door and unlatched the screen door.

"Is that you, Jem Finch?" she said. "You got your sister with you. I don't know—"

"Let 'em both in, Jessie," said Mrs. Dubose. Jessie admitted us and went off to the kitchen.

An oppressive odor met us when we crossed the threshold, an odor I had met many times in rain-rotted gray houses where there are coal-oil lamps, water dippers, and unbleached domestic sheets. It always made me afraid, expectant, watchful.

In the corner of the room was a brass bed, and in the bed was Mrs. Dubose. I wondered if Jem's activities had put her there, and for a moment I felt sorry for her. She was lying under a pile of quilts and looked almost friendly.

There was a marble-topped washstand by her bed; on it were a glass with a teaspoon in it, a red ear syringe, a box of absorbent cotton, and a steel alarm clock standing on three tiny legs.

"So you brought that dirty little sister of yours, did you?" was her greeting.

Jem said quietly, "My sister ain't dirty and I ain't scared of you," although I noticed his knees shaking.

I was expecting a tirade, but all she said was, "You may commence reading, Jeremy."

Jem sat down in a cane-bottom chair and opened *Ivanhoe*. I pulled up another one and sat beside him.

"Come closer," said Mrs. Dubose. "Come to the side of the bed."

We moved our chairs forward. This was the nearest I had ever been to her, and the thing I wanted most to do was move my chair back again.

She was horrible. Her face was the color of a dirty pillowcase, and the corners of her mouth glistened with wet, which inched like a glacier down the deep grooves enclosing her chin. Old-age liver spots dotted her cheeks, and her pale eyes had black pinpoint pupils. Her hands were knobby, and the cuticles were grown up over her fingernails. Her bottom plate was not in, and her upper lip protruded; from time to time she would draw her nether lip to her upper plate and carry her chin with it. This made the wet move faster.

I didn't look any more than I had to. Jem reopened *Ivanhoe* and began reading. I tried to keep up with him, but he read too fast. When Jem came to a word he didn't know, he skipped it, but Mrs. Dubose would catch him and make him spell it out. Jem read for perhaps twenty minutes, during which time I looked at the soot-stained mantelpiece, out the window, anywhere to keep from looking at her. As he read along, I noticed that Mrs. Dubose's corrections grew fewer and farther between, that Jem had even left one sentence dangling in mid-air. She was not listening.

I looked toward the bed.

Something had happened to her. She lay on her back, with the quilts up to her chin. Only her head and shoulders were visible. Her head moved slowly from side to side. From time to time she would open her mouth wide, and I could see her tongue undulate faintly. Cords of saliva would collect on her lips; she would draw them in, then open her mouth again. Her mouth seemed to have a private existence of its own. It worked separate and apart from the rest of her, out and in, like a clam hole at low tide. Occasionally it would say, "Pt," like some viscous substance coming to a boil.

I pulled Jem's sleeve.

He looked at me, then at the bed. Her head made its regular sweep toward us, and Jem said, "Mrs. Dubose, are you all right?" She did not hear him.

The alarm clock went off and scared us stiff. A minute later, nerves still tingling, Jem and I were on the sidewalk headed for home. We did not run away, Jessie sent us: before the clock wound down she was in the room pushing Jem and me out of it.

"Shoo," she said, "you all go home."

Jem hesitated at the door.

"It's time for her medicine," Jessie said. As the door swung shut behind us I saw Jessie walking quickly toward Mrs. Dubose's bed.

It was only three forty-five when we got home, so Jem and I drop-kicked in the back yard until it was time to meet Atticus. Atticus had two yellow pencils for me and a football magazine for Jem, which I suppose was a silent reward for our first day's session with Mrs. Dubose. Jem told him what happened.

"Did she frighten you?" asked Atticus.

"No sir," said Jem, "but she's so nasty. She has fits or somethin'. She spits a lot."

"She can't help that. When people are sick they don't look nice sometimes."

"She scared me," I said.

Atticus looked at me over his glasses. "You don't have to go with Jem, you know."

The next afternoon at Mrs. Dubose's was the same as the first, and so was the next, until gradually a pattern emerged: everything would begin normally—that is, Mrs. Dubose would hound Jem for a while on her favorite subjects, her camellias and our father's nigger-loving propensities; she would grow increasingly silent, then go away from us. The alarm clock would ring, Jessie would shoo us out, and the rest of the day was ours.

"Atticus," I said one evening, "what exactly is a nigger-lover?"

Atticus's face was grave. "Has somebody been calling you that?"

"No sir, Mrs. Dubose calls you that. She warms up every afternoon calling you that. Francis called me that last Christmas, that's where I first heard it."

"Is that the reason you jumped on him?" asked Atticus.

"Yes sir . . ."

"Then why are you asking me what it means?"

I tried to explain to Atticus that it wasn't so much what Francis said that had infuriated me as the way he had said it. "It was like he'd said snot-nose or somethin'."

"Scout," said Atticus, "nigger-lover is just one of those terms that don't mean anything—like snot-nose. It's hard to explain—ignorant, trashy people use it when they think somebody's favoring Negroes over and above themselves. It's slipped into usage with some people like ourselves, when they want a common, ugly term to label somebody."

"You aren't really a nigger-lover, then, are you?"

"I certainly am. I do my best to love everybody . . . I'm hard put, sometimes—baby, it's never an insult to be called what somebody thinks is a bad name. It just shows you how poor that person is, it doesn't hurt you. So don't let Mrs. Dubose get you down. She has enough troubles of her own."

One afternoon a month later Jem was ploughing his way through Sir Walter Scout, as Jem called him, and Mrs. Dubose was correcting him at every turn, when there was a knock on the door. "Come in!" she screamed.

Atticus came in. He went to the bed and took Mrs. Dubose's hand. "I was coming from the office and didn't see the children," he said. "I thought they might still be here."

Mrs. Dubose smiled at him. For the life of me I could not figure out how she could bring herself to speak to him when she seemed to hate him so. "Do you know what time it is, Atticus?" she said. "Exactly fourteen minutes past five. The alarm clock's set for five-thirty. I want you to know that."

It suddenly came to me that each day we had been staying a little longer at Mrs. Dubose's, that the alarm clock went off a few minutes later every day, and that she was well into one of her fits by the time it sounded. Today she had antagonized Jem for nearly two hours with no intention of having a fit, and I felt hopelessly trapped. The alarm clock was the signal for our release; if one day it did not ring, what would we do?

"I have a feeling that Jem's reading days are numbered," said Atticus.

"Only a week longer, I think," she said, "just to make sure . . ."

Jem rose. "But—"

Atticus put out his hand and Jem was silent. On the way home, Jem said he had to do it just for a month and the month was up and it wasn't fair.

"Just one more week, son," said Atticus.

"No," said Jem.

"Yes," said Atticus.

The following week found us back at Mrs. Dubose's. The alarm clock had ceased sounding, but Mrs. Dubose would release us with, "That'll do," so late in the afternoon Atticus would be home reading the paper when we returned. Although her fits had passed off, she was in every other way her old self: when Sir Walter Scott became involved in lengthy descriptions of moats and castles, Mrs. Dubose would become bored and pick on us:

"Jeremy Finch, I told you you'd live to regret tearing up my camellias. You regret it now, don't you?"

Jem would say he certainly did.

"Thought you could kill my Snow-on-the-Mountain, did you? Well, Jessie says the top's growing back out. Next time you'll know how to do it right, won't you? You'll pull it up by the roots, won't you?"

Jem would say he certainly would.

"Don't you mutter at me, boy! You hold up your head and say yes ma'am. Don't guess you feel like holding it up, though, with your father what he is."

Jem's chin would come up, and he would gaze at Mrs. Dubose with a face devoid of resentment. Through the weeks he had cultivated an expression of polite and detached interest, which he would present to her in answer to her most blood-curdling inventions.

At last the day came. When Mrs. Dubose said, "That'll do," one afternoon, she added, "And that's all. Good-day to you."

It was over. We bounded down the sidewalk on a spree of sheer relief, leaping and howling.

That spring was a good one: the days grew longer and gave us more playing time. Jem's mind was occupied mostly with the vital statistics of every college football player in the nation. Every night Atticus would read us the sports pages of the newspapers. Alabama might go to the Rose Bowl again this year, judging from its prospects, not one of whose names we could pronounce. Atticus was in the middle of Windy Seaton's column one evening when the telephone rang.

He answered it, then went to the hat rack in the hall. "I'm going down to Mrs. Dubose's for a while," he said. "I won't be long."

But Atticus stayed away until long past my bedtime. When he returned he was carrying a candy box. Atticus sat down in the livingroom and put the box on the floor beside his chair.

"What'd she want?" asked Jem.

We had not seen Mrs. Dubose for over a month. She was never on the porch any more when we passed.

"She's dead, son," said Atticus. "She died a few minutes ago."

"Oh," said Jem. "Well."

"Well is right," said Atticus. "She's not suffering any

more. She was sick for a long time. Son, didn't you know what her fits were?"

Jem shook his head.

"Mrs. Dubose was a morphine addict," said Atticus. "She took it as a pain-killer for years. The doctor put her on it. She'd have spent the rest of her life on it and died without so much agony, but she was too contrary—"

"Sir?" said Jem.

Atticus said, "Just before your escapade she called me to make her will. Dr. Reynolds told her she had only a few months left. Her business affairs were in perfect order but she said, 'There's still one thing out of order.'"

"What was that?" Jem was perplexed.

"She said she was going to leave this world beholden to nothing and nobody. Jem, when you're sick as she was, it's all right to take anything to make it easier, but it wasn't all right for her. She said she meant to break herself of it before she died, and that's what she did."

Jem said, "You mean that's what her fits were?"

"Yes, that's what they were. Most of the time you were reading to her I doubt if she heard a word you said. Her whole mind and body were concentrated on that alarm clock. If you hadn't fallen into her hands, I'd have made you go read to her anyway. It may have been some distraction. There was another reason—"

"Did she die free?" asked Jem.

"As the mountain air," said Atticus. "She was conscious to the last, almost. Conscious," he smiled, "and cantankerous. She still disapproved heartily of my doings, and said I'd probably spend the rest of my life bailing you out of jail. She had Jessie fix you this box—"

Atticus reached down and picked up the candy box. He handed it to Jem.

Jem opened the box. Inside, surrounded by wads of damp cotton, was a white, waxy, perfect camellia. It was a Snow-on-the-Mountain.

Jem's eyes nearly popped out of his head. "Old hell-devil, old hell-devil!" he screamed, flinging it down. "Why can't she leave me alone?"

In a flash Atticus was up and standing over him. Jem buried his face in Atticus's shirt front. "Sh-h," he said. "I think that was her way of telling you—everything's all right now, Jem, everything's all right. You know, she was a great lady.''

''A lady?'' Jem raised his head. His face was scarlet. ''After all those things she said about you, a lady?''

''She was. She had her own views about things, a lot different from mine, maybe . . . son, I told you that if you hadn't lost your head I'd have made you go read to her. I wanted you to see something about her—I wanted you to see what real courage is, instead of getting the idea that courage is a man with a gun in his hand. It's when you know you're licked before you begin but you begin anyway and you see it through no matter what. You rarely win, but sometimes you do. Mrs. Dubose won, all ninety-eight pounds of her. According to her views, she died beholden to nothing and nobody. She was the bravest person I ever knew.''

Jem picked up the candy box and threw it in the fire. He picked up the camellia, and when I went off to bed I saw him fingering the wide petals. Atticus was reading the paper.

Part Two

Part Two

12

Jem was twelve. He was difficult to live with, inconsistent, moody. His appetite was appalling, and he told me so many times to stop pestering him I consulted Atticus: "Reckon he's got a tapeworm?" Atticus said no, Jem was growing. I must be patient with him and disturb him as little as possible.

This change in Jem had come about in a matter of weeks. Mrs. Dubose was not cold in her grave—Jem had seemed grateful enough for my company when he went to read to her. Overnight, it seemed, Jem had acquired an alien set of values and was trying to impose them on me: several times he went so far as to tell me what to do. After one altercation when Jem hollered, "It's time you started bein' a girl and acting right!" I burst into tears and fled to Calpurnia.

"Don't you fret too much over Mister Jem—" she began.

"Mister Jem?"

"Yeah, he's just about Mister Jem now."

"He ain't that old," I said. "All he needs is somebody to beat him up, and I ain't big enough."

"Baby," said Calpurnia, "I just can't help it if Mister Jem's growin' up. He's gonna want to be off to himself a lot now, doin' whatever boys do, so you just come right on in the kitchen when you feel lonesome. We'll find lots of things to do in here."

The beginning of that summer boded well: Jem could do as he pleased; Calpurnia would do until Dill came. She seemed glad to see me when I appeared in the kitchen, and by watching her I began to think there was some skill involved in being a girl.

But summer came and Dill was not there. I received a letter and a snapshot from him. The letter said he had a new father whose picture was enclosed, and he would have to stay in Meridian because they planned to build a fishing boat. His father was a lawyer like Atticus, only much younger. Dill's new father had a pleasant face, which made me glad Dill had captured him, but I was crushed. Dill concluded by saying he would love me forever and not to worry, he would come get me and marry me as soon as he got enough money together, so please write.

The fact that I had a permanent fiancé was little compensation for his absence: I had never thought about it, but summer was Dill by the fishpool smoking string, Dill's eyes alive with complicated plans to make Boo Radley emerge; summer was the swiftness with which Dill would reach up and kiss me when Jem was not looking, the longings we sometimes felt each other feel. With him, life was routine; without him, life was unbearable. I stayed miserable for two days.

As if that were not enough, the state legislature was called into emergency session and Atticus left us for two weeks. The Governor was eager to scrape a few barnacles off the ship of state; there were sit-down strikes in Birmingham; bread lines in the cities grew longer, people in the country grew poorer. But these were events remote from the world of Jem and me.

We were surprised one morning to see a cartoon in the *Montgomery Advertiser* above the caption, "Maycomb's Finch." It showed Atticus barefooted and in short pants, chained to a desk: he was diligently writing on a slate while some frivolous-looking girls yelled, "Yoo-hoo!" at him.

"That's a compliment," explained Jem. "He spends his time doin' things that wouldn't get done if nobody did 'em."

"Huh?"

In addition to Jem's newly developed characteristics, he had acquired a maddening air of wisdom.

"Oh, Scout, it's like reorganizing the tax systems of the counties and things. That kind of thing's pretty dry to most men."

"How do you know?"

"Oh, go on and leave me alone. I'm readin' the paper."

Jem got his wish. I departed for the kitchen.

While she was shelling peas, Calpurnia suddenly said, "What am I gonna do about you all's church this Sunday?"

"Nothing, I reckon. Atticus left us collection."

Calpurnia's eyes narrowed and I could tell what was going through her mind. "Cal," I said, "you know we'll behave. We haven't done anything in church in years."

Calpurnia evidently remembered a rainy Sunday when we were both fatherless and teacherless. Left to its own devices, the class tied Eunice Ann Simpson to a chair and placed her in the furnace room. We forgot her, trooped upstairs to church, and were listening quietly to the sermon when a dreadful banging issued from the radiator pipes, persisting until someone investigated and brought forth Eunice Ann saying she didn't want to play Shadrach any more—Jem Finch said she wouldn't get burnt if she had enough faith, but it was hot down there.

"Besides, Cal, this isn't the first time Atticus has left us," I protested.

"Yeah, but he makes certain your teacher's gonna be there. I didn't hear him say this time—reckon he forgot it." Calpurnia scratched her head. Suddenly she smiled. "How'd you and Mister Jem like to come to church with me tomorrow?"

"Really?"

"How 'bout it?" grinned Calpurnia.

If Calpurnia had ever bathed me roughly before, it was nothing compared to her supervision of that Saturday night's routine. She made me soap all over twice, drew fresh water in the tub for each rinse; she stuck my head in the basin and washed it with Octagon soap and castile. She had trusted Jem for years, but that night she invaded his privacy and provoked an outburst: "Can't anybody take a bath in this house without the whole family lookin'?"

Next morning she began earlier than usual, to "go over our clothes." When Calpurnia stayed overnight with us she slept on a folding cot in the kitchen; that morning it was covered with our Sunday habiliments. She had put so much starch in my dress it came up like a tent when I sat down.

She made me wear a petticoat and she wrapped a pink sash tightly around my waist. She went over my patent-leather shoes with a cold biscuit until she saw her face in them.

"It's like we were goin' to Mardi Gras," said Jem "What's all this for, Cal?"

"I don't want anybody sayin' I don't look after my children," she muttered. "Mister Jem, you absolutely can't wear that tie with that suit. It's green."

" 'smatter with that?"

"Suit's blue. Can't you tell?"

"Hee hee," I howled, "Jem's color blind."

His face flushed angrily, but Calpurnia said, "Now you all quit that. You're gonna go to First Purchase with smiles on your faces."

First Purchase African M.E. Church was in the Quarters outside the southern town limits, across the old sawmill tracks. It was an ancient paint-peeled frame building, the only church in Maycomb with a steeple and bell, called First Purchase because it was paid for from the first earnings of freed slaves. Negroes worshiped in it on Sundays and white men gambled in it on weekdays.

The churchyard was brick-hard clay, as was the cemetery beside it. If someone died during a dry spell, the body was covered with chunks of ice until rain softened the earth. A few graves in the cemetery were marked with crumbling tombstones; newer ones were outlined with brightly colored glass and broken Coca-Cola bottles. Lightning rods guarding some graves denoted dead who rested uneasily; stumps of burned-out candles stood at the heads of infant graves. It was a happy cemetery.

The warm bittersweet smell of clean Negro welcomed us as we entered the churchyard—Hearts of Love hairdressing mingled with asafoetida, snuff, Hoyt's Cologne, Brown's Mule, peppermint, and lilac talcum.

When they saw Jem and me with Calpurnia, the men stepped back and took off their hats; the women crossed their arms at their waists, weekday gestures of respectful attention. They parted and made a small pathway to the church door for us. Calpurnia walked between Jem and me, responding to the greetings of her brightly clad neighbors.

"What you up to, Miss Cal?" said a voice behind us.

Calpurnia's hands went to our shoulders and we stopped and looked around: standing in the path behind us was a tall Negro woman. Her weight was on one leg; she rested her left elbow in the curve of her hip, pointing at us with upturned palm. She was bullet-headed with strange almond-shaped eyes, straight nose, and an Indian-bow mouth. She seemed seven feet high.

I felt Calpurnia's hand dig into my shoulder. "What you want, Lula?" she asked, in tones I had never heard her use. She spoke quietly, contemptuously.

"I wants to know why you bringin' white chillun to nigger church."

"They's my comp'ny," said Calpurnia. Again I thought her voice strange: she was talking like the rest of them.

"Yeah, an' I reckon you's comp'ny at the Finch house durin' the week."

A murmur ran through the crowd. "Don't you fret," Calpurnia whispered to me, but the roses on her hat trembled indignantly.

When Lula came up the pathway toward us Calpurnia said, "Stop right there, nigger."

Lula stopped, but she said, "You ain't got no business bringin' white chillun here—they got their church, we got our'n. It is our church, ain't it, Miss Cal?"

Calpurnia said, "It's the same God, ain't it?"

Jem said, "Let's go home, Cal, they don't want us here—"

I agreed: they did not want us here. I sensed, rather than saw, that we were being advanced upon. They seemed to be drawing closer to us, but when I looked up at Calpurnia there was amusement in her eyes. When I looked down the pathway again, Lula was gone. In her place was a solid mass of colored people.

One of them stepped from the crowd. It was Zeebo, the garbage collector. "Mister Jem," he said, "we're mighty glad to have you all here. Don't pay no 'tention to Lula, she's contentious because Reverend Sykes threatened to church her. She's a troublemaker from way back, got fancy ideas an' haughty ways—we're mighty glad to have you all."

With that, Calpurnia led us to the church door where we were greeted by Reverend Sykes, who led us to the front pew.

First Purchase was unceiled and unpainted within. Along its walls unlighted kerosene lamps hung on brass brackets; pine benches served as pews. Behind the rough oak pulpit a faded pink silk banner proclaimed God Is Love, the church's only decoration except a rotogravure print of Hunt's *The Light of the World*. There was no sign of piano, organ, hymn-books, church programs—the familiar ecclesiastical impedimenta we saw every Sunday. It was dim inside, with a damp coolness slowly dispelled by the gathering congregation. At each seat was a cheap cardboard fan bearing a garish Garden of Gethsemane, courtesy Tyndal's Hardware Co. (You-Name-It-We-Sell-It).

Calpurnia motioned Jem and me to the end of the row and placed herself between us. She fished in her purse, drew out her handkerchief, and untied the hard wad of change in its corner. She gave a dime to me and a dime to Jem. "We've got ours," he whispered. "You keep it," Calpurnia said, "you're my company." Jem's face showed brief indecision on the ethics of withholding his own dime, but his innate courtesy won and he shifted his dime to his pocket. I did likewise with no qualms.

"Cal," I whispered, "where are the hymn-books?"

"We don't have any," she said.

"Well how—?"

"Sh-h," she said. Reverend Sykes was standing behind the pulpit staring the congregation to silence. He was a short, stocky man in a black suit, black tie, white shirt, and a gold watch-chain that glinted in the light from the frosted windows.

He said, "Brethren and sisters, we are particularly glad to have company with us this morning. Mister and Miss Finch. You all know their father. Before I begin I will read some announcements."

Reverend Sykes shuffled some papers, chose one and held it at arm's length. "The Missionary Society meets in the home of Sister Annette Reeves next Tuesday. Bring your sewing."

He read from another paper. "You all know of Brother Tom Robinson's trouble. He has been a faithful member of

First Purchase since he was a boy. The collection taken up today and for the next three Sundays will go to Helen—his wife, to help her out at home.''

I punched Jem. ''That's the Tom Atticus's de—''

''Sh-h!''

I turned to Calpurnia but was hushed before I opened my mouth. Subdued, I fixed my attention upon Reverend Sykes, who seemed to be waiting for me to settle down. ''Will the music superintendent lead us in the first hymn,'' he said.

Zeebo rose from his pew and walked down the center aisle, stopping in front of us and facing the congregation. He was carrying a battered hymn-book. He opened it and said, ''We'll sing number two seventy-three.''

This was too much for me. ''How're we gonna sing it if there ain't any hymn-books?''

Calpurnia smiled. ''Hush baby,'' she whispered, ''you'll see in a minute.''

Zeebo cleared his throat and read in a voice like the rumble of distant artillery:

''There's a land beyond the river.''

Miraculously on pitch, a hundred voices sang out Zeebo's words. The last syllable, held to a husky hum, was followed by Zeebo saying,

''That we call the sweet forever.''

Music again swelled around us; the last note lingered and Zeebo met it with the next line: ''And we only reach that shore by faith's decree.''

The congregation hesitated, Zeebo repeated the line carefully, and it was sung. At the chorus Zeebo closed the book, a signal for the congregation to proceed without his help.

On the dying notes of ''Jubilee,'' Zeebo said, ''In that far-off sweet forever, just beyond the shining river.''

Line for line, voices followed in simple harmony until the hymn ended in a melancholy murmur.

I looked at Jem, who was looking at Zeebo from the corners of his eyes. I didn't believe it either, but we had both heard it.

Reverend Sykes then called on the Lord to bless the sick and the suffering, a procedure no different from our church practice, except Reverend Sykes directed the Deity's attention to several specific cases.

His sermon was a forthright denunciation of sin, an austere declaration of the motto on the wall behind him: he warned his flock against the evils of heady brews, gambling, and strange women. Bootleggers caused enough trouble in the Quarters, but women were worse. Again, as I had often met it in my own church, I was confronted with the Impurity of Women doctrine that seemed to preoccupy all clergymen.

Jem and I had heard the same sermon Sunday after Sunday, with only one exception. Reverend Sykes used his pulpit more freely to express his views on individual lapses from grace: Jim Hardy had been absent from church for five Sundays and he wasn't sick; Constance Jackson had better watch her ways—she was in grave danger for quarreling with her neighbors; she had erected the only spite fence in the history of the Quarters.

Reverend Sykes closed his sermon. He stood beside a table in front of the pulpit and requested the morning offering, a proceeding that was strange to Jem and me. One by one, the congregation came forward and dropped nickels and dimes into a black enameled coffee can. Jem and I followed suit, and received a soft, "Thank you, thank you," as our dimes clinked.

To our amazement, Reverend Sykes emptied the can onto the table and raked the coins into his hand. He straightened up and said, "This is not enough, we must have ten dollars."

The congregation stirred. "You all know what it's for—Helen can't leave those children to work while Tom's in jail. If everybody gives one more dime, we'll have it—" Reverend Sykes waved his hand and called to someone in the back of the church. "Alec, shut the doors. Nobody leaves here till we have ten dollars."

Calpurnia scratched in her handbag and brought forth a battered leather coin purse. "Naw Cal," Jem whispered, when she handed him a shiny quarter, "we can put ours in. Gimme your dime, Scout."

The church was becoming stuffy, and it occurred to me that Reverend Sykes intended to sweat the amount due out of his flock. Fans crackled, feet shuffled, tobacco-chewers were in agony.

Reverend Sykes startled me by saying sternly, "Carlow Richardson, I haven't seen you up this aisle yet."

A thin man in khaki pants came up the aisle and deposited a coin. The congregation murmured approval.

Reverend Sykes then said, "I want all of you with no children to make a sacrifice and give one more dime apiece. Then we'll have it."

Slowly, painfully, the ten dollars was collected. The door was opened, and the gust of warm air revived us. Zeebo lined *On Jordan's Stormy Banks*, and church was over.

I wanted to stay and explore, but Calpurnia propelled me up the aisle ahead of her. At the church door, while she paused to talk with Zeebo and his family, Jem and I chatted with Reverend Sykes. I was bursting with questions, but decided I would wait and let Calpurnia answer them.

"We were 'specially glad to have you all here," said Reverend Sykes. "This church has no better friend than your daddy."

My curiosity burst: "Why were you all takin' up collection for Tom Robinson's wife?"

"Didn't you hear why?" asked Reverend Sykes. "Helen's got three little'uns and she can't go out to work—"

"Why can't she take 'em with her, Reverend?" I asked. It was customary for field Negroes with tiny children to deposit them in whatever shade there was while their parents worked—usually the babies sat in the shade between two rows of cotton. Those unable to sit were strapped papoose-style on their mothers' backs, or resided in extra cotton bags.

Reverend Sykes hesitated. "To tell you the truth, Miss Jean Louise, Helen's finding it hard to get work these days . . . when it's picking time, I think Mr. Link Deas'll take her."

"Why not, Reverend?"

Before he could answer, I felt Calpurnia's hand on my shoulder. At its pressure I said, "We thank you for lettin' us come." Jem echoed me, and we made our way homeward.

"Cal, I know Tom Robinson's in jail an' he's done somethin' awful, but why won't folks hire Helen?" I asked.

Calpurnia, in her navy voile dress and tub of a hat, walked between Jem and me. "It's because of what folks say Tom's done," she said. "Folks aren't anxious to—to have anything to do with any of his family."

"Just what did he do, Cal?"

Calpurnia sighed. "Old Mr. Bob Ewell accused him of rapin' his girl an' had him arrested an' put in jail—"

"Mr. Ewell?" My memory stirred. "Does he have anything to do with those Ewells that come every first day of school an' then go home? Why, Atticus said they were absolute trash—I never heard Atticus talk about folks the way he talked about the Ewells. He said—"

"Yeah, those are the ones."

"Well, if everybody in Maycomb knows what kind of folks the Ewells are they'd be glad to hire Helen . . . what's rape, Cal?"

"It's somethin' you'll have to ask Mr. Finch about," she said. "He can explain it better than I can. You all hungry? The Reverend took a long time unwindin' this morning, he's not usually so tedious."

"He's just like our preacher," said Jem, "but why do you all sing hymns that way?"

"Linin'?" she asked.

"Is that what it is?"

"Yeah, it's called linin'. They've done it that way as long as I can remember."

Jem said it looked like they could save the collection money for a year and get some hymn-books.

Calpurnia laughed. "Wouldn't do any good," she said. "They can't read."

"Can't read?" I asked. "All those folks?"

"That's right," Calpurnia nodded. "Can't but about four folks in First Purchase read . . . I'm one of 'em."

"Where'd you go to school, Cal?" asked Jem.

"Nowhere. Let's see now, who taught me my letters? It was Miss Maudie Atkinson's aunt, old Miss Buford—"

"Are you that old?"

"I'm older than Mr. Finch, even." Calpurnia grinned. "Not sure how much, though. We started rememberin' one time, trying to figure out how old I was—I can remember back just a few years more'n he can, so I'm not much older, when you take off the fact that men can't remember as well as women."

"What's your birthday, Cal?"

"I just have it on Christmas, it's easier to remember that way—I don't have a real birthday."

"But Cal," Jem protested, "you don't look even near as old as Atticus."

"Colored folks don't show their ages so fast," she said.

"Maybe because they can't read. Cal, did you teach Zeebo?"

"Yeah, Mister Jem. There wasn't a school even when he was a boy. I made him learn, though."

Zeebo was Calpurnia's eldest son. If I had ever thought about it, I would have known that Calpurnia was of mature years—Zeebo had half-grown children—but then I had never thought about it.

"Did you teach him out of a primer, like us?" I asked.

"No, I made him get a page of the Bible every day, and there was a book Miss Buford taught me out of—bet you don't know where I got it," she said.

We didn't know.

Calpurnia said, "Your Granddaddy Finch gave it to me."

"Were you from the Landing?" Jem asked. "You never told us that."

"I certainly am, Mister Jem. Grew up down there between the Buford Place and the Landin'. I've spent all my days workin' for the Finches or the Bufords, an' I moved to Maycomb when your daddy and your mamma married."

"What was the book, Cal?" I asked.

"Blackstone's *Commentaries*."

Jem was thunderstruck. "You mean you taught Zeebo outa *that*?"

"Why yes sir, Mister Jem." Calpurnia timidly put her fingers to her mouth. "They were the only books I had. Your grandaddy said Mr. Blackstone wrote fine English—"

"That's why you don't talk like the rest of 'em," said Jem.

"The rest of who?"

"Rest of the colored folks. Cal, but you talked like they did in church. . . ."

That Calpurnia led a modest double life never dawned on me. The idea that she had a separate existence outside our household was a novel one, to say nothing of her having command of two languages.

"Cal," I asked, "why do you talk nigger-talk to the—to your folks when you know it's not right?"

"Well, in the first place I'm black—"

"That doesn't mean you hafta talk that way when you know better," said Jem.

Calpurnia tilted her hat and scratched her head, then pressed her hat down carefully over her ears. "It's right hard to say," she said. "Suppose you and Scout talked colored-folks' talk at home it'd be out of place, wouldn't it? Now what if I talked white-folks' talk at church, and with my neighbors? They'd think I was puttin' on airs to beat Moses."

"But Cal, you know better," I said.

"It's not necessary to tell all you know. It's not ladylike —in the second place, folks don't like to have somebody around knowin' more than they do. It aggravates 'em. You're not gonna change any of them by talkin' right, they've got to want to learn themselves, and when they don't want to learn there's nothing you can do but keep your mouth shut or talk their language."

"Cal, can I come to see you sometimes?"

She looked down at me. "See me, honey? You see me every day."

"Out to your house," I said. "Sometimes after work? Atticus can get me."

"Any time you want to," she said. "We'd be glad to have you."

We were on the sidewalk by the Radley Place.

"Look on the porch yonder," Jem said.

I looked over to the Radley Place, expecting to see its phantom occupant sunning himself in the swing. The swing was empty.

"I mean our porch," said Jem.

I looked down the street. Enarmored, upright, uncompromising, Aunt Alexandra was sitting in a rocking chair exactly as if she had sat there every day of her life.

13

"Put my bag in the front bedroom, Calpurnia," was the first thing Aunt Alexandra said. "Jean Louise, stop scratching your head," was the second thing she said.

Calpurnia picked up Aunty's heavy suitcase and opened the door. "I'll take it," said Jem, and took it. I heard the suitcase hit the bedroom floor with a thump. The sound had a dull permanence about it.

"Have you come for a visit, Aunty?" I asked. Aunt Alexandra's visits from the Landing were rare, and she traveled in state. She owned a bright green square Buick and a black chauffeur, both kept in an unhealthy state of tidiness, but today they were nowhere to be seen.

"Didn't your father tell you?" she asked.

Jem and I shook our heads.

"Probably he forgot. He's not in yet, is he?"

"Nome, he doesn't usually get back till late afternoon," said Jem.

"Well, your father and I decided it was time I came to stay with you for a while."

"For a while" in Maycomb meant anything from three days to thirty years. Jem and I exchanged glances.

"Jem's growing up now and you are too," she said to me. "We decided that it would be best for you to have some feminine influence. It won't be many years, Jean Louise, before you become interested in clothes and boys—"

I could have made several answers to this: Cal's a girl, it would be many years before I would be interested in boys, I would never be interested in clothes . . . but I kept quiet.

"What about Uncle Jimmy?" asked Jem. "Is he comin', too?"

"Oh no, he's staying at the Landing. He'll keep the place going."

The moment I said, "Won't you miss him?" I realized that this was not a tactful question. Uncle Jimmy present or Uncle Jimmy absent made not much difference, he never said anything. Aunt Alexandra ignored my question.

I could think of nothing else to say to her. In fact I could never think of anything to say to her, and I sat thinking of past painful conversations between us: How are you, Jean Louise? Fine, thank you ma'am, how are you? Very well, thank you, what have you been doing with yourself? Nothin'. Don't you do anything? Nome. Certainly you have friends? Yessum. Well what do you all do? Nothin'.

It was plain that Aunty thought me dull in the extreme, because I once heard her tell Atticus that I was sluggish.

There was a story behind all this, but I had no desire to extract it from her then. Today was Sunday, and Aunt Alexandra was positively irritable on the Lord's Day. I guess it was her Sunday corset. She was not fat, but solid, and she chose protective garments that drew up her bosom to giddy heights, pinched in her waist, flared out her rear, and managed to suggest that Aunt Alexandra's was once an hour-glass figure. From any angle, it was formidable.

The remainder of the afternoon went by in the gentle gloom that descends when relatives appear, but was dispelled when we heard a car turn in the driveway. It was Atticus, home from Montgomery. Jem, forgetting his dignity, ran with me to meet him. Jem seized his briefcase and bag, I jumped into his arms, felt his vague dry kiss and said, " 'd you bring me a book? 'd you know Aunty's here?"

Atticus answered both questions in the affirmative. "How'd you like for her to come live with us?"

I said I would like it very much, which was a lie, but one must lie under certain circumstances and at all times when one can't do anything about them.

"We felt it was time you children needed—well, it's like this, Scout," Atticus said. "Your aunt's doing me a favor as well as you all. I can't stay here all day with you, and the summer's going to be a hot one."

"Yes sir," I said, not understanding a word he said. I had an idea, however, that Aunt Alexandra's appearance on the scene was not so much Atticus's doing as hers. Aunty had a way of declaring What Is Best For The Family, and I suppose her coming to live with us was in that category.

Maycomb welcomed her. Miss Maudie Atkinson baked a Lane cake so loaded with shinny it made me tight; Miss Stephanie Crawford had long visits with Aunt Alexandra, consisting mostly of Miss Stephanie shaking her head and saying, "Uh, uh, uh." Miss Rachel next door had Aunty over for coffee in the afternoons, and Mr. Nathan Radley went so far as to come up in the front yard and say he was glad to see her.

When she settled in with us and life resumed its daily pace, Aunt Alexandra seemed as if she had always lived with us. Her Missionary Society refreshments added to her reputation as a hostess (she did not permit Calpurnia to make the delicacies required to sustain the Society through long reports on Rice Christians); she joined and became Secretary of the Maycomb Amanuensis Club. To all parties present and participating in the life of the county, Aunt Alexandra was one of the last of her kind: she had river-boat, boarding-school manners; let any moral come along and she would uphold it; she was born in the objective case; she was an incurable gossip. When Aunt Alexandra went to school, self-doubt could not be found in any textbook, so she knew not its meaning. She was never bored, and given the slightest chance she would exercise her royal prerogative: she would arrange, advise, caution, and warn.

She never let a chance escape her to point out the shortcomings of other tribal groups to the greater glory of our own, a habit that amused Jem rather than annoyed him: "Aunty better watch how she talks—scratch most folks in Maycomb and they're kin to us."

Aunt Alexandra, in underlining the moral of young Sam Merriweather's suicide, said it was caused by a morbid streak in the family. Let a sixteen-year-old girl giggle in the choir and Aunty would say, "It just goes to show you, all the Penfield women are flighty." Everybody in Maycomb, it seemed, had a Streak: a Drinking Streak, a Gambling Streak, a Mean Streak, a Funny Streak.

Once, when Aunty assured us that Miss Stephanie Crawford's tendency to mind other people's business was hereditary, Atticus said, "Sister, when you stop to think about it, our generation's practically the first in the Finch family not to marry its cousins. Would you say the Finches have an Incestuous Streak?"

Aunty said no, that's where we got our small hands and feet.

I never understood her preoccupation with heredity. Somewhere, I had received the impression that Fine Folks were people who did the best they could with the sense they had, but Aunt Alexandra was of the opinion, obliquely expressed, that the longer a family had been squatting on one patch of land the finer it was.

"That makes the Ewells fine folks, then," said Jem. The tribe of which Burris Ewell and his brethren consisted had lived on the same plot of earth behind the Maycomb dump, and had thrived on county welfare money for three generations.

Aunt Alexandra's theory had something behind it, though. Maycomb was an ancient town. It was twenty miles east of Finch's Landing, awkwardly inland for such an old town. But Maycomb would have been closer to the river had it not been for the nimble-wittedness of one Sinkfield, who in the dawn of history operated an inn where two pig-trails met, the only tavern in the territory. Sinkfield, no patriot, served and supplied ammunition to Indians and settlers alike, neither knowing or caring whether he was a part of the Alabama Territory or the Creek Nation so long as business was good. Business was excellent when Governor William Wyatt Bibb, with a view to promoting the newly created county's domestic tranquility, dispatched a team of surveyors to locate its exact center and there establish its seat of government. The surveyors, Sinkfield's guests, told their host that he was in the territorial confines of Maycomb County, and showed him the probable spot where the county seat would be built. Had not Sinkfield made a bold stroke to preserve his holdings, Maycomb would have sat in the middle of Winston Swamp, a place totally devoid of interest. Instead, Maycomb grew and sprawled out from its hub, Sinkfield's Tavern, because Sinkfield reduced his guests to myopic drunkenness one evening, induced them to bring forward their maps and charts, lop off a little here, add a bit there, and adjust the center of the county to meet his requirements. He sent them packing next day armed with their charts and five quarts of shinny in their saddlebags—two apiece and one for the Governor.

Because its primary reason for existence was government, Maycomb was spared the grubbiness that distinguished most Alabama towns its size. In the beginning its buildings were solid, its courthouse proud, its streets graciously wide. Maycomb's proportion of professional people ran high: one went there to have his teeth pulled, his wagon fixed, his heart listened to, his money deposited, his soul saved, his mules vetted. But the ultimate wisdom of Sinkfield's maneuver is open to question. He placed the young town too far away from the only kind of public transportation in those days— river-boat—and it took a man from the north end of the county two days to travel to Maycomb for store-bought goods. As a result the town remained the same size for a hundred years, an island in a patchwork sea of cottonfields and timberland.

Although Maycomb was ignored during the War Between the States, Reconstruction rule and economic ruin forced the town to grow. It grew inward. New people so rarely settled there, the same families married the same families until the members of the community looked faintly alike. Occasionally someone would return from Montgomery or Mobile with an outsider, but the result caused only a ripple in the quiet stream of family resemblance. Things were more or less the same during my early years.

There was indeed a caste system in Maycomb, but to my mind it worked this way: the older citizens, the present generation of people who had lived side by side for years and years, were utterly predictable to one another: they took for granted attitudes, character shadings, even gestures, as having been repeated in each generation and refined by time. Thus the dicta No Crawford Minds His Own Business, Every Third Merriweather Is Morbid, The Truth Is Not in the Delafields, All the Bufords Walk Like That, were simply guides to daily living: never take a check from a Delafield without a discreet call to the bank; Miss Maudie Atkinson's shoulder stoops because she was a Buford; if Mrs. Grace Merriweather sips gin out of Lydia E. Pinkham bottles it's nothing unusual— her mother did the same.

Aunt Alexandra fitted into the world of Maycomb like a

hand into a glove, but never into the world of Jem and me. I so often wondered how she could be Atticus's and Uncle Jack's sister that I revived half-remembered tales of changelings and mandrake roots that Jem had spun long ago.

These were abstract speculations for the first month of her stay, as she had little to say to Jem or me, and we saw her only at mealtimes and at night before we went to bed. It was summer and we were outdoors. Of course some afternoons when I would run inside for a drink of water, I would find the livingroom overrun with Maycomb ladies, sipping, whispering, fanning, and I would be called: "Jean Louise, come speak to these ladies."

When I appeared in the doorway, Aunty would look as if she regretted her request; I was usually mud-splashed or covered with sand.

"Speak to your Cousin Lily," she said one afternoon, when she had trapped me in the hall.

"Who?" I said.

"Your Cousin Lily Brooke," said Aunt Alexandra.

"She our cousin? I didn't know that."

Aunt Alexandra managed to smile in a way that conveyed a gentle apology to Cousin Lily and firm disapproval to me. When Cousin Lily Brooke left I knew I was in for it.

It was a sad thing that my father had neglected to tell me about the Finch Family, or to install any pride into his children. She summoned Jem, who sat warily on the sofa beside me. She left the room and returned with a purple-covered book on which *Meditations of Joshua S. St. Clair* was stamped in gold.

"Your cousin wrote this," said Aunt Alexandra. "He was a beautiful character."

Jem examined the small volume. "Is this the Cousin Joshua who was locked up for so long?"

Aunt Alexandra said, "How did you know that?"

"Why, Atticus said he went round the bend at the University. Said he tried to shoot the president. Said Cousin Joshua said he wasn't anything but a sewer-inspector and tried to shoot him with an old flintlock pistol, only it just blew up in his hand. Atticus said it cost the family five hundred dollars to get him out of that one—"

Aunt Alexandra was standing stiff as a stork. "That's all," she said. "We'll see about this."

Before bedtime I was in Jem's room trying to borrow a book, when Atticus knocked and entered. He sat on the side of Jem's bed, looked at us soberly, then he grinned.

"Er—h'rm," he said. He was beginning to preface some things he said with a throaty noise, and I thought he must at last be getting old, but he looked the same. "I don't exactly know how to say this," he began.

"Well, just say it," said Jem. "Have we done something?"

Our father was actually fidgeting. "No, I just want to explain to you that—your Aunt Alexandra asked me . . . son, you know you're a Finch, don't you?"

"That's what I've been told." Jem looked out of the corners of his eyes. His voice rose uncontrollably, "Atticus, what's the matter?"

Atticus crossed his knees and folded his arms. "I'm trying to tell you the facts of life."

Jem's disgust deepened. "I know all that stuff," he said.

Atticus suddenly grew serious. In his lawyer's voice, without a shade of inflection, he said: "Your aunt has asked me to try and impress upon you and Jean Louise that you are not from run-of-the-mill people, that you are the product of several generations' gentle breeding——" Atticus paused, watching me locate an elusive redbug on my leg.

"Gentle breeding," he continued, when I had found and scratched it, "and that you should try to live up to your name——" Atticus persevered in spite of us: "She asked me to tell you you must try to behave like the little lady and gentleman that you are. She wants to talk to you about the family and what it's meant to Maycomb County through the years, so you'll have some idea of who you are, so you might be moved to behave accordingly," he concluded at a gallop.

Stunned, Jem and I looked at each other, then at Atticus, whose collar seemed to worry him. We did not speak to him.

Presently I picked up a comb from Jem's dresser and ran its teeth along the edge.

"Stop that noise," Atticus said.

His curtness stung me. The comb was midway in its journey, and I banged it down. For no reason I felt myself beginning to cry, but I could not stop. This was not my father. My father never thought these thoughts. My father never spoke so. Aunt Alexandra had put him up to this, somehow. Through my tears I saw Jem standing in a similar pool of isolation, his head cocked to one side.

There was nowhere to go, but I turned to go and met Atticus's vest front. I buried my head in it and listened to the small internal noises that went on behind the light blue cloth: his watch ticking, the faint crackle of his starched shirt, the soft sound of his breathing.

"Your stomach's growling," I said.

"I know it," he said.

"You better take some soda."

"I will," he said.

"Atticus, is all this behavin' an' stuff gonna make things different? I mean are you—?"

I felt his hand on the back of my head. "Don't you worry about anything," he said. "It's not time to worry."

When I heard that, I knew he had come back to us. The blood in my legs began to flow again, and I raised my head. "You really want us to do all that? I can't remember everything Finches are supposed to do. . . ."

"I don't want you to remember it. Forget it."

He went to the door and out of the room, shutting the door behind him. He nearly slammed it, but caught himself at the last minute and closed it softly. As Jem and I stared, the door opened again and Atticus peered around. His eyebrows were raised, his glasses had slipped. "Get more like Cousin Joshua every day, don't I? Do you think I'll end up costing the family five hundred dollars?"

I know now what he was trying to do, but Atticus was only a man. It takes a woman to do that kind of work.

14

Although we heard no more about the Finch family from Aunt Alexandra, we heard plenty from the town. On Saturdays, armed with our nickels, when Jem permitted me to accompany him (he was now positively allergic to my presence when in public), we would squirm our way through sweating sidewalk crowds and sometimes hear, "There's his chillun," or, "Yonder's some Finches." Turning to face our accusers, we would see only a couple of farmers studying the enema bags in the Mayco Drugstore window. Or two dumpy countrywomen in straw hats sitting in a Hoover cart.

"They c'n go loose and rape up the countryside for all of 'em who run this county care," was one obscure observation we met head on from a skinny gentleman when he passed us. Which reminded me that I had a question to ask Atticus.

"What's rape?" I asked him that night.

Atticus looked around from behind his paper. He was in his chair by the window. As we grew older, Jem and I thought it generous to allow Atticus thirty minutes to himself after supper.

He sighed, and said rape was carnal knowledge of a female by force and without consent.

"Well if that's all it is why did Calpurnia dry me up when I asked her what it was?"

Atticus looked pensive. "What's that again?"

"Well, I asked Calpurnia comin' from church that day what it was and she said ask you but I forgot to and now I'm askin' you."

His paper was now in his lap. "Again, please," he said.

I told him in detail about our trip to church with Calpurnia. Atticus seemed to enjoy it, but Aunt Alexandra, who was sitting in a corner quietly sewing, put down her embroidery and stared at us.

"You all were coming back from Calpurnia's church that Sunday?"

Jem said, "Yessum, she took us."

I remembered something. "Yessum, and she promised me I could come out to her house some afternoon. Atticus, I'll go next Sunday if it's all right, can I? Cal said she'd come get me if you were off in the car."

"You may *not*."

Aunt Alexandra said it. I wheeled around, startled, then turned back to Atticus in time to catch his swift glance at her, but it was too late. I said, "I didn't ask you!"

For a big man, Atticus could get up and down from a chair faster than anyone I ever knew. He was on his feet. "Apologize to your aunt," he said.

"I didn't ask her, I asked you—"

Atticus turned his head and pinned me to the wall with his good eye. His voice was deadly: "First, apologize to your aunt."

"I'm sorry, Aunty," I muttered.

"Now then," he said. "Let's get this clear: you do as Calpurnia tells you, you do as I tell you, and as long as your aunt's in this house, you will do as she tells you. Understand?"

I understood, pondered a while, and concluded that the only way I could retire with a shred of dignity was to go to the bathroom, where I stayed long enough to make them think I had to go. Returning, I lingered in the hall to hear a fierce discussion going on in the livingroom. Through the door I could see Jem on the sofa with a football magazine in front of his face, his head turning as if its pages contained a live tennis match.

". . . you've got to do something about her," Aunty was saying. "You've let things go on too long, Atticus, too long."

"I don't see any harm in letting her go out there. Cal'd look after her there as well as she does here."

Who was the "her" they were talking about? My heart sank: me. I felt the starched walls of a pink cotton penitentiary closing in on me, and for the second time in my life I thought of running away. Immediately.

"Atticus, it's all right to be soft-hearted, you're an easy

man, but you have a daughter to think of. A daughter who's growing up."

"That's what I am thinking of."

"And don't try to get around it. You've got to face it sooner or later and it might as well be tonight. We don't need her now."

Atticus's voice was even: "Alexandra, Calpurnia's not leaving this house until she wants to. You may think otherwise, but I couldn't have got along without her all these years. She's a faithful member of this family and you'll simply have to accept things the way they are. Besides, sister, I don't want you working your head off for us—you've no reason to do that. We still need Cal as much as we ever did."

"But Atticus—"

"Besides, I don't think the children've suffered one bit from her having brought them up. If anything, she's been harder on them in some ways than a mother would have been . . . she's never let them get away with anything, she's never indulged them the way most colored nurses do. She tried to bring them up according to her lights, and Cal's lights are pretty good—and another thing, the children love her."

I breathed again. It wasn't me, it was only Calpurnia they were talking about. Revived, I entered the livingroom. Atticus had retreated behind his newspaper and Aunt Alexandra was worrying her embroidery. Punk, punk, punk, her needle broke the taut circle. She stopped, and pulled the cloth tighter: punk-punk-punk. She was furious.

Jem got up and padded across the rug. He motioned me to follow. He led me to his room and closed the door. His face was grave.

"They've been fussing, Scout."

Jem and I fussed a great deal these days, but I had never heard of or seen anyone quarrel with Atticus. It was not a comfortable sight.

"Scout, try not to antagonize Aunty, hear?"

Atticus's remarks were still rankling, which made me miss the request in Jem's question. My feathers rose again. "You tryin' to tell me what to do?"

"Naw, it's—he's got a lot on his mind now, without us worrying him."

"Like what?" Atticus didn't appear to have anything especially on his mind.

"It's this Tom Robinson case that's worryin' him to death—"

I said Atticus didn't worry about anything. Besides, the case never bothered us except about once a week and then it didn't last.

"That's because you can't hold something in your mind but a little while," said Jem. "It's different with grown folks, we—"

His maddening superiority was unbearable these days. He didn't want to do anything but read and go off by himself. Still, everything he read he passed along to me, but with this difference: formerly, because he thought I'd like it; now, for my edification and instruction.

"Jee crawling hova, Jem! Who do you think you are?"

"Now I mean it, Scout, you antagonize Aunty and I'll—I'll spank you."

With that, I was gone. "You damn morphodite, I'll kill you!" He was sitting on the bed, and it was easy to grab his front hair and land one on his mouth. He slapped me and I tried another left, but a punch in the stomach sent me sprawling on the floor. It nearly knocked the breath out of me, but it didn't matter because I knew he was fighting, he was fighting me back. We were still equals.

"Ain't so high and mighty now, are you!" I screamed, sailing in again. He was still on the bed and I couldn't get a firm stance, so I threw myself at him as hard as I could, hitting, pulling, pinching, gouging. What had begun as a fistfight became a brawl. We were still struggling when Atticus separated us.

"That's all," he said. "Both of you go to bed right now."

"Taah!" I said at Jem. He was being sent to bed at my bedtime.

"Who started it?" asked Atticus, in resignation.

"Jem did. He was tryin' to tell me what to do. I don't have to mind *him* now, do I?"

Atticus smiled. "Let's leave it at this: you mind Jem whenever he can make you. Fair enough?"

Aunt Alexandra was present but silent, and when she went down the hall with Atticus we heard her say, ". . . just one of the things I've been telling you about," a phrase that united us again.

Ours were adjoining rooms; as I shut the door between them Jem said, "Night, Scout."

"Night," I murmured, picking my way across the room to turn on the light. As I passed the bed I stepped on something warm, resilient, and rather smooth. It was not quite like hard rubber, and I had the sensation that it was alive. I also heard it move.

I switched on the light and looked at the floor by the bed. Whatever I had stepped on was gone. I tapped on Jem's door.

"What," he said.

"How does a snake feel?"

"Sort of rough. Cold. Dusty. Why?"

"I think there's one under my bed. Can you come look?"

"Are you bein' funny?" Jem opened the door. He was in his pajama bottoms. I noticed not without satisfaction that the mark of my knuckles was still on his mouth. When he saw I meant what I said, he said, "If you think I'm gonna put my face down to a snake you've got another think comin'. Hold on a minute."

He went to the kitchen and fetched the broom. "You better get up on the bed," he said.

"You reckon it's really one?" I asked. This was an occasion. Our houses had no cellars; they were built on stone blocks a few feet above the ground, and the entry of reptiles was not unknown but was not commonplace. Miss Rachel Haverford's excuse for a glass of neat whiskey every morning was that she never got over the fright of finding a rattler coiled in her bedroom closet, on her washing, when she went to hang up her negligee.

Jem made a tentative swipe under the bed. I looked over the foot to see if a snake would come out. None did. Jem made a deeper swipe.

"Do snakes grunt?"

"It ain't a snake," Jem said. "It's somebody."

Suddenly a filthy brown package shot from under the bed. Jem raised the broom and missed Dill's head by an inch when it appeared.

"God Almighty." Jem's voice was reverent.

We watched Dill emerge by degrees. He was a tight fit.

He stood up and eased his shoulders, turned his feet in their ankle sockets, rubbed the back of his neck. His circulation restored, he said, "Hey."

Jem petitioned God again. I was speechless.

"I'm 'bout to perish," said Dill. "Got anything to eat?"

In a dream, I went to the kitchen. I brought him back some milk and half a pan of corn bread left over from supper. Dill devoured it, chewing with his front teeth, as was his custom.

I finally found my voice. "How'd you get here?"

By an involved route. Refreshed by food, Dill recited this narrative: having been bound in chains and left to die in the basement (there were basements in Meridian) by his new father, who disliked him, and secretly kept alive on raw field peas by a passing farmer who heard his cries for help (the good man poked a bushel pod by pod through the ventilator), Dill worked himself free by pulling the chains from the wall. Still in wrist manacles, he wandered two miles out of Meridian where he discovered a small animal show and was immediately engaged to wash the camel. He traveled with the show all over Mississippi until his infallible sense of direction told him he was in Abbott County, Alabama, just across the river from Maycomb. He walked the rest of the way.

"How'd you get here?" asked Jem.

He had taken thirteen dollars from his mother's purse, caught the nine o'clock from Meridian and got off at Maycomb Junction. He had walked ten or eleven of the fourteen miles to Maycomb, off the highway in the scrub bushes lest the authorities be seeking him, and had ridden the remainder of the way clinging to the backboard of a cotton wagon. He had been under the bed for two hours, he thought; he had heard us in the diningroom, and the clink of forks on plates nearly drove him crazy. He thought Jem and I would never go to bed; he had considered emerging and helping me beat Jem, as Jem had grown far taller, but he knew Mr. Finch would break it up soon, so he thought it best to stay where he was. He was worn out, dirty beyond belief, and home.

"They must not know you're here," said Jem. "We'd know if they were lookin' for you. . . ."

"Think they're still searchin' all the picture shows in Meridian." Dill grinned.

"You oughta let your mother know where you are," said Jem. "You oughta let her know you're here. . . ."

Dill's eyes flickered at Jem, and Jem looked at the floor. Then he rose and broke the remaining code of our childhood. He went out of the room and down the hall. "Atticus," his voice was distant, "can you come here a minute, sir?"

Beneath its sweat-streaked dirt Dill's face went white. I felt sick. Atticus was in the doorway.

He came to the middle of the room and stood with his hands in his pockets, looking down at Dill.

I finally found my voice: "It's okay, Dill. When he wants you to know somethin', he tells you."

Dill looked at me. "I mean it's all right," I said. "You know he wouldn't bother you, you know you ain't scared of Atticus."

"I'm not scared . . ." Dill muttered.

"Just hungry, I'll bet." Atticus's voice had its usual pleasant dryness. "Scout, we can do better than a pan of cold corn bread, can't we? You fill this fellow up and when I get back we'll see what we can see."

"Mr. Finch, don't tell Aunt Rachel, don't make me go back, *please* sir! I'll run off again—!"

"Whoa, son," said Atticus. "Nobody's about to make you go anywhere but to bed pretty soon. I'm just going over to tell Miss Rachel you're here and ask her if you could spend the night with us—you'd like that, wouldn't you? And for goodness' sake put some of the county back where it belongs, the soil erosion's bad enough as it is."

Dill stared at my father's retreating figure.

"He's tryin' to be funny," I said. "He means take a bath. See there, I told you he wouldn't bother you."

Jem was standing in a corner of the room, looking like the traitor he was. "Dill, I had to tell him," he said. "You can't run three hundred miles off without your mother knowin'."

We left him without a word.

Dill ate, and ate, and ate. He hadn't eaten since last night. He used all his money for a ticket, boarded the train as he had done many times, coolly chatted with the conductor, to whom Dill was a familiar sight, but he had not the nerve to invoke the rule on small children traveling a distance alone if you've lost your money the conductor will lend you enough for dinner and your father will pay him back at the end of the line.

Dill made his way through the leftovers and was reaching for a can of pork and beans in the pantry when Miss Rachel's Do-oo Je-sus went off in the hall. He shivered like a rabbit.

He bore with fortitude her Wait Till I Get You Home, Your Folks Are Out of Their Minds Worryin', was quite calm during That's All the Harris in You Coming Out, smiled at her Reckon You Can Stay One Night, and returned the hug at long last bestowed upon him.

Atticus pushed up his glasses and rubbed his face.

"Your father's tired," said Aunt Alexandra, her first words in hours, it seemed. She had been there, but I suppose struck dumb most of the time. "You children get to bed now."

We left them in the diningroom, Atticus still mopping his face. "From rape to riot to runaways," we heard him chuckle. "I wonder what the next two hours will bring."'

Since things appeared to have worked out pretty well, Dill and I decided to be civil to Jem. Besides, Dill had to sleep with him so we might as well speak to him.

I put on my pajamas, read for a while and found myself suddenly unable to keep my eyes open. Dill and Jem were quiet; when I turned off my reading lamp there was no strip of light under the door to Jem's room.

I must have slept a long time, for when I was punched awake the room was dim with the light of the setting moon.

"Move over, Scout."

"He thought he had to," I mumbled. "Don't stay mad with him."

Dill got in bed beside me. "I ain't," he said. "I just wanted to sleep with you. Are you waked up?"

By this time I was, but lazily so. "Why'd you do it?"

No answer. "I said why'd you run off? Was he really hateful like you said?"

"Naw . . ."

"Didn't you all build that boat like you wrote you were gonna?"

"He just said we would. We never did."

I raised up on my elbow, facing Dill's outline. "It's no reason to run off. They don't get around to doin' what they say they're gonna do half the time. . . ."

"That wasn't it, he—they just wasn't interested in me."

This was the weirdest reason for flight I had ever heard. "How come?"

"Well, they stayed gone all the time, and when they were home, even, they'd get off in a room by themselves."

"What'd they do in there?"

"Nothin', just sittin' and readin'—but they didn't want me with 'em."

I pushed the pillow to the headboard and sat up. "You know something? I was fixin' to run off tonight because there they all were. You don't want 'em around you all the time, Dill—"

Dill breathed his patient breath, a half-sigh.

"—good night, Atticus's gone all day and sometimes half the night and off in the legislature and I don't know what— you don't want 'em around all the time, Dill, you couldn't do anything if they were."

"That's not it."

As Dill explained, I found myself wondering what life would be if Jem were different, even from what he was now; what I would do if Atticus did not feel the necessity of my presence, help and advice. Why, he couldn't get along a day without me. Even Calpurnia couldn't get along unless I was there. They needed me.

"Dill, you ain't telling me right—your folks couldn't do without you. They must be just mean to you. Tell you what to do about that—"

Dill's voice went on steadily in the darkness: "The thing is, what I'm tryin' to say is—they *do* get on a lot better without me, I can't help them any. They ain't mean. They buy me everything I want, but it's now-you've-got-it-go-play-with-it. You've got a roomful of things. I-got-you-that-book-so-go-read-it." Dill tried to deepen his voice. "You're not a boy. Boys get out and play baseball with other boys, they don't hang around the house worryin' their folks."

Dill's voice was his own again: "Oh, they ain't mean. They kiss you and hug you good night and good mornin' and good-bye and tell you they love you—Scout, let's get us a baby."

"Where?"

There was a man Dill had heard of who had a boat that he

rowed across to a foggy island where all these babies were; you could order one—

"That's a lie. Aunty said God drops 'em down the chimney. At least that's what I think she said." For once, Aunty's diction had not been too clear.

"Well that ain't so. You get babies from each other. But there's this man, too—he has all these babies just waitin' to wake up, he breathes life into 'em. . . ."

Dill was off again. Beautiful things floated around in his dreamy head. He could read two books to my one, but he preferred the magic of his own inventions. He could add and subtract faster than lightning, but he preferred his own twilight world, a world where babies slept, waiting to be gathered like morning lilies. He was slowly talking himself to sleep and taking me with him, but in the quietness of his foggy island there rose the faded image of a gray house with sad brown doors.

"Dill?"

"Mm?"

"Why do you reckon Boo Radley's never run off?"

Dill sighed a long sigh and turned away from me.

"Maybe he doesn't have anywhere to run off to. . . ."

15

After many telephone calls, much pleading on behalf of the defendant, and a long forgiving letter from his mother, it was decided that Dill could stay. We had a week of peace together. After that, little, it seemed. A nightmare was upon us.

It began one evening after supper. Dill was over; Aunt Alexandra was in her chair in the corner, Atticus was in his; Jem and I were on the floor reading. It had been a placid week: I had minded Aunty; Jem had outgrown the treehouse, but helped Dill and me construct a new rope ladder for it; Dill had hit upon a foolproof plan to make Boo Radley come out at no cost to ourselves (place a trail of lemon drops from the back door to the front yard and he'd follow it, like an ant). There was a knock on the front door, Jem answered it and said it was Mr. Heck Tate.

"Well, ask him to come in," said Atticus.

"I already did. There's some men outside in the yard, they want you to come out."

In Maycomb, grown men stood outside in the front yard for only two reasons: death and politics. I wondered who had died. Jem and I went to the front door, but Atticus called, "Go back in the house."

Jem turned out the livingroom lights and pressed his nose to a window screen. Aunt Alexandra protested. "Just for a second, Aunty, let's see who it is," he said.

Dill and I took another window. A crowd of men was standing around Atticus. They all seemed to be talking at once.

". . . movin' him to the county jail tomorrow," Mr. Tate was saying, "I don't look for any trouble, but I can't guarantee there won't be any. . . ."

"Don't be foolish, Heck," Atticus said. "This is Maycomb."

". . . said I was just uneasy."

"Heck, we've gotten one postponement of this case just to make sure there's nothing to be uneasy about. This is Saturday," Atticus said. "Trial'll probably be Monday. You can keep him one night, can't you? I don't think anybody in Maycomb'll begrudge me a client, with times this hard."

There was a murmur of glee that died suddenly when Mr. Link Deas said, "Nobody around here's up to anything, it's that Old Sarum bunch I'm worried about . . . can't you get a—what is it, Heck?"

"Change of venue," said Mr. Tate. "Not much point in that, now is it?"

Atticus said something inaudible. I turned to Jem, who waved me to silence.

"—besides," Atticus was saying, "you're not scared of that crowd, are you?"

". . . know how they do when they get shinnied up."

"They don't usually drink on Sunday, they go to church most of the day . . ." Atticus said.

"This is a special occasion, though . . ." someone said.

They murmured and buzzed until Aunty said if Jem didn't turn on the livingroom lights he would disgrace the family. Jem didn't hear her.

"—don't see why you touched it in the first place," Mr. Link Deas was saying. "You've got everything to lose from this, Atticus. I mean everything."

"Do you really think so?"

This was Atticus's dangerous question. "Do you really think you want to move there, Scout?" Bam, bam, bam, and the checkerboard was swept clean of my men. "Do you really think that, son? Then read this." Jem would struggle the rest of an evening through the speeches of Henry W. Grady.

"Link, that boy might go to the chair, but he's not going till the truth's told." Atticus's voice was even. "And you know what the truth is."

There was a murmur among the group of men, made more ominous when Atticus moved back to the bottom front step and the men drew nearer to him.

Suddenly Jem screamed, "Atticus, the telephone's ringing!"

The men jumped a little and scattered; they were people we saw every day: merchants, in-town farmers; Dr. Reynolds was there; so was Mr. Avery.

"Well, answer it, son," called Atticus.

Laughter broke them up. When Atticus switched on the overhead light in the livingroom he found Jem at the window, pale except for the vivid mark of the screen on his nose.

"Why on earth are you all sitting in the dark?" he asked.

Jem watched him go to his chair and pick up the evening paper. I sometimes think Atticus subjected every crisis of his life to tranquil evaluation behind *The Mobile Register*, *The Birmingham News* and *The Montgomery Advertiser*.

"They were after you, weren't they?" Jem went to him. "They wanted to get you, didn't they?"

Atticus lowered the paper and gazed at Jem. "What have you been reading?" he asked. Then he said gently, "No son, those were our friends."

"It wasn't a—a gang?" Jem was looking from the corners of his eyes.

Atticus tried to stifle a smile but didn't make it. "No, we

don't have mobs and that nonsense in Maycomb. I've never heard of a gang in Maycomb."

"Ku Klux got after some Catholics one time."

"Never heard of any Catholics in Maycomb either," said Atticus, "you're confusing that with something else. Way back about nineteen-twenty there was a Klan, but it was a political organization more than anything. Besides, they couldn't find anybody to scare. They paraded by Mr. Sam Levy's house one night, but Sam just stood on his porch and told 'em things had come to a pretty pass, he'd sold 'em the very sheets on their backs. Sam made 'em so ashamed of themselves they went away."

The Levy family met all criteria for being Fine Folks: they did the best they could with the sense they had, and they had been living on the same plot of ground in Maycomb for five generations.

"The Ku Klux's gone," said Atticus. "It'll never come back."

I walked home with Dill and returned in time to overhear Atticus saying to Aunty, ". . . in favor of Southern womanhood as much as anybody, but not for preserving polite fiction at the expense of human life," a pronouncement that made me suspect they had been fussing again.

I sought Jem and found him in his room, on the bed deep in thought. "Have they been at it?" I asked.

"Sort of. She won't let him alone about Tom Robinson. She almost said Atticus was disgracin' the family. Scout . . . I'm scared."

"Scared'a what?"

"Scared about Atticus. Somebody might hurt him." Jem preferred to remain mysterious; all he would say to my questions was go on and leave him alone.

Next day was Sunday. In the interval between Sunday School and Church when the congregation stretched its legs, I saw Atticus standing in the yard with another knot of men. Mr. Heck Tate was present, and I wondered if he had seen the light. He never went to church. Even Mr. Underwood was there. Mr. Underwood had no use for any organization but *The Maycomb Tribune*, of which he was the sole owner, editor, and printer. His days were spent at his linotype, where he refreshed himself occasionally from an ever-present gallon jug of cherry wine. He rarely gathered news; people brought it to him. It was said that he made up every edition of *The Maycomb Tribune* out of his own head and wrote it down on the linotype. This was believable. Something must have been up to haul Mr. Underwood out.

I caught Atticus coming in the door, and he said that they'd moved Tom Robinson to the Maycomb jail. He also said, more to himself than to me, that if they'd kept him there in the first place there wouldn't have been any fuss. I watched him take his seat on the third row from the front, and I heard him rumble, "Nearer my God to thee," some notes behind the rest of us. He never sat with Aunty, Jem and me. He liked to be by himself in church.

The fake peace that prevailed on Sundays was made more irritating by Aunt Alexandra's presence. Atticus would flee to his office directly after dinner, where if we sometimes looked in on him, we would find him sitting back in his swivel chair reading. Aunt Alexandra composed herself for a two-hour nap and dared us to make any noise in the yard, the neighborhood was resting. Jem in his old age had taken to his room with a stack of football magazines. So Dill and I spent our Sundays creeping around in Deer's Pasture.

Shooting on Sundays was prohibited, so Dill and I kicked Jem's football around the pasture for a while, which was no fun. Dill asked if I'd like to have a poke at Boo Radley. I said I didn't think it'd be nice to bother him, and spent the rest of the afternoon filling Dill in on last winter's events. He was considerably impressed.

We parted at suppertime, and after our meal Jem and I were settling down to a routine evening, when Atticus did something that interested us: he came into the livingroom carrying a long electrical extension cord. There was a light bulb on the end.

"I'm going out for a while," he said. "You folks'll be in bed when I come back, so I'll say good night now."

With that, he put his hat on and went out the back door.

"He's takin' the car," said Jem.

Our father had a few peculiarities: one was, he never ate desserts; another was that he liked to walk. As far back as I could remember, there was always a Chevrolet in excellent condition in the carhouse, and Atticus put many miles on it in business trips, but in Maycomb he walked to and from his office four times a day, covering about two miles. He said his only exercise was walking. In Maycomb, if one went for a walk with no definite purpose in mind, it was correct to believe one's mind incapable of definite purpose.

Later on, I bade my aunt and brother good night and was well into a book when I heard Jem rattling around in his room. His go-to-bed noises were so familiar to me that I knocked on his door: "Why ain't you going to bed?"

"I'm goin' downtown for a while." He was changing his pants.

"Why? It's almost ten o'clock, Jem."

He knew it, but he was going anyway.

"Then I'm goin' with you. If you say no you're not, I'm goin' anyway, hear?"

Jem saw that he would have to fight me to keep me home, and I suppose he thought a fight would antagonize Aunty, so he gave in with little grace.

I dressed quickly. We waited until Aunty's light went out, and we walked quietly down the back steps. There was no moon tonight.

"Dill'll wanta come," I whispered.

"So he will," said Jem gloomily.

We leaped over the driveway wall, cut through Miss Rachel's side yard and went to Dill's window. Jem whistled bobwhite. Dill's face appeared at the screen, disappeared, and five minutes later he unhooked the screen and crawled out. An old campaigner, he did not speak until we were on the sidewalk. "What's up?"

"Jem's got the look-arounds," an affliction Calpurnia said all boys caught at his age.

"I've just got this feeling," Jem said, "just this feeling."

We went by Mrs. Dubose's house, standing empty and shuttered, her camellias grown up in weeds and johnson grass. There were eight more houses to the post office corner.

The south side of the square was deserted. Giant monkey-puzzle bushes bristled on each corner, and between them an iron hitching rail glistened under the street lights. A light shone in the county toilet, otherwise that side of the court-house was dark. A larger square of stores surrounded the courthouse square; dim lights burned from deep within them.

Atticus's office was in the courthouse when he began his law practice, but after several years of it he moved to quieter quarters in the Maycomb Bank building. When we rounded the corner of the square, we saw the car parked in front of the bank. "He's in there," said Jem.

But he wasn't. His office was reached by a long hallway. Looking down the hall, we should have seen *Atticus Finch, Attorney-at-Law* in small sober letters against the light from behind his door. It was dark.

Jem peered in the bank door to make sure. He turned the knob. The door was locked. "Let's go up the street. Maybe he's visitin' Mr. Underwood."

Mr. Underwood not only ran *The Maycomb Tribune* office, he lived in it. That is, above it. He covered the courthouse and jailhouse news simply by looking out his upstairs win-dow. The office building was on the northwest corner of the square, and to reach it we had to pass the jail.

The Maycomb jail was the most venerable and hideous of the county's buildings. Atticus said it was like something Cousin Joshua St. Clair might have designed. It was certainly someone's dream. Starkly out of place in a town of square-faced stores and steep-roofed houses, the Maycomb jail was a miniature Gothic joke one cell wide and two cells high, complete with tiny battlements and flying buttresses. Its fan-tasy was heightened by its red brick façade and the thick steel bars at its ecclesiastical windows. It stood on no lonely hill, but was wedged between Tyndal's Hardware Store and *The Maycomb Tribune* office. The jail was Maycomb's only con-versation piece: its detractors said it looked like a Victorian privy; its supporters said it gave the town a good solid re-spectable look, and no stranger would ever suspect that it was full of niggers.

As we walked up the sidewalk, we saw a solitary light burning in the distance. "That's funny," said Jem, "jail doesn't have an outside light."

"Looks like it's over the door," said Dill.

A long extension cord ran between the bars of a second-floor window and down the side of the building. In the light from its bare bulb, Atticus was sitting propped against the front door. He was sitting in one of his office chairs, and he was reading, oblivious of the nightbugs dancing over his head.

I made to run, but Jem caught me. "Don't go to him," he said, "he might not like it. He's all right, let's go home. I just wanted to see where he was."

We were taking a short cut across the square when four dusty cars came in from the Meridian highway, moving slowly in a line. They went around the square, passed the bank building, and stopped in front of the jail.

Nobody got out. We saw Atticus look up from his newspaper. He closed it, folded it deliberately, dropped it in his lap, and pushed his hat to the back of his head. He seemed to be expecting them.

"Come on," whispered Jem. We streaked across the square, across the street, until we were in the shelter of the Jitney Jungle door. Jem peeked up the sidewalk. "We can get closer," he said. We ran to Tyndal's Hardware door—near enough, at the same time discreet.

In ones and twos, men got out of the cars. Shadows became substance as lights revealed solid shapes moving toward the jail door. Atticus remained where he was. The men hid him from view.

"He in there, Mr. Finch?" a man said.

"He is," we heard Atticus answer, "and he's asleep. Don't wake him up."

In obedience to my father, there followed what I later realized was a sickeningly comic aspect of an unfunny situation: the men talked in near-whispers.

"You know what we want," another man said. "Get aside from the door, Mr. Finch."

"You can turn around and go home again, Walter," Atticus said pleasantly. "Heck Tate's around somewhere."

"The hell he is," said another man. "Heck's bunch's so deep in the woods they won't get out till mornin'."

"Indeed? Why so?"

"Called 'em off on a snipe hunt," was the succinct answer. "Didn't you think a'that, Mr. Finch?"

"Thought about it, but didn't believe it. Well then," my father's voice was still the same, "that changes things, doesn't it?"

"It do," another deep voice said. Its owner was a shadow.

"Do you really think so?"

This was the second time I heard Atticus ask that question in two days, and it meant somebody's man would get jumped. This was too good to miss. I broke away from Jem and ran as fast as I could to Atticus.

Jem shrieked and tried to catch me, but I had a lead on him and Dill. I pushed my way through dark smelly bodies and burst into the circle of light.

"H-ey, Atticus!"

I thought he would have a fine surprise, but his face killed my joy. A flash of plain fear was going out of his eyes, but returned when Dill and Jem wriggled into the light.

There was a smell of stale whiskey and pigpen about, and when I glanced around I discovered that these men were strangers. They were not the people I saw last night. Hot embarrassment shot through me: I had leaped triumphantly into a ring of people I had never seen before.

Atticus got up from his chair, but he was moving slowly, like an old man. He put the newspaper down very carefully, adjusting its creases with lingering fingers. They were trembling a little.

"Go home, Jem," he said. "Take Scout and Dill home."

We were accustomed to prompt, if not always cheerful acquiescence to Atticus's instructions, but from the way he stood Jem was not thinking of budging.

"Go home, I said."

Jem shook his head. As Atticus's fists went to his hips, so did Jem's, and as they faced each other I could see little resemblance between them: Jem's soft brown hair and eyes, his oval face and snug-fitting ears were our mother's, contrasting oddly with Atticus's graying black hair and square-cut features, but they were somehow alike. Mutual defiance made them alike.

"Son, I said go home."

Jem shook his head.

"I'll send him home," a burly man said, and grabbed Jem roughly by the collar. He yanked Jem nearly off his feet.

"Don't you touch him!" I kicked the man swiftly. Bare-footed, I was surprised to see him fall back in real pain. I intended to kick his shin, but aimed too high.

"That'll do, Scout." Atticus put his hand on my shoulder. "Don't kick folks. No—" he said, as I was pleading justification.

"Ain't nobody gonna do Jem that way," I said.

"All right, Mr. Finch, get 'em outa here," someone growled. "You got fifteen seconds to get 'em outa here."

In the midst of this strange assembly, Atticus stood trying to make Jem mind him. "I ain't going," was his steady answer to Atticus's threats, requests, and finally, "Please Jem, take them home."

I was getting a bit tired of that, but felt Jem had his own reasons for doing as he did, in view of his prospects once Atticus did get him home. I looked around the crowd. It was a summer's night, but the men were dressed, most of them, in overalls and denim shirts buttoned up to the collars. I thought they must be cold-natured, as their sleeves were unrolled and buttoned at the cuffs. Some wore hats pulled firmly down over their ears. They were sullen-looking, sleepy-eyed men who seemed unused to late hours. I sought once more for a familiar face, and at the center of the semi-circle I found one.

"Hey, Mr. Cunningham."

The man did not hear me, it seemed.

"Hey, Mr. Cunningham. How's your entailment gettin' along?"

Mr. Walter Cunningham's legal affairs were well known to me; Atticus had once described them at length. The big man blinked and hooked his thumbs in his overall straps. He seemed uncomfortable; he cleared his throat and looked away. My friendly overture had fallen flat.

Mr. Cunningham wore no hat, and the top half of his forehead was white in contrast to his sunscorched face, which led me to believe that he wore one most days. He shifted his feet, clad in heavy work shoes.

"Don't you remember me, Mr. Cunningham? I'm Jean Louise Finch. You brought us some hickory nuts one time, remember?" I began to sense the futility one feels when unacknowledged by a chance acquaintance.

"I go to school with Walter," I began again. "He's your boy, ain't he? Ain't he, sir?"

Mr. Cunningham was moved to a faint nod. He did know me, after all.

"He's in my grade," I said, "and he does right well. He's a good boy," I added, "a real nice boy. We brought him home for dinner one time. Maybe he told you about me, I beat him up one time but he was real nice about it. Tell him hey for me, won't you?"

Atticus had said it was the polite thing to talk to people about what they were interested in, not about what you were interested in. Mr. Cunningham displayed no interest in his son, so I tackled his entailment once more in a last-ditch effort to make him feel at home.

"Entailments are bad," I was advising him, when I slowly awoke to the fact that I was addressing the entire aggregation. The men were all looking at me, some had their mouths half-open. Atticus had stopped poking at Jem: they were standing together beside Dill. Their attention amounted to fascination. Atticus's mouth, even, was half-open, an attitude he had once described as uncouth. Our eyes met and he shut it.

"Well, Atticus, I was just sayin' to Mr. Cunningham that entailments are bad an' all that, but you said not to worry, it takes a long time sometimes . . . that you all'd ride it out together . . ." I was slowly drying up, wondering what idiocy I had committed. Entailments seemed all right enough for livingroom talk.

I began to feel sweat gathering at the edges of my hair; I could stand anything but a bunch of people looking at me. They were quite still.

"What's the matter?" I asked.

Atticus said nothing. I looked around and up at Mr. Cunningham, whose face was equally impassive. Then he did a peculiar thing. He squatted down and took me by both shoulders.

"I'll tell him you said hey, little lady," he said.

Then he straightened up and waved a big paw. "Let's clear out," he called. "Let's get going, boys."

As they had come, in ones and twos the men shuffled back to their ramshackle cars. Doors slammed, engines coughed, and they were gone.

I turned to Atticus, but Atticus had gone to the jail and was leaning against it with his face to the wall. I went to him and pulled his sleeve. "Can we go home now?" He nodded, produced his handkerchief, gave his face a going-over and blew his nose violently.

"Mr. Finch?"

A soft husky voice came from the darkness above: "They gone?"

Atticus stepped back and looked up. "They've gone," he said. "Get some sleep, Tom. They won't bother you any more."

From a different direction, another voice cut crisply through the night: "You're damn tootin' they won't. Had you covered all the time, Atticus."

Mr. Underwood and a double-barreled shotgun were leaning out his window above *The Maycomb Tribune* office.

It was long past my bedtime and I was growing quite tired; it seemed that Atticus and Mr. Underwood would talk for the rest of the night, Mr. Underwood out the window and Atticus up at him. Finally Atticus returned, switched off the light above the jail door, and picked up his chair.

"Can I carry it for you, Mr. Finch?" asked Dill. He had not said a word the whole time.

"Why, thank you, son."

Walking toward the office, Dill and I fell into step behind Atticus and Jem. Dill was encumbered by the chair, and his pace was slower. Atticus and Jem were well ahead of us, and I assumed that Atticus was giving him hell for not going home, but I was wrong. As they passed under a streetlight, Atticus reached out and massaged Jem's hair, his one gesture of affection.

16

Jem heard me. He thrust his head around the connecting door. As he came to my bed Atticus's light flashed on. We stayed where we were until it went off; we heard him turn over, and we waited until he was still again.

Jem took me to his room and put me in bed beside him. "Try to go to sleep," he said. "It'll be all over after tomorrow, maybe."

We had come in quietly, so as not to wake Aunty. Atticus killed the engine in the driveway and coasted to the carhouse; we went in the back door and to our rooms without a word. I was very tired, and was drifting into sleep when the memory of Atticus calmly folding his newspaper and pushing back his hat became Atticus standing in the middle of an empty waiting street, pushing up his glasses. The full meaning of the night's events hit me and I began crying. Jem was awfully nice about it: for once he didn't remind me that people nearly nine years old didn't do things like that.

Everybody's appetite was delicate this morning, except Jem's: he ate his way through three eggs. Atticus watched in frank admiration; Aunt Alexandra sipped coffee and radiated waves of disapproval. Children who slipped out at night were a disgrace to the family. Atticus said he was right glad his disgraces had come along, but Aunty said, "Nonsense, Mr. Underwood was there all the time."

"You know, it's a funny thing about Braxton," said Atticus. "He despises Negroes, won't have one near him."

Local opinion held Mr. Underwood to be an intense, profane little man, whose father in a fey fit of humor christened Braxton Bragg, a name Mr. Underwood had done his best to live down. Atticus said naming people after Confederate generals made slow steady drinkers.

Calpurnia was serving Aunt Alexandra more coffee, and she shook her head at what I thought was a pleading winning look. "You're still too little," she said. "I'll tell you when you ain't." I said it might help my stomach. "All right," she said, and got a cup from the sideboard. She poured one tablespoonful of coffee into it and filled the cup to the brim with milk. I thanked her by sticking out my tongue at it, and looked up to catch Aunty's warning frown. But she was frowning at Atticus.

She waited until Calpurnia was in the kitchen, then she said, "Don't talk like that in front of them."

"Talk like what in front of whom?" he asked.

"Like that in front of Calpurnia. You said Braxton Underwood despises Negroes right in front of her."

"Well, I'm sure Cal knows it. Everybody in Maycomb knows it."

I was beginning to notice a subtle change in my father these days, that came out when he talked with Aunt Alexandra. It was a quiet digging in, never outright irritation. There was a faint starchiness in his voice when he said, "Anything fit to say at the table's fit to say in front of Calpurnia. She knows what she means to this family."

"I don't think it's a good habit, Atticus. It encourages them. You know how they talk among themselves. Everything that happens in this town's out to the Quarters before sundown."

My father put down his knife. "I don't know of any law that says they can't talk. Maybe if we didn't give them so much to talk about they'd be quiet. Why don't you drink your coffee, Scout?"

I was playing in it with the spoon. "I thought Mr. Cunningham was a friend of ours. You told me a long time ago he was."

"He still is."

"But last night he wanted to hurt you."

Atticus placed his fork beside his knife and pushed his plate aside. "Mr. Cunningham's basically a good man," he said, "he just has his blind spots along with the rest of us."

Jem spoke. "Don't call that a blind spot. He'da killed you last night when he first went there."

"He might have hurt me a little," Atticus conceded, "but son, you'll understand folks a little better when you're older. A mob's always made up of people, no matter what. Mr. Cunningham was part of a mob last night, but he was still a man. Every mob in every little Southern town is always made up of people you know—doesn't say much for them, does it?"

"I'll say not," said Jem.

"So it took an eight-year-old child to bring 'em to their senses, didn't it?" said Atticus. "That proves something—that a gang of wild animals *can* be stopped, simply because they're still human. Hmp, maybe we need a police force of children . . . you children last night made Walter Cunningham stand in my shoes for a minute. That was enough."

Well, I hoped Jem would understand folks a little better

when he was older; I wouldn't. "First day Walter comes back to school'll be his last," I affirmed.

"You will not touch him," Atticus said flatly. "I don't want either of you bearing a grudge about this thing, no matter what happens."

"You see, don't you," said Aunt Alexandra, "what comes of things like this. Don't say I haven't told you."

Atticus said he'd never say that, pushed out his chair and got up. "There's a day ahead, so excuse me. Jem, I don't want you and Scout downtown today, please."

As Atticus departed, Dill came bounding down the hall into the diningroom. "It's all over town this morning," he announced, "all about how we held off a hundred folks with our bare hands. . . ."

Aunt Alexandra stared him to silence. "It was not a hundred folks," she said, "and nobody held anybody off. It was just a nest of those Cunninghams, drunk and disorderly."

"Aw, Aunty, that's just Dill's way," said Jem. He signaled us to follow him.

"You all stay in the yard today," she said, as we made our way to the front porch.

It was like Saturday. People from the south end of the county passed our house in a leisurely but steady stream.

Mr. Dolphus Raymond lurched by on his thoroughbred. "Don't see how he stays in the saddle," murmured Jem. "How c'n you stand to get drunk 'fore eight in the morning?"

A wagonload of ladies rattled past us. They wore cotton sunbonnets and dresses with long sleeves. A bearded man in a wool hat drove them. "Yonder's some Mennonites," Jem said to Dill. "They don't have buttons." They lived deep in the woods, did most of their trading across the river, and rarely came to Maycomb. Dill was interested. "They've all got blue eyes," Jem explained, "and the men can't shave after they marry. Their wives like for 'em to tickle 'em with their beards."

Mr. X Billups rode by on a mule and waved to us. "He's a funny man," said Jem. "X's his name, not his initial. He was in court one time and they asked him his name. He said X Billups. Clerk asked him to spell it and he said X. Asked him again and he said X. They kept at it till he wrote X on a sheet of paper and held it up for everybody to see. They asked him where he got his name and he said that's the way his folks signed him up when he was born."

As the county went by us, Jem gave Dill the histories and general attitudes of the more prominent figures: Mr. Tensaw Jones voted the straight Prohibition ticket; Miss Emily Davis dipped snuff in private; Mr. Byron Waller could play the violin; Mr. Jake Slade was cutting his third set of teeth.

A wagonload of unusually stern-faced citizens appeared. When they pointed to Miss Maudie Atkinson's yard, ablaze with summer flowers, Miss Maudie herself came out on the porch. There was an odd thing about Miss Maudie—on her porch she was too far away for us to see her features clearly, but we could always catch her mood by the way she stood. She was now standing arms akimbo, her shoulders drooping a little, her head cocked to one side, her glasses winking in the sunlight. We knew she wore a grin of the uttermost wickedness.

The driver of the wagon slowed down his mules, and a shrill-voiced woman called out: "He that cometh in vanity departeth in darkness!"

Miss Maudie answered: "A merry heart maketh a cheerful countenance!"

I guess that the foot-washers thought that the Devil was quoting Scripture for his own purposes, as the driver speeded his mules. Why they objected to Miss Maudie's yard was a mystery, heightened in my mind because for someone who spent all the daylight hours outdoors, Miss Maudie's command of Scripture was formidable.

"You goin' to court this morning?" asked Jem. We had strolled over.

"I am not," she said. "I have no business with the court this morning."

"Aren't you goin' down to watch?" asked Dill.

"I am not. 't's morbid, watching a poor devil on trial for his life. Look at all those folks, it's like a Roman carnival."

"They hafta try him in public, Miss Maudie," I said. "Wouldn't be right if they didn't."

"I'm quite aware of that," she said. "Just because it's public, I don't have to go, do I?"

Miss Stephanie Crawford came by. She wore a hat and gloves. "Um, um, um," she said. "Look at all those folks —you'd think William Jennings Bryan was speakin'."

"And where are you going, Stephanie?" inquired Miss Maudie.

"To the Jitney Jungle."

Miss Maudie said she'd never seen Miss Stephanie go to the Jitney Jungle in a hat in her life.

"Well," said Miss Stephanie, "I thought I might just look in at the courthouse, to see what Atticus's up to."

"Better be careful he doesn't hand you a subpoena."

We asked Miss Maudie to elucidate: she said Miss Stephanie seemed to know so much about the case she might as well be called on to testify.

We held off until noon, when Atticus came home to dinner and said they'd spent the morning picking the jury. After dinner, we stopped by for Dill and went to town.

It was a gala occasion. There was no room at the public hitching rail for another animal, mules and wagons were parked under every available tree. The courthouse square was covered with picnic parties sitting on newspapers, washing down biscuit and syrup with warm milk from fruit jars. Some people were gnawing on cold chicken and cold fried pork chops. The more affluent chased their food with drugstore Coca-Cola in bulb-shaped soda glasses. Greasy-faced children popped-the-whip through the crowd, and babies lunched at their mothers' breasts.

In a far corner of the square, the Negroes sat quietly in the sun, dining on sardines, crackers, and the more vivid flavors of Nehi Cola. Mr. Dolphus Raymond sat with them.

"Jem," said Dill, "he's drinkin' out of a sack."

Mr. Dolphus Raymond seemed to be so doing: two yellow drugstore straws ran from his mouth to the depths of a brown paper bag.

"Ain't ever seen anybody do that," murmured Dill. "How does he keep what's in it in it?"

Jem giggled. "He's got a Co-Cola bottle full of whiskey in there. That's so's not to upset the ladies. You'll see him sip it all afternoon, he'll step out for a while and fill it back up."

"Why's he sittin' with the colored folks?"

"Always does. He likes 'em better'n he likes us, I reckon. Lives by himself way down near the county line. He's got a colored woman and all sorts of mixed chillun. Show you some of 'em if we see 'em.''

"He doesn't look like trash," said Dill.

"He's not, he owns all one side of the riverbank down there, and he's from a real old family to boot."

"Then why does he do like that?"

"That's just his way," said Jem. "They say he never got over his weddin'. He was supposed to marry one of the— the Spencer ladies, I think. They were gonna have a huge weddin', but they didn't—after the rehearsal the bride went upstairs and blew her head off. Shotgun. She pulled the trigger with her toes."

"Did they ever know why?"

"No," said Jem, "nobody ever knew quite why but Mr. Dolphus. They said it was because she found out about his colored woman, he reckoned he could keep her and get married too. He's been sorta drunk ever since. You know, though, he's real good to those chillun—"

"Jem," I asked, "what's a mixed child?"

"Half white, half colored. You've seen 'em, Scout. You know that red-kinky-headed one that delivers for the drugstore. He's half white. They're real sad."

"Sad, how come?"

"They don't belong anywhere. Colored folks won't have 'em because they're half white; white folks won't have 'em 'cause they're colored, so they're just in-betweens, don't belong anywhere. But Mr. Dolphus, now, they say he's shipped two of his up north. They don't mind 'em up north. Yonder's one of 'em."

A small boy clutching a Negro woman's hand walked toward us. He looked all Negro to me: he was rich chocolate with flaring nostrils and beautiful teeth. Sometimes he would skip happily, and the Negro woman tugged his hand to make him stop.

Jem waited until they passed us. "That's one of the little ones," he said.

"How can you tell?" asked Dill. "He looked black to me."

"You can't sometimes, not unless you know who they are. But he's half Raymond, all right."

"But how can you *tell*?" I asked.

"I told you, Scout, you just hafta know who they are."

"Well how do you know we ain't Negroes?"

"Uncle Jack Finch says we really don't know. He says as far as he can trace back the Finches we ain't, but for all he knows we mighta come straight out of Ethiopia durin' the Old Testament."

"Well if we came out durin' the Old Testament it's too long ago to matter."

"That's what I thought," said Jem, "but around here once you have a drop of Negro blood, that makes you all black. Hey, look—"

Some invisible signal had made the lunchers on the square rise and scatter bits of newspaper, cellophane, and wrapping paper. Children came to mothers, babies were cradled on hips as men in sweat-stained hats collected their families and herded them through the courthouse doors. In the far corner of the square the Negroes and Mr. Dolphus Raymond stood up and dusted their breeches. There were few women and children among them, which seemed to dispel the holiday mood. They waited patiently at the doors behind the white families.

"Let's go in," said Dill.

"Naw, we better wait till they get in, Atticus might not like it if he sees us," said Jem.

The Maycomb County courthouse was faintly reminiscent of Arlington in one respect: the concrete pillars supporting its south roof were too heavy for their light burden. The pillars were all that remained standing when the original courthouse burned in 1856. Another courthouse was built around them. It is better to say, built in spite of them. But for the south porch, the Maycomb County courthouse was early Victorian, presenting an unoffensive vista when seen from the north. From the other side, however, Greek revival columns clashed with a big nineteenth-century clock tower housing a rusty unreliable instrument, a view indicating a people determined to preserve every physical scrap of the past.

To reach the courtroom, on the second floor, one passed sundry sunless county cubbyholes: the tax assessor, the tax collector, the county clerk, the county solicitor, the circuit clerk, the judge of probate lived in cool dim hutches that smelled of decaying record books mingled with old damp cement and stale urine. It was necessary to turn on the lights in the daytime; there was always a film of dust on the rough floorboards. The inhabitants of these offices were creatures of their environment: little gray-faced men, they seemed untouched by wind or sun.

We knew there was a crowd, but we had not bargained for the multitudes in the first-floor hallway. I got separated from Jem and Dill, but made my way toward the wall by the stairwell, knowing Jem would come for me eventually. I found myself in the middle of the Idlers' Club and made myself as unobtrusive as possible. This was a group of white-shirted, khaki-trousered, suspendered old men who had spent their lives doing nothing and passed their twilight days doing same on pine benches under the live oaks on the square. Attentive critics of courthouse business, Atticus said they knew as much law as the Chief Justice, from long years of observation. Normally, they were the court's only spectators, and today they seemed resentful of the interruption of their comfortable routine. When they spoke, their voices sounded casually important. The conversation was about my father.

". . . thinks he knows what he's doing," one said.

"Oh-h now, I wouldn't say that," said another. "Atticus Finch's a deep reader, a mighty deep reader."

"He reads all right, that's all he does." The club snickered.

"Lemme tell you somethin' now, Billy," a third said, "you know the court appointed him to defend this nigger."

"Yeah, but Atticus aims to defend him. That's what I don't like about it."

This was news, news that put a different light on things: Atticus had to, whether he wanted to or not. I thought it odd that he hadn't said anything to us about it—we could have used it many times in defending him and ourselves. He had to, that's why he was doing it, equaled fewer fights and less fussing. But did that explain the town's attitude? The court appointed Atticus to defend him. Atticus aimed to defend him. That's what they didn't like about it. It was confusing.

The Negroes, having waited for the white people to go upstairs, began to come in. "Whoa now, just a minute," said a club member, holding up his walking stick. "Just don't start up them there stairs yet awhile."

The club began its stiff-jointed climb and ran into Dill and Jem on their way down looking for me. They squeezed past and Jem called, "Scout, come on, there ain't a seat left. We'll hafta stand up."

"Looka there, now," he said irritably, as the black people surged upstairs. The old men ahead of them would take most of the standing room. We were out of luck and it was my fault, Jem informed me. We stood miserably by the wall.

"Can't you all get in?"

Reverend Sykes was looking down at us, black hat in hand.

"Hey, Reverend," said Jem. "Naw, Scout here messed us up."

"Well, let's see what we can do."

Reverend Sykes edged his way upstairs. In a few moments he was back. "There's not a seat downstairs. Do you all reckon it'll be all right if you all came to the balcony with me?"

"Gosh yes," said Jem. Happily, we sped ahead of Reverend Sykes to the courtroom floor. There, we went up a covered staircase and waited at the door. Reverend Sykes came puffing behind us, and steered us gently through the black people in the balcony. Four Negroes rose and gave us their front-row seats.

The Colored balcony ran along three walls of the courtroom like a second-story veranda, and from it we could see everything.

The jury sat to the left, under long windows. Sunburned, lanky, they seemed to be all farmers, but this was natural: townfolk rarely sat on juries, they were either struck or excused. One or two of the jury looked vaguely like dressed-up Cunninghams. At this stage they sat straight and alert.

The circuit solicitor and another man, Atticus and Tom Robinson sat at tables with their backs to us. There was a brown book and some yellow tablets on the solicitor's table; Atticus's was bare.

Just inside the railing that divided the spectators from the court, the witnesses sat on cowhide-bottomed chairs. Their backs were to us.

Judge Taylor was on the bench, looking like a sleepy old

shark, his pilot fish writing rapidly below in front of him. Judge Taylor looked like most judges I had ever seen: amiable, white-haired, slightly ruddy-faced, he was a man who ran his court with an alarming informality—he sometimes propped his feet up, he often cleaned his fingernails with his pocket knife. In long equity hearings, especially after dinner, he gave the impression of dozing, an impression dispelled forever when a lawyer once deliberately pushed a pile of books to the floor in a desperate effort to wake him up. Without opening his eyes, Judge Taylor murmured, "Mr. Whitley, do that again and it'll cost you one hundred dollars."

He was a man learned in the law, and although he seemed to take his job casually, in reality he kept a firm grip on any proceedings that came before him. Only once was Judge Taylor ever seen at a dead standstill in open court, and the Cunninghams stopped him. Old Sarum, their stamping grounds, was populated by two families separate and apart in the beginning, but unfortunately bearing the same name. The Cunninghams married the Coninghams until the spelling of the names was academic—academic until a Cunningham disputed a Coningham over land titles and took to the law. During a controversy of this character, Jeems Cunningham testified that his mother spelled it Cunningham on deeds and things, but she was really a Coningham, she was an uncertain speller, a seldom reader, and was given to looking far away sometimes when she sat on the front gallery in the evening. After nine hours of listening to the eccentricities of Old Sarum's inhabitants, Judge Taylor threw the case out of court. When asked upon what grounds, Judge Taylor said, "Champertous connivance," and declared he hoped to God the litigants were satisfied by each having had their public say. They were. That was all they had wanted in the first place.

Judge Taylor had one interesting habit. He permitted smoking in his courtroom but did not himself indulge: sometimes, if one was lucky, one had the privilege of watching him put a long dry cigar into his mouth and munch it slowly up. Bit by bit the dead cigar would disappear, to reappear some hours later as a flat slick mess, its essence extracted and mingling with Judge Taylor's digestive juices. I once asked Atticus how Mrs. Taylor stood to kiss him, but Atticus said they didn't kiss much.

The witness stand was to the right of Judge Taylor, and when we got to our seats Mr. Heck Tate was already on it.

17

"Jem," I said, **"are those the Ewells sittin' down yonder?"**

"Hush," said Jem, "Mr. Heck Tate's testifyin'."

Mr. Tate had dressed for the occasion. He wore an ordinary business suit, which made him look somehow like every other man: gone were his high boots, lumber jacket, and bullet-studded belt. From that moment he ceased to terrify me. He was sitting forward in the witness chair, his hands clasped between his knees, listening attentively to the circuit solicitor.

The solicitor, a Mr. Gilmer, was not well known to us. He was from Abbottsville; we saw him only when court convened, and that rarely, for court was of no special interest to Jem and me. A balding, smooth-faced man, he could have been anywhere between forty and sixty. Although his back was to us, we knew he had a slight cast in one of his eyes which he used to his advantage: he seemed to be looking at a person when he was actually doing nothing of the kind, thus he was hell on juries and witnesses. The jury, thinking themselves under close scrutiny, paid attention; so did the witnesses, thinking likewise.

". . . in your own words, Mr. Tate," Mr. Gilmer was saying.

"Well," said Mr. Tate, touching his glasses and speaking to his knees, "I was called—"

"Could you say it to the jury, Mr. Tate? Thank you. Who called you?"

Mr. Tate said, "I was fetched by Bob—by Mr. Bob Ewell yonder, one night—"

"What night, sir?"

Mr. Tate said, "It was the night of November twenty-first. I was just leaving my office to go home when B—Mr. Ewell came in, very excited he was, and said get out to his house quick, some nigger'd raped his girl."

"Did you go?"

"Certainly. Got in the car and went out as fast as I could."

"And what did you find?"

"Found her lying on the floor in the middle of the front room, one on the right as you go in. She was pretty well beat up, but I heaved her to her feet and she washed her face in a bucket in the corner and said she was all right. I asked her who hurt her and she said it was Tom Robinson—"

Judge Taylor, who had been concentrating on his fingernails, looked up as if he were expecting an objection, but Atticus was quiet.

"—asked her if he beat her like that, she said yes he had. Asked her if he took advantage of her and she said yes he did. So I went down to Robinson's house and brought him back. She identified him as the one, so I took him in. That's all there was to it."

"Thank you," said Mr. Gilmer.

Judge Taylor said, "Any questions, Atticus?"

"Yes," said my father. He was sitting behind his table; his chair was skewed to one side, his legs were crossed and one arm was resting on the back of his chair.

"Did you call a doctor, Sheriff? Did anybody call a doctor?" asked Atticus.

"No sir," said Mr. Tate.

"Didn't call a doctor?"

"No sir," repeated Mr. Tate.

"Why not?" There was an edge to Atticus's voice.

"Well I can tell you why I didn't. It wasn't necessary, Mr. Finch. She was mighty banged up. Something sho' happened, it was obvious."

"But you didn't call a doctor? While you were there did anyone send for one, fetch one, carry her to one?"

"No sir—"

Judge Taylor broke in. "He's answered the question three times, Atticus. He didn't call a doctor."

Atticus said, "I just wanted to make sure, Judge," and the judge smiled.

Jem's hand, which was resting on the balcony rail, tightened around it. He drew in his breath suddenly. Glancing below, I saw no corresponding reaction, and wondered if Jem was trying to be dramatic. Dill was watching peacefully, and so was Reverend Sykes beside him. "What is it?" I whispered, and got a terse, "Sh-h!"

"Sheriff," Atticus was saying, "you say she was mighty banged up. In what way?"

"Well—"

"Just describe her injuries, Heck."

"Well, she was beaten around the head. There was already bruises comin' on her arms, and it happened about thirty minutes before—"

"How do you know?"

Mr. Tate grinned. "Sorry, that's what they said. Anyway, she was pretty bruised up when I got there, and she had a black eye comin'."

"Which eye?"

Mr. Tate blinked and ran his hands through his hair. "Let's see," he said softly, then he looked at Atticus as if he considered the question childish. "Can't you remember?" Atticus asked.

Mr. Tate pointed to an invisible person five inches in front of him and said, "Her left."

"Wait a minute, Sheriff," said Atticus. "Was it her left facing you or her left looking the same way you were?"

Mr. Tate said, "Oh yes, that'd make it her right. It was her right eye, Mr. Finch. I remember now, she was bunged up on that side of her face. . . ."

Mr. Tate blinked again, as if something had suddenly been made plain to him. Then he turned his head and looked around at Tom Robinson. As if by instinct, Tom Robinson raised his head.

Something had been made plain to Atticus also, and it brought him to his feet. "Sheriff, please repeat what you said."

"It was her right eye, I said."

"No . . ." Atticus walked to the court reporter's desk and bent down to the furiously scribbling hand. It stopped, flipped back the shorthand pad, and the court reporter said, " 'Mr. Finch. I remember now she was bunged up on that side of the face.' "

Atticus looked up at Mr. Tate. "Which side again, Heck?"

"The right side, Mr. Finch, but she had more bruises—you wanta hear about 'em?"

Atticus seemed to be bordering on another question, but he thought better of it and said, "Yes, what were her other injuries?" As Mr. Tate answered, Atticus turned and looked at Tom Robinson as if to say this was something they hadn't bargained for.

". . . her arms were bruised, and she showed me her neck. There were definite finger marks on her gullet—"

"All around her throat? At the back of her neck?"

"I'd say they were all around, Mr. Finch."

"You would?"

"Yes sir, she had a small throat, anybody could'a reached around it with—"

"Just answer the question yes or no, please, Sheriff," said Atticus dryly, and Mr. Tate fell silent.

Atticus sat down and nodded to the circuit solicitor, who shook his head at the judge, who nodded to Mr. Tate, who rose stiffly and stepped down from the witness stand.

Below us, heads turned, feet scraped the floor, babies were shifted to shoulders, and a few children scampered out of the courtroom. The Negroes behind us whispered softly among themselves; Dill was asking Reverend Sykes what it was all about, but Reverend Sykes said he didn't know. So far, things were utterly dull: nobody had thundered, there were no arguments between opposing counsel, there was no drama; a grave disappointment to all present, it seemed. Atticus was proceeding amiably, as if he were involved in a title dispute. With his infinite capacity for calming turbulent seas, he could make a rape case as dry as a sermon. Gone was the terror in my mind of stale whiskey and barnyard smells, of sleepy-eyed sullen men, of a husky voice calling in the night, "Mr. Finch? They gone?" Our nightmare had gone with daylight, everything would come out all right.

All the spectators were as relaxed as Judge Taylor, except Jem. His mouth was twisted into a purposeful half-grin, and his eyes happy about, and he said something about corroborating evidence, which made me sure he was showing off.

". . . Robert E. Lee Ewell!"

In answer to the clerk's booming voice, a little bantam

cock of a man rose and strutted to the stand, the back of his neck reddening at the sound of his name. When he turned around to take the oath, we saw that his face was as red as his neck. We also saw no resemblance to his namesake. A shock of wispy new-washed hair stood up from his forehead; his nose was thin, pointed, and shiny; he had no chin to speak of—it seemed to be part of his crepey neck.

"—so help me God," he crowed.

Every town the size of Maycomb had families like the Ewells. No economic fluctuations changed their status—people like the Ewells lived as guests of the county in prosperity as well as in the depths of a depression. No truant officers could keep their numerous offspring in school; no public health officer could free them from congenital defects, various worms, and the diseases indigenous to filthy surroundings.

Maycomb's Ewells lived behind the town garbage dump in what was once a Negro cabin. The cabin's plank walls were supplemented with sheets of corrugated iron, its roof shingled with tin cans hammered flat, so only its general shape suggested its original design: square, with four tiny rooms opening onto a shotgun hall, the cabin rested uneasily upon four irregular lumps of limestone. Its windows were merely open spaces in the walls, which in the summertime were covered with greasy strips of cheesecloth to keep out the varmints that feasted on Maycomb's refuse.

The varmints had a lean time of it, for the Ewells gave the dump a thorough gleaning every day, and the fruits of their industry (those that were not eaten) made the plot of ground around the cabin look like the playhouse of an insane child: what passed for a fence was bits of tree-limbs, broomsticks and tool shafts, all tipped with rusty hammer-heads, snaggletoothed rake heads, shovels, axes and grubbing hoes, held on with pieces of barbed wire. Enclosed by this barricade was a dirty yard containing the remains of a Model-T Ford (on blocks), a discarded dentist's chair, an ancient icebox, plus lesser items: old shoes, worn-out table radios, picture frames, and fruit jars, under which scrawny orange chickens pecked hopefully.

One corner of the yard, though, bewildered Maycomb. Against the fence, in a line, were six chipped-enamel slop jars holding brilliant red geraniums, cared for as tenderly as if they belonged to Miss Maudie Atkinson, had Miss Maudie deigned to permit a geranium on her premises. People said they were Mayella Ewell's.

Nobody was quite sure how many children were on the place. Some people said six, others said nine; there were always several dirty-faced ones at the windows when anyone passed by. Nobody had occasion to pass by except at Christmas, when the churches delivered baskets, and when the mayor of Maycomb asked us to please help the garbage collector by dumping our own trees and trash.

Atticus took us with him last Christmas when he complied with the mayor's request. A dirt road ran from the highway past the dump, down to a small Negro settlement some five hundred yards beyond the Ewells'. It was necessary either to back out to the highway or go the full length of the road and turn around; most people turned around in the Negroes' front yards. In the frosty December dusk, their cabins looked neat and snug with pale blue smoke rising from the chimneys and doorways glowing amber from the fires inside. There were delicious smells about: chicken, bacon frying crisp as the twilight air. Jem and I detected squirrel cooking, but it took an old countryman like Atticus to identify possum and rabbit, aromas that vanished when we rode back past the Ewell residence.

All the little man on the witness stand had that made him any better than his nearest neighbors was, that if scrubbed with lye soap in very hot water, his skin was white.

"Mr. Robert Ewell?" asked Mr. Gilmer.

"That's m'name, cap'n," said the witness.

Mr. Gilmer's back stiffened a little, and I felt sorry for him. Perhaps I'd better explain something now. I've heard that lawyers' children, on seeing their parents in court in the heat of argument, get the wrong idea: they think opposing counsel to be the personal enemies of their parents, they suffer agonies, and are surprised to see them often go out arm-in-arm with their tormenters during the first recess. This was not true of Jem and me. We acquired no traumas from watching our father win or lose. I'm sorry that I can't provide any drama in this respect; if I did, it would not be true. We could tell, however, when debate became more acrimonious than professional, but this was from watching lawyers other than our father. I never heard Atticus raise his voice in my life, except to a deaf witness. Mr. Gilmer was doing his job, as Atticus was doing his. Besides, Mr. Ewell was Mr. Gilmer's witness, and he had no business being rude to him of all people.

"Are you the father of Mayella Ewell?" was the next question.

"Well, if I ain't I can't do nothing about it now, her ma's dead," was the answer.

Judge Taylor stirred. He turned slowly in his swivel chair and looked benignly at the witness. "Are you the father of Mayella Ewell?" he asked, in a way that made the laughter below us stop suddenly.

"Yes sir," Mr. Ewell said meekly.

Judge Taylor went on in tones of good will: "This the first time you've ever been in court? I don't recall ever seeing you here." At the witness's affirmative nod he continued, "Well, let's get something straight. There will be no more audibly obscene speculations on any subject from anybody in this courtroom as long as I'm sitting here. Do you understand?"

Mr. Ewell nodded, but I don't think he did. Judge Taylor sighed and said, "All right, Mr. Gilmer?"

"Thank you, sir. Mr. Ewell, would you tell us in your own words what happened on the evening of November twenty-first, please?"

Jem grinned and pushed his hair back. Just-in-your own words was Mr. Gilmer's trademark. We often wondered who else's words Mr. Gilmer was afraid his witness might employ.

"Well, the night of November twenty-one I was comin' in from the woods with a load o'kindlin' and just as I got to the fence I heard Mayella screamin' like a stuck hog inside the house—"

Here Judge Taylor glanced sharply at the witness and must have decided his speculations devoid of evil intent, for he subsided sleepily.

"What time was it, Mr. Ewell?"

"Just 'fore sundown. Well, I was sayin' Mayella was screamin' fit to beat Jesus—" another glance from the bench silenced Mr. Ewell.

"Yes? She was screaming?" said Mr. Gilmer.

Mr. Ewell looked confusedly at the judge. "Well, Mayella

was raisin' this holy racket so I dropped m'load and run as fast as I could but I run into th' fence, but when I got distangled I run up to th' window and I seen—'' Mr. Ewell's face grew scarlet. He stood up and pointed his finger at Tom Robinson. ''—I seen that black nigger yonder ruttin' on my Mayella!''

So serene was Judge Taylor's court, that he had few occasions to use his gavel, but he hammered fully five minutes. Atticus was on his feet at the bench saying something to him, Mr. Heck Tate as first officer of the county stood in the middle aisle quelling the packed courtroom. Behind us, there was an angry muffled groan from the colored people.

Reverend Sykes leaned across Dill and me, pulling at Jem's elbow. ''Mr. Jem,'' he said, ''you better take Miss Jean Louise home. Mr. Jem, you hear me?''

Jem turned his head. ''Scout, go home. Dill, you'n'Scout go home.''

''You gotta make me first,'' I said, remembering Atticus's blessed dictum.

Jem scowled furiously at me, then said to Reverend Sykes, ''I think it's okay, Reverend, she doesn't understand it.''

I was mortally offended. ''I most certainly do, I c'n understand anything you can.''

''Aw hush. She doesn't understand it, Reverend, she ain't nine yet.''

Reverend Sykes's black eyes were anxious. ''Mr. Finch know you all are here? This ain't fit for Miss Jean Louise or you boys either.''

Jem shook his head. ''He can't see us this far away. It's all right, Reverend.''

I knew Jem would win, because I knew nothing could make him leave now. Dill and I were safe, for a while: Atticus could see us from where he was, if he looked.

As Judge Taylor banged his gavel, Mr. Ewell was sitting smugly in the witness chair, surveying his handiwork. With one phrase he had turned happy picknickers into a sulky, tense, murmuring crowd, being slowly hypnotized by gavel taps lessening in intensity until the only sound in the courtroom was a dim pink-pink-pink: the judge might have been rapping the bench with a pencil.

In possession of his court once more, Judge Taylor leaned

back in his chair. He looked suddenly weary; his age was showing, and I thought about what Atticus had said—he and Mrs. Taylor didn't kiss much—he must have been nearly seventy.

"There has been a request," Judge Taylor said, "that this courtroom be cleared of spectators, or at least of women and children, a request that will be denied for the time being. People generally see what they look for, and hear what they listen for, and they have the right to subject their children to it, but I can assure you of one thing: you will receive what you see and hear in silence or you will leave this courtroom, but you won't leave it until the whole boiling of you come before me on contempt charges. Mr. Ewell, you will keep your testimony within the confines of Christian English usage, if that is possible. Proceed, Mr. Gilmer."

Mr. Ewell reminded me of a deaf-mute. I was sure he had never heard the words Judge Taylor directed at him—his mouth struggled silently with them—but their import registered on his face. Smugness faded from it, replaced by a dogged earnestness that fooled Judge Taylor not at all: as long as Mr. Ewell was on the stand, the judge kept his eyes on him, as if daring him to make a false move.

Mr. Gilmer and Atticus exchanged glances. Atticus was sitting down again, his fist rested on his cheek and we could not see his face. Mr. Gilmer looked rather desperate. A question from Judge Taylor made him relax: "Mr. Ewell, did you see the defendant having sexual intercourse with your daughter?"

"Yes, I did."

The spectators were quiet, but the defendant said something. Atticus whispered to him, and Tom Robinson was silent.

"You say you were at the window?" asked Mr. Gilmer.

"Yes sir."

"How far is it from the ground?"

" 'bout three foot."

"Did you have a clear view of the room?"

"Yes sir."

"How did the room look?"

"Well, it was all slung about, like there was a fight."

"What did you do when you saw the defendant?"

"Well, I run around the house to get in, but he run out the front door just ahead of me. I sawed who he was, all right. I was too distracted about Mayella to run after'im. I run in the house and she was lyin' on the floor squallin'—"

"Then what did you do?"

"Why, I run for Tate quick as I could. I knowed who it was, all right, lived down yonder in that nigger-nest, passed the house every day. Jedge, I've asked this county for fifteen years to clean out that nest down yonder, they're dangerous to live around 'sides devaluin' my property—"

"Thank you, Mr. Ewell," said Mr. Gilmer hurriedly.

The witness made a hasty descent from the stand and ran smack into Atticus, who had risen to question him. Judge Taylor permitted the court to laugh.

"Just a minute, sir," said Atticus genially. "Could I ask you a question or two?"

Mr. Ewell backed up into the witness chair, settled himself, and regarded Atticus with haughty suspicion, an expression common to Maycomb County witnesses when confronted by opposing counsel.

"Mr. Ewell," Atticus began, "folks were doing a lot of running that night. Let's see, you say you ran to the house, you ran to the window, you ran inside, you ran to Mayella, you ran for Mr. Tate. Did you, during all this running, run for a doctor?"

"Wadn't no need to. I seen what happened."

"But there's one thing I don't understand," said Atticus. "Weren't you concerned with Mayella's condition?"

"I most positively was," said Mr. Ewell. "I seen who done it."

"No, I mean her physical condition. Did you not think the nature of her injuries warranted immediate medical attention?"

"What?"

"Didn't you think she should have had a doctor, immediately?"

The witness said he never thought of it, he had never called a doctor to any of his'n in his life, and if he had it would have cost him five dollars. "That all?" he asked.

"Not quite," said Atticus casually. "Mr. Ewell, you heard the sheriff's testimony, didn't you?"

"How's that?"

"You were in the courtroom when Mr. Heck Tate was on the stand, weren't you? You heard everything he said, didn't you?"

Mr. Ewell considered the matter carefully, and seemed to decide that the question was safe.

"Yes," he said.

"Do you agree with his description of Mayella's injuries?"

"How's that?"

Atticus looked around at Mr. Gilmer and smiled. Mr. Ewell seemed determined not to give the defense the time of day.

"Mr. Tate testified that her right eye was blackened, that she was beaten around the—"

"Oh yeah," said the witness. "I hold with everything Tate said."

"You do?" asked Atticus mildly. "I just want to make sure." He went to the court reporter, said something, and the reporter entertained us for some minutes by reading Mr. Tate's testimony as if it were stock-market quotations: ". . . which eye her left oh yes that'd make it her right it was her right eye Mr. Finch I remember now she was bunged." He flipped the page. "Up on that side of the face Sheriff please repeat what you said it was her right eye I said—"

"Thank you, Bert," said Atticus. "You heard it again, Mr. Ewell. Do you have anything to add to it? Do you agree with the sheriff?"

"I holds with Tate. Her eye was blacked and she was mighty beat up."

The little man seemed to have forgotten his previous humiliation from the bench. It was becoming evident that he thought Atticus an easy match. He seemed to grow ruddy again; his chest swelled, and once more he was a red little rooster. I thought he'd burst his shirt at Atticus's next question:

"Mr. Ewell, can you read and write?"

Mr. Gilmer interrupted. "Objection," he said. "Can't see what witness's literacy has to do with the case, irrelevant'-n'immaterial."

Judge Taylor was about to speak but Atticus said, "Judge, if you'll allow the question plus another one you'll soon see."

"All right, let's see," said Judge Taylor, "but make sure we see, Atticus. Overruled."

Mr. Gilmer seemed as curious as the rest of us as to what bearing the state of Mr. Ewell's education had on the case.

"I'll repeat the question," said Atticus. "Can you read and write?"

"I most positively can."

"Will you write your name and show us?"

"I most positively will. How do you think I sign my relief checks?"

Mr. Ewell was endearing himself to his fellow citizens. The whispers and chuckles below us probably had to do with what a card he was.

I was becoming nervous. Atticus seemed to know what he was doing—but it seemed to me that he'd gone frog-sticking without a light. Never, never, never, on cross-examination ask a witness a question you don't already know the answer to, was a tenet I absorbed with my baby-food. Do it, and you'll often get an answer you don't want, an answer that might wreck your case.

Atticus was reaching into the inside pocket of his coat. He drew out an envelope, then reached into his vest pocket and unclipped his fountain pen. He moved leisurely, and had turned so that he was in full view of the jury. He unscrewed the fountain-pen cap and placed it gently on his table. He shook the pen a little, then handed it with the envelope to the witness. "Would you write your name for us?" he asked. "Clearly now, so the jury can see you do it."

Mr. Ewell wrote on the back of the envelope and looked up complacently to see Judge Taylor staring at him as if he were some fragrant gardenia in full bloom on the witness stand, to see Mr. Gilmer half-sitting, half-standing at his table. The jury was watching him, one man was leaning forward with his hands over the railing.

"What's so interestin'?" he asked.

"You're left-handed, Mr. Ewell," said Judge Taylor. Mr. Ewell turned angrily to the judge and said he didn't see what his being left-handed had to do with it, that he was a Christfearing man and Atticus Finch was taking advantage of him. Tricking lawyers like Atticus Finch took advantage of him all the time with their tricking ways. He had told them what happened, he'd say it again and again—which he did. Nothing Atticus asked him after that shook his story, that he'd looked through the window, then ran the nigger off, then ran for the sheriff. Atticus finally dismissed him.

Mr. Gilmer asked him one more question. "About your writing with your left hand, are you ambidextrous, Mr. Ewell?"

"I most positively am not, I can use one hand good as the other. One hand good as the other," he added, glaring at the defense table.

Jem seemed to be having a quiet fit. He was pounding the balcony rail softly, and once he whispered, "We've got him."

I didn't think so: Atticus was trying to show, it seemed to me, that Mr. Ewell could have beaten up Mayella. That much I could follow. If her right eye was blacked and she was beaten mostly on the right side of the face, it would tend to show that a left-handed person did it. Sherlock Holmes and Jem Finch would agree. But Tom Robinson could easily be left-handed, too. Like Mr. Heck Tate, I imagined a person facing me, went through a swift mental pantomime, and concluded that he might have held her with his right hand and pounded her with his left. I looked down at him. His back was to us, but I could see his broad shoulders and bull-thick neck. He could easily have done it. I thought Jem was counting his chickens.

18

But someone was booming again.

"Mayella Violet Ewell—!"

A young girl walked to the witness stand. As she raised her hand and swore that the evidence she gave would be the truth, the whole truth, and nothing but the truth so help her God, she seemed somehow fragile-looking, but when she sat facing us in the witness chair she became what she was, a thick-bodied girl accustomed to strenuous labor.

In Maycomb County, it was easy to tell when someone bathed regularly, as opposed to yearly lavations: Mr. Ewell had a scalded look; as if an overnight soaking had deprived him of protective layers of dirt, his skin appeared to be sensitive to the elements. Mayella looked as if she tried to keep clean, and I was reminded of the row of red geraniums in the Ewell yard.

Mr. Gilmer asked Mayella to tell the jury in her own words what happened on the evening of November twenty-first of last year, just in her own words, please.

Mayella sat silently.

"Where were you at dusk on that evening?" began Mr. Gilmer patiently.

"On the porch."

"Which porch?"

"Ain't but one, the front porch."

"What were you doing on the porch?"

"Nothin'."

Judge Taylor said, "Just tell us what happened. You can do that, can't you?"

Mayella stared at him and burst into tears. She covered her mouth with her hands and sobbed. Judge Taylor let her cry for a while, then he said, "That's enough now. Don't be 'fraid of anybody here, as long as you tell the truth. All this is strange to you, I know, but you've nothing to be ashamed of and nothing to fear. What are you scared of?"

Mayella said something behind her hands. "What was that?" asked the judge.

"Him," she sobbed, pointing at Atticus.

"Mr. Finch?"

She nodded vigorously, saying, "Don't want him doin' me like he done Papa, tryin' to make him out lefthanded . . ."

Judge Taylor scratched his thick white hair. It was plain that he had never been confronted with a problem of this kind. "How old are you?" he asked.

"Nineteen-and-a-half," Mayella said.

Judge Taylor cleared his throat and tried unsuccessfully to

speak in soothing tones. "Mr. Finch has no idea of scaring you," he growled, "and if he did, I'm here to stop him. That's one thing I'm sitting up here for. Now you're a big girl, so you just sit up straight and tell the—tell us what happened to you. You can do that, can't you?"

I whispered to Jem, "Has she got good sense?"

Jem was squinting down at the witness stand. "Can't tell yet," he said. "She's got enough sense to get the judge sorry for her, but she might be just—oh, I don't know."

Mollified, Mayella gave Atticus a final terrified glance and said to Mr. Gilmer, "Well sir, I was on the porch and—and he came along and, you see, there was this old chiffarobe in the yard Papa'd brought in to chop up for kindlin'—Papa told me to do it while he was off in the woods but I wadn't feelin' strong enough then, so he came by—"

"Who is 'he'?"

Mayella pointed to Tom Robinson. "I'll have to ask you to be more specific, please," said Mr. Gilmer. "The reporter can't put down gestures very well."

"That'n yonder," she said. "Robinson."

"Then what happened?"

"I said come here, nigger, and bust up this chiffarobe for me, I gotta nickel for you. He coulda done it easy enough, he could. So he come in the yard an' I went in the house to get him the nickel and I turned around an 'fore I knew it he was on me. Just run up behind me, he did. He got me round the neck, cussin' me an' sayin' dirt—I fought'n'hollered, but he had me round the neck. He hit me agin an' agin—"

Mr. Gilmer waited for Mayella to collect herself: she had twisted her handkerchief into a sweaty rope; when she opened it to wipe her face it was a mass of creases from her hot hands. She waited for Mr. Gilmer to ask another question, but when he didn't, she said, "—he chunked me on the floor an' choked me'n took advantage of me."

"Did you scream?" asked Mr. Gilmer. "Did you scream and fight back?"

"Reckon I did, hollered for all I was worth, kicked and hollered loud as I could."

"Then what happened?"

"I don't remember too good, but next thing I knew Papa was in the room a'standing over me hollerin' who done it, who done it? Then I sorta fainted an' the next thing I knew Mr. Tate was pullin' me up offa the floor and leadin' me to the water bucket.''

Apparently Mayella's recital had given her confidence, but it was not her father's brash kind: there was something stealthy about hers, like a steady-eyed cat with a twitchy tail.

"You say you fought him off as hard as you could? Fought him tooth and nail?" asked Mr. Gilmer.

"I positively did," Mayella echoed her father.

"You are positive that he took full advantage of you?"

Mayella's face contorted, and I was afraid that she would cry again. Instead, she said, "He done what he was after."

Mr. Gilmer called attention to the hot day by wiping his head with his hand. "That's all for the time being," he said pleasantly, "but you stay there. I expect big bad Mr. Finch has some questions to ask you."

"State will not prejudice the witness against counsel for the defense," murmured Judge Taylor primly, "at least not at this time."

Atticus got up grinning but instead of walking to the witness stand, he opened his coat and hooked his thumbs in his vest, then he walked slowly across the room to the windows. He looked out, but didn't seem especially interested in what he saw, then he turned and strolled back to the witness stand. From long years of experience, I could tell he was trying to come to a decision about something.

"Miss Mayella," he said, smiling, "I won't try to scare you for a while, not yet. Let's just get acquainted. How old are you?"

"Said I was nineteen, said it to the judge yonder." Mayella jerked her head resentfully at the bench.

"So you did, so you did, ma'am. You'll have to bear with me, Miss Mayella, I'm getting along and can't remember as well as I used to. I might ask you things you've already said before, but you'll give me an answer, won't you? Good."

I could see nothing in Mayella's expression to justify Atticus's assumption that he had secured her wholehearted co-operation. She was looking at him furiously.

"Won't answer a word you say long as you keep on mockin' me," she said.

"Ma'am?" asked Atticus, startled.

"Long's you keep on makin' fun o'me."

Judge Taylor said, "Mr. Finch is not making fun of you. What's the matter with you?"

Mayella looked from under lowered eyelids at Atticus, but she said to the judge: "Long's he keeps on callin' me ma'am an sayin' Miss Mayella. I don't hafta take his sass, I ain't called upon to take it."

Atticus resumed his stroll to the windows and let Judge Taylor handle this one. Judge Taylor was not the kind of figure that ever evoked pity, but I did feel a pang for him as he tried to explain. "That's just Mr. Finch's way," he told Mayella. "We've done business in this court for years and years, and Mr. Finch is always courteous to everybody. He's not trying to mock you, he's trying to be polite. That's just his way."

The judge leaned back. "Atticus, let's get on with these proceedings, and let the record show that the witness has not been sassed, her views to the contrary."

I wondered if anybody had ever called her "ma'am," or "Miss Mayella" in her life; probably not, as she took offense to routine courtesy. What on earth was her life like? I soon found out.

"You say you're nineteen," Atticus resumed. "How many sisters and brothers have you?" He walked from the windows back to the stand.

"Seb'm," she said, and I wondered if they were all like the specimen I had seen the first day I started to school.

"You the eldest? The oldest?"

"Yes."

"How long has your mother been dead?"

"Don't know—long time."

"Did you ever go to school?"

"Read'n'write good as Papa yonder."

Mayella sounded like a Mr. Jingle in a book I had been reading.

"How long did you go to school?"

"Two year—three year—dunno."

Slowly but surely I began to see the pattern of Atticus's questions: from questions that Mr. Gilmer did not deem sufficiently irrelevant or immaterial to object to, Atticus was quietly building up before the jury a picture of the Ewells' home life. The jury learned the following things: their relief check was far from enough to feed the family, and there was strong suspicion that Papa drank it up anyway—he sometimes went off in the swamp for days and came home sick; the weather was seldom cold enough to require shoes, but when it was, you could make dandy ones from strips of old tires; the family hauled its water in buckets from a spring that ran out at one end of the dump—they kept the surrounding area clear of trash—and it was everybody for himself as far as keeping clean went: if you wanted to wash you hauled your own water; the younger children had perpetual colds and suffered from chronic ground-itch; there was a lady who came around sometimes and asked Mayella why she didn't stay in school—she wrote down the answer; with two members of the family reading and writing, there was no need for the rest of them to learn—Papa needed them at home.

"Miss Mayella," said Atticus, in spite of himself, "a nineteen-year-old girl like you must have friends. Who are your friends?"

The witness frowned as if puzzled. "Friends?"

"Yes, don't you know anyone near your age, or older, or younger? Boys and girls? Just ordinary friends?"

Mayella's hostility, which had subsided to grudging neutrality, flared again. "You makin' fun o'me agin, Mr. Finch?"

Atticus let her question answer his.

"Do you love your father, Miss Mayella?" was his next.

"Love him, whatcha mean?"

"I mean, is he good to you, is he easy to get along with?"

"He does tollable, 'cept when—"

"Except when?"

Mayella looked at her father, who was sitting with his chair tipped against the railing. He sat up straight and waited for her to answer.

"Except when nothin'," said Mayella. "I said he does tollable."

Mr. Ewell leaned back again.

"Except when he's drinking?" asked Atticus so gently that Mayella nodded.

"Does he ever go after you?"

"How you mean?"

"When he's—riled, has he ever beaten you?"

Mayella looked around, down at the court reporter, up at the judge. "Answer the question, Miss Mayella," said Judge Taylor.

"My paw's never touched a hair o'my head in my life," she declared firmly. "He never touched me."

Atticus's glasses had slipped a little, and he pushed them up on his nose. "We've had a good visit, Miss Mayella, and now I guess we'd better get to the case. You say you asked Tom Robinson to come chop up a—what was it?"

"A chiffarobe, a old dresser full of drawers on one side."

"Was Tom Robinson well known to you?"

"Whaddya mean?"

"I mean did you know who he was, where he lived?"

Mayella nodded. "I knowed who he was, he passed the house every day."

"Was this the first time you asked him to come inside the fence?"

Mayella jumped slightly at the question. Atticus was making his slow pilgrimage to the windows, as he had been doing: he would ask a question, then look out, waiting for an answer. He did not see her involuntary jump, but it seemed to me that he knew she had moved. He turned around and raised his eyebrows. "Was—" he began again.

"Yes it was."

"Didn't you ever ask him to come inside the fence before?"

She was prepared now. "I did not, I certainly did not."

"One did not's enough," said Atticus serenely. "You never asked him to do odd jobs for you before?"

"I mighta," conceded Mayella. "There was several niggers around."

"Can you remember any other occasions?"

"No."

"All right, now to what happened. You said Tom Robinson was behind you in the room when you turned around, that right?"

"Yes."

"You said he 'got you around the neck cussing and saying dirt'—is that right?"

" 't's right."

Atticus's memory had suddenly become accurate. "You say 'he caught me and choked me and took advantage of me'—is that right?"

"That's what I said."

"Do you remember him beating you about the face?"

The witness hesitated.

"You seem sure enough that he choked you. All this time you were fighting back, remember? You 'kicked and hollered as loud as you could.' Do you remember him beating you about the face?"

Mayella was silent. She seemed to be trying to get something clear to herself. I thought for a moment she was doing Mr. Heck Tate's and my trick of pretending there was a person in front of us. She glanced at Mr. Gilmer.

"It's an easy question, Miss Mayella, so I'll try again. Do you remember him beating you about the face?" Atticus's voice had lost its comfortableness; he was speaking in his arid, detached professional voice. "Do you remember him beating you about the face?"

"No, I don't recollect if he hit me. I mean yes I do, he hit me."

"Was your last sentence your answer?"

"Huh? Yes, he hit—I just don't remember, I just don't remember . . . it all happened so quick."

Judge Taylor looked sternly at Mayella. "Don't you cry, young woman—" he began, but Atticus said, "Let her cry if she wants to, Judge. We've got all the time in the world."

Mayella sniffed wrathfully and looked at Atticus. "I'll answer any question you got—get me up here an' mock me, will you? I'll answer any question you got—"

"That's fine," said Atticus. "There're only a few more. Miss Mayella, not to be tedious, you've testified that the defendant hit you, grabbed you around the neck, choked you, and took advantage of you. I want you to be sure you have the right man. Will you identify the man who raped you?"

"I will, that's him right yonder."

Atticus turned to the defendant. "Tom, stand up. Let Miss Mayella have a good long look at you. Is this the man, Miss Mayella?"

Tom Robinson's powerful shoulders rippled under his thin shirt. He rose to his feet and stood with his right hand on the back of his chair. He looked oddly off balance, but it was not from the way he was standing. His left arm was fully twelve inches shorter than his right, and hung dead at his side. It ended in a small shriveled hand, and from as far away as the balcony I could see that it was no use to him.

"Scout," breathed Jem. "Scout, look! Reverend, he's crippled!"

Reverend Sykes leaned across me and whispered to Jem. "He got it caught in a cotton gin, caught it in Mr. Dolphus Raymond's cotton gin when he was a boy . . . like to bled to death . . . tore all the muscles loose from his bones—"

Atticus said, "Is this the man who raped you?"

"It most certainly is."

Atticus's next question was one word long. "How?"

Mayella was raging. "I don't know how he done it, but he done it—I said it all happened so fast I—"

"Now let's consider this calmly—" began Atticus, but Mr. Gilmer interrupted with an objection: he was not irrelevant or immaterial, but Atticus was browbeating the witness.

Judge Taylor laughed outright. "Oh sit down, Horace, he's doing nothing of the sort. If anything, the witness's browbeating Atticus."

Judge Taylor was the only person in the courtroom who laughed. Even the babies were still, and I suddenly wondered if they had been smothered at their mothers' breasts.

"Now," said Atticus, "Miss Mayella, you've testified that the defendant choked and beat you—you didn't say that he sneaked up behind you and knocked you cold, but you turned around and there he was—" Atticus was back behind his table, and he emphasized his words by tapping his knuckles on it. "—do you wish to reconsider any of your testimony?"

"You want me to say something that didn't happen?"

"No ma'am, I want you to say something that did happen. Tell us once more, please, what happened?"

"I told'ja what happened."

"You testified that you turned around and there he was. He choked you then?"

"Yes."

"Then he released your throat and hit you?"

"I said he did."

"He blacked your left eye with his right fist?"

"I ducked and it—it glanced, that's what it did. I ducked and it glanced off." Mayella had finally seen the light.

"You're becoming suddenly clear on this point. A while ago you couldn't remember too well, could you?"

"I said he hit me."

"All right. He choked you, he hit you, then he raped you, that right?"

"It most certainly is."

"You're a strong girl, what were you doing all the time, just standing there?"

"I told'ja I hollered'n'kicked'n'fought—"

Atticus reached up and took off his glasses, turned his good right eye to the witness, and rained questions on her. Judge Taylor said, "One question at a time, Atticus. Give the witness a chance to answer."

"All right, why didn't you run?"

"I tried . . ."

"Tried to? What kept you from it?"

"I—he slung me down. That's what he did, he slung me down'n got on top of me."

"You were screaming all this time?"

"I certainly was."

"Then why didn't the other children hear you? Where were they? At the dump?"

"Where were they?"

No answer.

"Why didn't your screams make them come running? The dump's closer than the woods, isn't it?"

No answer.

"Or didn't you scream until you saw your father in the window? You didn't think to scream until then, did you?"

No answer.

"Did you scream first at your father instead of at Tom Robinson? Was that it?"

No answer.

"Who beat you up? Tom Robinson or your father?"

No answer.

"What did your father see in the window, the crime of rape or the best defense to it? Why don't you tell the truth, child, didn't Bob Ewell beat you up?"

When Atticus turned away from Mayella he looked like

his stomach hurt, but Mayella's face was a mixture of terror and fury. Atticus sat down wearily and polished his glasses with his handkerchief.

Suddenly Mayella became articulate. "I got somethin' to say," she said.

Atticus raised his head. "Do you want to tell us what happened?"

But she did not hear the compassion in his invitation. "I got somethin' to say an' then I ain't gonna say no more. That nigger yonder took advantage of me an' if you fine fancy gentlemen don't wanta do nothin' about it then you're all yellow stinkin' cowards, stinkin' cowards, the lot of you. Your fancy airs don't come to nothin'—your ma'amin' and Miss Mayellerin' don't come to nothin', Mr. Finch—"

Then she burst into real tears. Her shoulders shook with angry sobs. She was as good as her word. She answered no more questions, even when Mr. Gilmer tried to get her back on the track. I guess if she hadn't been so poor and ignorant, Judge Taylor would have put her under the jail for the contempt she had shown everybody in the courtroom. Somehow, Atticus had hit her hard in a way that was not clear to me, but it gave him no pleasure to do so. He sat with his head down, and I never saw anybody glare at anyone with the hatred Mayella showed when she left the stand and walked by Atticus's table.

When Mr. Gilmer told Judge Taylor that the state rested, Judge Taylor said, "It's time we all did. We'll take ten minutes."

Atticus and Mr. Gilmer met in front of the bench and whispered, then they left the courtroom by a door behind the witness stand, which was a signal for us all to stretch. I discovered that I had been sitting on the edge of the long bench, and I was somewhat numb. Jem got up and yawned, Dill did likewise, and Reverend Sykes wiped his face on his hat. The temperature was an easy ninety, he said.

Mr. Braxton Underwood, who had been sitting quietly in a chair reserved for the Press, soaking up testimony with his sponge of a brain, allowed his bitter eyes to rove over the colored balcony, and they met mine. He gave a snort and looked away.

"Jem," I said, "Mr. Underwood's seen us."

"That's okay. He won't tell Atticus, he'll just put it on the social side of the *Tribune*." Jem turned back to Dill, explaining, I suppose, the finer points of the trial to him, but I wondered what they were. There had been no lengthy debates between Atticus and Mr. Gilmer on any points; Mr. Gilmer seemed to be prosecuting almost reluctantly; witnesses had been led by the nose as asses are, with few objections. But Atticus had once told us that in Judge Taylor's court any lawyer who was a strict constructionist on evidence usually wound up receiving strict instructions from the bench. He distilled this for me to mean that Judge Taylor might look lazy and operate in his sleep, but he was seldom reversed, and that was the proof of the pudding. Atticus said he was a good judge.

Presently Judge Taylor returned and climbed into his swivel chair. He took a cigar from his vest pocket and examined it thoughtfully. I punched Dill. Having passed the judge's inspection, the cigar suffered a vicious bite. "We come down sometimes to watch him," I explained. "It's gonna take him the rest of the afternoon, now. You watch." Unaware of public scrutiny from above, Judge Taylor disposed of the severed end by propelling it expertly to his lips and saying, "Fhluck!" He hit a spittoon so squarely we could hear it slosh. "Bet he was hell with a spitball," murmured Dill.

As a rule, a recess meant a general exodus, but today people weren't moving. Even the Idlers who had failed to shame younger men from their seats had remained standing along the walls. I guess Mr. Heck Tate had reserved the county toilet for court officials.

Atticus and Mr. Gilmer returned, and Judge Taylor looked at his watch. "It's gettin' on to four," he said, which was intriguing, as the courthouse clock must have struck the hour at least twice. I had not heard it or felt its vibrations.

"Shall we try to wind up this afternoon?" asked Judge Taylor. "How 'bout it, Atticus?"

"I think we can," said Atticus.

"How many witnesses you got?"

"One."

"Well, call him."

19

Thomas Robinson reached around, ran his fingers under his left arm and lifted it. He guided his arm to the Bible and his rubber-like left hand sought contact with the black binding. As he raised his right hand, the useless one slipped off the Bible and hit the clerk's table. He was trying again when Judge Taylor growled, "That'll do, Tom." Tom took the oath and stepped into the witness chair. Atticus very quickly induced him to tell us:

Tom was twenty-five years of age; he was married with three children; he had been in trouble with the law before: he once received thirty days for disorderly conduct.

"It must have been disorderly," said Atticus. "What did it consist of?"

"Got in a fight with another man, he tried to cut me."

"Did he succeed?"

"Yes suh, a little, not enough to hurt. You see, I—" Tom moved his left shoulder.

"Yes," said Atticus. "You were both convicted?"

"Yes suh, I had to serve 'cause I couldn't pay the fine. Other fellow paid his'n."

Dill leaned across me and asked Jem what Atticus was doing. Jem said Atticus was showing the jury that Tom had nothing to hide.

"Were you acquainted with Mayella Violet Ewell?" asked Atticus.

"Yes suh, I had to pass her place goin' to and from the field every day."

"Whose field?"

"I picks for Mr. Link Deas."

"Were you picking cotton in November?"

"No suh, I works in his yard fall an' wintertime. I works pretty steady for him all year round, he's got a lot of pecan trees'n things."

"You say you had to pass the Ewell place to get to and from work. Is there any other way to go?"

"No suh, none's I know of."

"Tom, did she ever speak to you?"

"Why, yes suh, I'd tip m'hat when I'd go by, and one day she asked me to come inside the fence and bust up a chiffarobe for her."

"When did she ask you to chop up the—the chiffarobe?"

"Mr. Finch, it was way last spring. I remember it because it was choppin' time and I had my hoe with me. I said I didn't have nothin' but this hoe, but she said she had a hatchet. She give me the hatchet and I broke up the chiffarobe. She said, 'I reckon I'll hafta give you a nickel, won't I?' an' I said, 'No ma'am, there ain't no charge.' Then I went home. Mr. Finch, that was way last spring, way over a year ago."

"Did you ever go on the place again?"

"Yes suh."

"When?"

"Well, I went lots of times."

Judge Taylor instinctively reached for his gavel, but let his hand fall. The murmur below us died without his help.

"Under what circumstances?"

"Please, suh?"

"Why did you go inside the fence lots of times?"

Tom Robinson's forehead relaxed. "She'd call me in, suh. Seemed like every time I passed by yonder she'd have some little somethin' for me to do—choppin' kindlin', totin' water for her. She watered them red flowers every day—"

"Were you paid for your services?"

"No suh, not after she offered me a nickel the first time. I was glad to do it, Mr. Ewell didn't seem to help her none, and neither did the chillun, and I knowed she didn't have no nickels to spare."

"Where were the other children?"

"They was always around, all over the place. They'd watch me work, some of 'em, some of 'em'd set in the window."

"Would Miss Mayella talk to you?"

"Yes sir, she talked to me."

As Tom Robinson gave his testimony, it came to me that Mayella Ewell must have been the loneliest person in the world. She was even lonelier than Boo Radley, who had not been out of the house in twenty-five years. When Atticus asked had she any friends, she seemed not to know what he meant, then she thought he was making fun of her. She was as sad, I thought, as what Jem called a mixed child: white people wouldn't have anything to do with her because she lived among pigs; Negroes wouldn't have anything to do with her because she was white. She couldn't live like Mr. Dolphus Raymond, who preferred the company of Negroes, because she didn't own a riverbank and she wasn't from a fine old family. Nobody said, "That's just their way," about the Ewells. Maycomb gave them Christmas baskets, welfare money, and the back of its hand. Tom Robinson was probably the only person who was ever decent to her. But she said he took advantage of her, and when she stood up she looked at him as if he were dirt beneath her feet.

"Did you ever," Atticus interrupted my meditations, "at any time, go on the Ewell property—did you ever set foot on the Ewell property without an express invitation from one of them?"

"No suh, Mr. Finch, I never did. I wouldn't do that, suh."

Atticus sometimes said that one way to tell whether a witness was lying or telling the truth was to listen rather than watch: I applied his test—Tom denied it three times in one breath, but quietly, with no hint of whining in his voice, and I found myself believing him in spite of his protesting too much. He seemed to be a respectable Negro, and a respectable Negro would never go up into somebody's yard of his own volition.

"Tom, what happened to you on the evening of November twenty-first of last year?"

Below us, the spectators drew a collective breath and leaned forward. Behind us, the Negroes did the same.

Tom was a black-velvet Negro, not shiny, but soft black velvet. The whites of his eyes shone in his face, and when he spoke we saw flashes of his teeth. If he had been whole, he would have been a fine specimen of a man.

"Mr. Finch," he said, "I was goin' home as usual that evenin', an' when I passed the Ewell place Miss Mayella were on the porch, like she said she were. It seemed real quiet like, an' I didn't quite know why. I was studyin' why, just passin' by, when she says for me to come there and help her a minute. Well, I went inside the fence an' looked around for some kindlin' to work on, but I didn't see none, and she says, 'Naw, I got somethin' for you to do in the house. Th' old door's off its hinges an' fall's comin' on pretty fast.' I said you got a screwdriver, Miss Mayella? She said she sho' had. Well, I went up the steps an' she motioned me to come inside, and I went in the front room an' looked at the door. I said Miss Mayella, this door look all right. I pulled it back'n forth and those hinges was all right. Then she shet the door in my face. Mr. Finch, I was wonderin' why it was so quiet like, an' it come to me that there weren't a chile on the place, not a one of 'em, and I said Miss Mayella, where the chillun?''

Tom's black velvet skin had begun to shine, and he ran his hand over his face.

"I say where the chillun?'' he continued, ''an' she says —she was laughin', sort of—she says they all gone to town to get ice creams. She says, 'took me a slap year to save seb'm nickels, but I done it. They all gone to town.' ''

Tom's discomfort was not from the humidity. ''What did you say then, Tom?'' asked Atticus.

"I said somethin' like, why Miss Mayella, that's right smart o'you to treat 'em. An' she said, 'You think so?' I don't think she understood what I was thinkin'—I meant it was smart of her to save like that, an' nice of her to treat 'em.''

"I understand you, Tom. Go on,'' said Atticus.

"Well, I said I best be goin', I couldn't do nothin' for her, an' she says oh yes I could, an' I ask her what, and she says to just step on that chair yonder an' git that box down from on top of the chiffarobe.''

"Not the same chiffarobe you busted up?'' asked Atticus.

The witness smiled. ''Naw suh, another one. Most as tall as the room. So I done what she told me, an' I was just reachin' when the next thing I knows she—she'd grabbed me round the legs, grabbed me round th' legs, Mr. Finch. She scared me so bad I hopped down an' turned the chair over—that was the only thing, only furniture, 'sturbed in that room, Mr. Finch, when I left it. I swear 'fore God.''

"What happened after you turned the chair over?''

Tom Robinson had come to a dead stop. He glanced at

Atticus, then at the jury, then at Mr. Underwood sitting across the room.

"Tom, you're sworn to tell the whole truth. Will you tell it?"

Tom ran his hand nervously over his mouth.

"What happened after that?"

"Answer the question," said Judge Taylor. One-third of his cigar had vanished.

"Mr. Finch, I got down offa that chair an' turned around an' she sorta jumped on me."

"Jumped on you? Violently?"

"No suh, she—she hugged me. She hugged me round the waist."

This time Judge Taylor's gavel came down with a bang, and as it did the overhead lights went on in the courtroom. Darkness had not come, but the afternoon sun had left the windows. Judge Taylor quickly restored order.

"Then what did she do?"

The witness swallowed hard. "She reached up an' kissed me 'side of th' face. She says she never kissed a grown man before an' she might as well kiss a nigger. She says what her papa do to her don't count. She says, 'Kiss me back, nigger.' I say Miss Mayella lemme outa here an' tried to run but she got her back to the door an' I'da had to push her. I didn't wanta harm her, Mr. Finch, an' I say lemme pass, but just when I say it Mr. Ewell yonder hollered through th' window."

"What did he say?"

Tom Robinson swallowed again, and his eyes widened. "Somethin' not fittin' to say—not fittin' for these folks'n chillun to hear—"

"What did he say, Tom? You *must* tell the jury what he said."

Tom Robinson shut his eyes tight. "He says you goddamn whore, I'll kill ya."

"Then what happened?"

"Mr. Finch, I was runnin' so fast I didn't know what happened."

"Tom, did you rape Mayella Ewell?"

"I did not, suh."

"Did you harm her in any way?"

"I did not, suh."

"Did you resist her advances?"

"Mr. Finch, I tried. I tried to 'thout bein' ugly to her. I didn't wanta be ugly, I didn't wanta push her or nothin'."

It occurred to me that in their own way, Tom Robinson's manners were as good as Atticus's. Until my father explained it to me later, I did not understand the subtlety of Tom's predicament: he would not have dared strike a white woman under any circumstances and expect to live long, so he took the first opportunity to run—a sure sign of guilt.

"Tom, go back once more to Mr. Ewell," said Atticus. "Did he say anything to you?"

"Not anything, suh. He mighta said somethin', but I weren't there—"

"That'll do," Atticus cut in sharply. "What you did hear, who was he talking to?"

"Mr. Finch, he were talkin' and lookin' at Miss Mayella."

"Then you ran?"

"I sho' did, suh."

"Why did you run?"

"I was scared, suh."

"Why were you scared?"

"Mr. Finch, if you was a nigger like me, you'd be scared, too."

Atticus sat down. Mr. Gilmer was making his way to the witness stand, but before he got there Mr. Link Deas rose from the audience and announced:

"I just want the whole lot of you to know one thing right now. That boy's worked for me eight years an' I ain't had a speck o'trouble outa him. Not a speck."

"*Shut your mouth, sir!*" Judge Taylor was wide awake and roaring. He was also pink in the face. His speech was miraculously unimpaired by his cigar. "Link Deas," he yelled, "if you have anything you want to say you can say it under oath and at the proper time, but until then you get out of this room, you hear me? Get out of this room, sir, you hear me? I'll be damned if I'll listen to this case again!"

Judge Taylor looked daggers at Atticus, as if daring him to speak, but Atticus had ducked his head and was laughing into his lap. I remembered something he had said about Judge Taylor's ex cathedra remarks sometimes exceeding his duty, but that few lawyers ever did anything about them. I looked at Jem, but Jem shook his head. "It ain't like one of the jurymen got up and started talking," he said. "I think it'd be different then. Mr. Link was just disturbin' the peace or something."

Judge Taylor told the reporter to expunge anything he happened to have written down after Mr. Finch if you were a nigger like me you'd be scared too, and told the jury to disregard the interruption. He looked suspiciously down the middle aisle and waited, I suppose, for Mr. Link Deas to effect total departure. Then he said, "Go ahead, Mr. Gilmer."

"You were given thirty days once for disorderly conduct, Robinson?" asked Mr. Gilmer.

"Yes suh."

"What'd the nigger look like when you got through with him?"

"He beat me, Mr. Gilmer."

"Yes, but you were convicted, weren't you?"

Atticus raised his head. "It was a misdemeanor and it's in the record, Judge." I thought he sounded tired.

"Witness'll answer, though," said Judge Taylor, just as wearily.

"Yes suh, I got thirty days."

I knew that Mr. Gilmer would sincerely tell the jury that anyone who was convicted of disorderly conduct could easily have had it in his heart to take advantage of Mayella Ewell, that was the only reason he cared. Reasons like that helped.

"Robinson, you're pretty good at busting up chiffarobes and kindling with one hand, aren't you?"

"Yes, suh, I reckon so."

"Strong enough to choke the breath out of a woman and sling her to the floor?"

"I never done that, suh."

"But you are strong enough to?"

"I reckon so, suh."

"Had your eye on her a long time, hadn't you, boy?"

"No suh, I never looked at her."

"Then you were mighty polite to do all that chopping and hauling for her, weren't you, boy?"

"I was just tryin' to help her out, suh."

"That was mighty generous of you, you had chores at home after your regular work, didn't you?"

"Yes suh."

"Why didn't you do them instead of Miss Ewell's?"

"I done 'em both, suh."

"You must have been pretty busy. Why?"

"Why what, suh?"

"Why were you so anxious to do that woman's chores?" Tom Robinson hesitated, searching for an answer. "Looked like she didn't have nobody to help her, like I says—"

"With Mr. Ewell and seven children on the place, boy?"

"Well, I says it looked like they never help her none—"

"You did all this chopping and work from sheer goodness, boy?"

"Tried to help her, I says."

Mr. Gilmer smiled grimly at the jury. "You're a mighty good fellow, it seems—did all this for not one penny?"

"Yes, suh. I felt right sorry for her, she seemed to try more'n the rest of 'em—"

"*You* felt sorry for *her*, you felt *sorry* for her?" Mr. Gilmer seemed ready to rise to the ceiling.

The witness realized his mistake and shifted uncomfortably in the chair. But the damage was done. Below us, nobody liked Tom Robinson's answer. Mr. Gilmer paused a long time to let it sink in.

"Now you went by the house as usual, last November twenty-first," he said, "and she asked you to come in and bust up a chiffarobe?"

"No suh."

"Do you deny that you went by the house?"

"No suh—she said she had somethin' for me to do inside the house—"

"She says she asked you to bust up a chiffarobe, is that right?"

"No suh, it ain't."

"Then you say she's lying, boy?"

Atticus was on his feet, but Tom Robinson didn't need him. "I don't say she's lyin', Mr. Gilmer, I say she's mistaken in her mind."

To the next ten questions, as Mr. Gilmer reviewed Mayella's version of events, the witness's steady answer was that she was mistaken in her mind.

"Didn't Mr. Ewell run you off the place, boy?"

"No suh, I don't think he did."

"Don't think, what do you mean?"

"I mean I didn't stay long enough for him to run me off."

"You're very candid about this, why did you run so fast?"

"I says I was scared, suh."

"If you had a clear conscience, why were you scared?"

"Like I says before, it weren't safe for any nigger to be in a—fix like that."

"But you weren't in a fix—you testified that you were resisting Miss Ewell. Were you so scared that she'd hurt you, you ran, a big buck like you?"

"No suh, I's scared I'd be in court, just like I am now."

"Scared of arrest, scared you'd have to face up to what you did?"

"No suh, scared I'd hafta face up to what I didn't do."

"Are you being impudent to me, boy?"

"No suh, I didn't go to be."

This was as much as I heard of Mr. Gilmer's cross-examination, because Jem made me take Dill out. For some reason Dill had started crying and couldn't stop; quietly at first, then his sobs were heard by several people in the balcony. Jem said if I didn't go with him he'd make me, and Reverend Sykes said I'd better go, so I went. Dill had seemed to be all right that day, nothing wrong with him, but I guessed he hadn't fully recovered from running away.

"Ain't you feeling good?" I asked, when we reached the bottom of the stairs.

Dill tried to pull himself together as we ran down the south steps. Mr. Link Deas was a lonely figure on the top step. "Anything happenin', Scout?" he asked as we went by. "No sir," I answered over my shoulder. "Dill here, he's sick."

"Come on out under the trees," I said. "Heat got you, I expect." We chose the fattest live oak and we sat under it.

"It was just him I couldn't stand," Dill said.

"Who, Tom?"

"That old Mr. Gilmer doin' him thataway, talking so hateful to him—"

"Dill, that's his job. Why, if we didn't have prosecutors —well, we couldn't have defense attorneys, I reckon."

Dill exhaled patiently. "I know all that, Scout. It was the way he said it made me sick, plain sick."

"He's supposed to act that way, Dill, he was cross—"

"He didn't act that way when—"

"Dill, those were his own witnesses."

"Well, Mr. Finch didn't act that way to Mayella and old man Ewell when he cross-examined them. The way that man called him 'boy' all the time an' sneered at him, an' looked around at the jury every time he answered—"

"Well, Dill, after all he's just a Negro."

"I don't care one speck. It ain't right, somehow it ain't right to do 'em that way. Hasn't anybody got any business talkin' like that—it just makes me sick."

"That's just Mr. Gilmer's way, Dill, he does 'em all that way. You've never seen him get good'n down on one yet. Why, when—well, today Mr. Gilmer seemed to me like he wasn't half trying. They do 'em all that way, most lawyers, I mean."

"Mr. Finch doesn't."

"He's not an example, Dill, he's—" I was trying to grope in my memory for a sharp phrase of Miss Maudie Atkinson's. I had it: "He's the same in the courtroom as he is on the public streets."

"That's not what I mean," said Dill.

"I know what you mean, boy," said a voice behind us. We thought it came from the tree-trunk, but it belonged to Mr. Dolphus Raymond. He peered around the trunk at us. "You aren't thin-hided, it just makes you sick, doesn't it?"

20

"Come on round here, son, I got something that'll settle your stomach."

As Mr. Dolphus Raymond was an evil man I accepted his invitation reluctantly, but I followed Dill. Somehow, I didn't think Atticus would like it if we became friendly with Mr. Raymond, and I knew Aunt Alexandra wouldn't.

"Here," he said, offering Dill his paper sack with straws in it. "Take a good sip, it'll quieten you."

Dill sucked on the straws, smiled, and pulled at length.

"Hee hee," said Mr. Raymond, evidently taking delight in corrupting a child.

"Dill, you watch out, now," I warned.

Dill released the straws and grinned. "Scout, it's nothing but Coca-Cola."

Mr. Raymond sat up against the tree-trunk. He had been lying on the grass. "You little folks won't tell on me now, will you? It'd ruin my reputation if you did."

"You mean all you drink in that sack's Coca-Cola? Just plain Coca-Cola?"

"Yes ma'am," Mr. Raymond nodded. I liked his smell: it was of leather, horses, cottonseed. He wore the only English riding boots I had ever seen. "That's all I drink, most of the time."

"Then you just pretend you're half—? I beg your pardon, sir," I caught myself. "I didn't mean to be—"

Mr. Raymond chuckled, not at all offended, and I tried to frame a discreet question: "Why do you do like you do?"

"Wh—oh yes, you mean why do I pretend? Well, it's very simple," he said. "Some folks don't—like the way I live. Now I could say the hell with 'em, I don't care if they don't like it. I do say I don't care if they don't like it, right enough—but I don't say the hell with 'em, see?"

Dill and I said, "No sir."

"I try to give 'em a reason, you see. It helps folks if they can latch onto a reason. When I come to town, which is seldom, if I weave a little and drink out of this sack, folks can say Dolphus Raymond's in the clutches of whiskey—that's why he won't change his ways. He can't help himself, that's why he lives the way he does."

"That ain't honest, Mr. Raymond, making yourself out badder'n you are already—"

"It ain't honest but it's mighty helpful to folks. Secretly, Miss Finch, I'm not much of a drinker, but you see they could never, never understand that I live like I do because that's the way I want to live.''

I had a feeling that I shouldn't be here listening to this sinful man who had mixed children and didn't care who knew it, but he was fascinating. I had never encountered a being who deliberately perpetrated fraud against himself. But why had he entrusted us with his deepest secret? I asked him why.

''Because you're children and you can understand it,'' he said, ''and because I heard that one—''

He jerked his head at Dill: ''Things haven't caught up with that one's instinct yet. Let him get a little older and he won't get sick and cry. Maybe things'll strike him as being—not quite right, say, but he won't cry, not when he gets a few years on him.''

''Cry about what, Mr. Raymond?'' Dill's maleness was beginning to assert itself.

''Cry about the simple hell people give other people— without even thinking. Cry about the hell white people give colored folks, without even stopping to think that they're people, too.''

''Atticus says cheatin' a colored man is ten times worse than cheatin' a white man,'' I muttered. ''Says it's the worst thing you can do.''

Mr. Raymond said, ''I don't reckon it's—Miss Jean Louise, you don't know your pa's not a run-of-the-mill man, it'll take a few years for that to sink in—you haven't seen enough of the world yet. You haven't even seen this town, but all you gotta do is step back inside the courthouse.''

Which reminded me that we were missing nearly all of Mr. Gilmer's cross-examination. I looked at the sun, and it was dropping fast behind the store-tops on the west side of the square. Between two fires, I could not decide which I wanted to jump into: Mr. Raymond or the 5th Judicial Circuit Court. ''C'mon, Dill,'' I said. ''You all right, now?''

''Yeah. Glad t've metcha, Mr. Raymond, and thanks for the drink, it was mighty settlin'.''

We raced back to the courthouse, up the steps, up two flights of stairs, and edged our way along the balcony rail. Reverend Sykes had saved our seats.

The courtroom was still, and again I wondered where the babies were. Judge Taylor's cigar was a brown speck in the center of his mouth; Mr. Gilmer was writing on one of the yellow pads on his table, trying to outdo the court reporter, whose hand was jerking rapidly. "Shoot," I muttered, "we missed it."

Atticus was halfway through his speech to the jury. He had evidently pulled some papers from his briefcase that rested beside his chair, because they were on his table. Tom Robinson was toying with them.

". . . absence of any corroborative evidence, this man was indicted on a capital charge and is now on trial for his life. . . ."

I punched Jem. "How long's he been at it?"

"He's just gone over the evidence," Jem whispered, "and we're gonna win, Scout. I don't see how we can't. He's been at it 'bout five minutes. He made it as plain and easy as— well, as I'da explained it to you. You could've understood it, even."

"Did Mr. Gilmer—?"

"Sh-h. Nothing new, just the usual. Hush now."

We looked down again. Atticus was speaking easily, with the kind of detachment he used when he dictated a letter. He walked slowly up and down in front of the jury, and the jury seemed to be attentive: their heads were up, and they followed Atticus's route with what seemed to be appreciation. I guess it was because Atticus wasn't a thunderer.

Atticus paused, then he did something he didn't ordinarily do. He unhitched his watch and chain and placed them on the table, saying, "With the court's permission—"

Judge Taylor nodded, and then Atticus did something I never saw him do before or since, in public or in private: he unbuttoned his vest, unbuttoned his collar, loosened his tie, and took off his coat. He never loosened a scrap of his clothing until he undressed at bedtime, and to Jem and me, this was the equivalent of him standing before us stark naked. We exchanged horrified glances.

Atticus put his hands in his pockets, and as he returned to the jury, I saw his gold collar button and the tips of his pen and pencil winking in the light.

"Gentlemen," he said. Jem and I again looked at each other: Atticus might have said, "Scout." His voice had lost its aridity, its detachment, and he was talking to the jury as if they were folks on the post office corner.

"Gentlemen," he was saying, "I shall be brief, but I would like to use my remaining time with you to remind you that this case is not a difficult one, it requires no minute sifting of complicated facts, but it does require you to be sure beyond all reasonable doubt as to the guilt of the defendant. To begin with, this case should never have come to trial. This case is as simple as black and white.

"The state has not produced one iota of medical evidence to the effect that the crime Tom Robinson is charged with ever took place. It has relied instead upon the testimony of two witnesses whose evidence has not only been called into serious question on cross-examination, but has been flatly contradicted by the defendant. The defendant is not guilty, but somebody in this courtroom is.

"I have nothing but pity in my heart for the chief witness for the state, but my pity does not extend so far as to her putting a man's life at stake, which she has done in an effort to get rid of her own guilt.

"I say guilt, gentlemen, because it was guilt that motivated her. She has committed no crime, she has merely broken a rigid and time-honored code of our society, a code so severe that whoever breaks it is hounded from our midst as unfit to live with. She is the victim of cruel poverty and ignorance, but I cannot pity her: she is white. She knew full well the enormity of her offense, but because her desires were stronger than the code she was breaking, she persisted in breaking it. She persisted, and her subsequent reaction is something that all of us have known at one time or another. She did something every child has done—she tried to put the evidence of her offense away from her. But in this case she was no child hiding stolen contraband: she struck out at her victim—of necessity she must put him away from her—he must be removed from her presence, from this world. She must destroy the evidence of her offense.

"What was the evidence of her offense? Tom Robinson, a human being. She must put Tom Robinson away from her. Tom Robinson was her daily reminder of what she did. What did she do? She tempted a Negro.

"She was white, and she tempted a Negro. She did something that in our society is unspeakable: she kissed a black man. Not an old Uncle, but a strong young Negro man. No code mattered to her before she broke it, but it came crashing down on her afterwards.

"Her father saw it, and the defendant has testified as to his remarks. What did her father do? We don't know, but there is circumstantial evidence to indicate that Mayella Ewell was beaten savagely by someone who led almost exclusively with his left. We do know in part what Mr. Ewell did: he did what any God-fearing, persevering, respectable white man would do under the circumstances—he swore out a warrant, no doubt signing it with his left hand, and Tom Robinson now sits before you, having taken the oath with the only good hand he possesses—his right hand.

"And so a quiet, respectable, humble Negro who had the unmitigated temerity to 'feel sorry' for a white woman has had to put his word against two white people's. I need not remind you of their appearance and conduct on the stand—you saw them for yourselves. The witnesses for the state, with the exception of the sheriff of Maycomb County, have presented themselves to you gentlemen, to this court, in the cynical confidence that their testimony would not be doubted, confident that you gentlemen would go along with them on the assumption—the evil assumption—that *all* Negroes lie, that *all* Negroes are basically immoral beings, that *all* Negro men are not to be trusted around our women, an assumption one associates with minds of their caliber.

"Which, gentlemen, we know is in itself a lie as black as Tom Robinson's skin, a lie I do not have to point out to you. You know the truth, and the truth is this: some Negroes lie, some Negroes are immoral, some Negro men are not to be trusted around women—black or white. But this is a truth that applies to the human race and to no particular race of men. There is not a person in this courtroom who has never told a lie, who has never done an immoral thing, and there is no man living who has never looked upon a woman without desire."

Atticus paused and took out his handkerchief. Then he took off his glasses and wiped them, and we saw another "first":

we had never seen him sweat—he was one of those men whose faces never perspired, but now it was shining tan.

"One more thing, gentlemen, before I quit. Thomas Jefferson once said that all men are created equal, a phrase that the Yankees and the distaff side of the Executive branch in Washington are fond of hurling at us. There is a tendency in this year of grace, 1935, for certain people to use this phrase out of context, to satisfy all conditions. The most ridiculous example I can think of is that the people who run public education promote the stupid and idle along with the industrious—because all men are created equal, educators will gravely tell you, the children left behind suffer terrible feelings of inferiority. We know all men are not created equal in the sense some people would have us believe—some people are smarter than others, some people have more opportunity because they're born with it, some men make more money than others, some ladies make better cakes than others—some people are born gifted beyond the normal scope of most men.

"But there is one way in this country in which all men are created equal—there is one human institution that makes a pauper the equal of a Rockefeller, the stupid man the equal of an Einstein, and the ignorant man the equal of any college president. That institution, gentlemen, is a court. It can be the Supreme Court of the United States or the humblest J.P. court in the land, or this honorable court which you serve. Our courts have their faults, as does any human institution, but in this country our courts are the great levelers, and in our courts all men are created equal.

"I'm no idealist to believe firmly in the integrity of our courts and in the jury system—that is no ideal to me, it is a living, working reality. Gentlemen, a court is no better than each man of you sitting before me on this jury. A court is only as sound as its jury, and a jury is only as sound as the men who make it up. I am confident that you gentlemen will review without passion the evidence you have heard, come to a decision, and restore this defendant to his family. In the name of God, do your duty."

Atticus's voice had dropped, and as he turned away from the jury he said something I did not catch. He said it more to himself than to the court. I punched Jem. "What'd he say?"

" 'In the name of God, believe him,' I think that's what he said."

Dill suddenly reached over me and tugged at Jem. "Looka yonder!"

We followed his finger with sinking hearts. Calpurnia was making her way up the middle aisle, walking straight toward Atticus.

21

She stopped shyly at the railing and waited to get Judge Taylor's attention. She was in a fresh apron and she carried an envelope in her hand.

Judge Taylor saw her and said, "It's Calpurnia, isn't it?"

"Yes sir," she said. "Could I just pass this note to Mr. Finch, please sir? It hasn't got anything to do with—with the trial."

Judge Taylor nodded and Atticus took the envelope from Calpurnia. He opened it, read its contents and said, "Judge, I—this note is from my sister. She says my children are missing, haven't turned up since noon . . . I . . . could you—"

"I know where they are, Atticus." Mr. Underwood spoke up. "They're right up yonder in the colored balcony—been there since precisely one-eighteen P.M."

Our father turned around and looked up. "Jem, come down from there," he called. Then he said something to the Judge we didn't hear. We climbed across Reverend Sykes and made our way to the staircase.

Atticus and Calpurnia met us downstairs. Calpurnia looked peeved, but Atticus looked exhausted.

Jem was jumping in excitement. "We've won, haven't we?"

"I've no idea," said Atticus shortly. "You've been here

all afternoon? Go home with Calpurnia and get your supper—and stay home.''

"Aw, Atticus, let us come back," pleaded Jem. "Please let us hear the verdict, *please* sir."

"The jury might be out and back in a minute, we don't know—" but we could tell Atticus was relenting. "Well, you've heard it all, so you might as well hear the rest. Tell you what, you all can come back when you've eaten your supper—eat slowly, now, you won't miss anything important—and if the jury's still out, you can wait with us. But I expect it'll be over before you get back."

"You think they'll acquit him that fast?" asked Jem.

Atticus opened his mouth to answer, but shut it and left us.

I prayed that Reverend Sykes would save our seats for us, but stopped praying when I remembered that people got up and left in droves when the jury was out—tonight, they'd overrun the drugstore, the O.K. Café and the hotel, that is, unless they had brought their suppers too.

Calpurnia marched us home: "—skin every one of you alive, the very idea, you children listenin' to all that! Mister Jem, don't you know better'n to take your little sister to that trial? Miss Alexandra'll absolutely have a stroke of paralysis when she finds out! Ain't fittin' for children to hear. . . ."

The streetlights were on, and we glimpsed Calpurnia's indignant profile as we passed beneath them. "Mister Jem, I thought you was gettin' some kinda head on your shoulders—the very idea, she's your little sister! The very *idea*, sir! You oughta be perfectly ashamed of yourself—ain't you got any sense at all?"

I was exhilarated. So many things had happened so fast I felt it would take years to sort them out, and now here was Calpurnia giving her precious Jem down the country—what new marvels would the evening bring?

Jem was chuckling. "Don't you want to hear about it, Cal?"

"Hush your mouth, sir! When you oughta be hangin' your head in shame you go along laughin'—" Calpurnia revived a series of rusty threats that moved Jem to little remorse, and she sailed up the front steps with her classic, "If Mr. Finch don't wear you out, I will—get in that house, sir!"

Jem went in grinning, and Calpurnia nodded tacit consent to having Dill in to supper. "You all call Miss Rachel right now and tell her where you are," she told him. "She's run distracted lookin' for you—you watch out she don't ship you back to Meridian first thing in the mornin'."

Aunt Alexandra met us and nearly fainted when Calpurnia told her where we were. I guess it hurt her when we told her Atticus said we could go back, because she didn't say a word during supper. She just rearranged food on her plate, looking at it sadly while Calpurnia served Jem, Dill and me with a vengeance. Calpurnia poured milk, dished out potato salad and ham, muttering, " 'shamed of yourselves," in varying degrees of intensity. "Now you all eat slow," was her final command.

Reverend Sykes had saved our places. We were surprised to find that we had been gone nearly an hour, and were equally surprised to find the courtroom exactly as we had left it, with minor changes: the jury box was empty, the defendant was gone; Judge Taylor had been gone, but he reappeared as we were seating ourselves.

"Nobody's moved, hardly," said Jem.

"They moved around some when the jury went out," said Reverend Sykes. "The menfolk down there got the womenfolk their suppers, and they fed their babies."

"How long have they been out?" asked Jem.

" 'bout thirty minutes. Mr. Finch and Mr. Gilmer did some more talkin', and Judge Taylor charged the jury."

"How was he?" asked Jem.

"What say? Oh, he did right well. I ain't complainin' one bit—he was mighty fair-minded. He sorta said if you believe this, then you'll have to return one verdict, but if you believe this, you'll have to return another one. I thought he was leanin' a little to our side—" Reverend Sykes scratched his head.

Jem smiled. "He's not supposed to lean, Reverend, but don't fret, we've won it," he said wisely. "Don't see how any jury could convict on what we heard—"

"Now don't you be so confident, Mr. Jem, I ain't ever seen any jury decide in favor of a colored man over a white man. . . ." But Jem took exception to Reverend Sykes, and we were subjected to a lengthy review of the evidence with

Jem's ideas on the law regarding rape: it wasn't rape if she let you, but she had to be eighteen—in Alabama, that is—and Mayella was nineteen. Apparently you had to kick and holler, you had to be overpowered and stomped on, preferably knocked stone cold. If you were under eighteen, you didn't have to go through all this.

"Mr. Jem," Reverend Sykes demurred, "this ain't a polite thing for little ladies to hear . . ."

"Aw, she doesn't know what we're talkin' about," said Jem. "Scout, this is too old for you, ain't it?"

"It most certainly is not, I know every word you're saying." Perhaps I was too convincing, because Jem hushed and never discussed the subject again.

"What time is it, Reverend?" he asked.

"Gettin' on toward eight."

I looked down and saw Atticus strolling around with his hands in his pockets: he made a tour of the windows, then walked by the railing over to the jury box. He looked in it, inspected Judge Taylor on his throne, then went back to where he started. I caught his eye and waved to him. He acknowledged my salute with a nod, and resumed his tour.

Mr. Gilmer was standing at the windows talking to Mr. Underwood. Bert, the court reporter, was chain-smoking: he sat back with his feet on the table.

But the officers of the court, the ones present—Atticus, Mr. Gilmer, Judge Taylor sound asleep, and Bert, were the only ones whose behavior seemed normal. I had never seen a packed courtroom so still. Sometimes a baby would cry out fretfully, and a child would scurry out, but the grown people sat as if they were in church. In the balcony, the Negroes sat and stood around us with biblical patience.

The old courthouse clock suffered its preliminary strain and struck the hour, eight deafening bongs that shook our bones.

When it bonged eleven times I was past feeling: tired from fighting sleep, I allowed myself a short nap against Reverend Sykes's comfortable arm and shoulder. I jerked awake and made an honest effort to remain so, by looking down and concentrating on the heads below: there were sixteen bald ones, fourteen men that could pass for redheads, forty heads varying between brown and black, and—I remembered something Jem had once explained to me when he went through a brief period of psychical research: he said if enough people—a stadium full, maybe—were to concentrate on one thing, such as setting a tree afire in the woods, that the tree would ignite of its own accord. I toyed with the idea of asking everyone below to concentrate on setting Tom Robinson free, but thought if they were as tired as I, it wouldn't work.

Dill was sound asleep, his head on Jem's shoulder, and Jem was quiet.

"Ain't it a long time?" I asked him.

"Sure is, Scout," he said happily.

"Well, from the way you put it, it'd just take five minutes."

Jem raised his eyebrows. "There are things you don't understand," he said, and I was too weary to argue.

But I must have been reasonably awake, or I would not have received the impression that was creeping into me. It was not unlike one I had last winter, and I shivered, though the night was hot. The feeling grew until the atmosphere in the courtroom was exactly the same as a cold February morning, when the mockingbirds were still, and the carpenters had stopped hammering on Miss Maudie's new house, and every wood door in the neighborhood was shut as tight as the doors of the Radley Place. A deserted, waiting, empty street, and the courtroom was packed with people. A steaming summer night was no different from a winter morning. Mr. Heck Tate, who had entered the courtroom and was talking to Atticus, might have been wearing his high boots and lumber jacket. Atticus had stopped his tranquil journey and had put his foot onto the bottom rung of a chair; as he listened to what Mr. Tate was saying, he ran his hand slowly up and down his thigh. I expected Mr. Tate to say any minute, "Take him, Mr. Finch. . . ."

But Mr. Tate said, "This court will come to order," in a voice that rang with authority, and the heads below us jerked up. Mr. Tate left the room and returned with Tom Robinson. He steered Tom to his place beside Atticus, and stood there. Judge Taylor had roused himself to sudden alertness and was sitting up straight, looking at the empty jury box.

What happened after that had a dreamlike quality: in a dream I saw the jury return, moving like underwater swimmers, and Judge Taylor's voice came from far away and was tiny. I saw something only a lawyer's child could be expected to see, could be expected to watch for, and it was like watching Atticus walk into the street, raise a rifle to his shoulder and pull the trigger, but watching all the time knowing that the gun was empty.

A jury never looks at a defendant it has convicted, and when this jury came in, not one of them looked at Tom Robinson. The foreman handed a piece of paper to Mr. Tate who handed it to the clerk who handed it to the judge. . . .

I shut my eyes. Judge Taylor was polling the jury: "Guilty . . . guilty . . . guilty . . . guilty . . ." I peeked at Jem: his hands were white from gripping the balcony rail, and his shoulders jerked as if each "guilty" was a separate stab between them.

Judge Taylor was saying something. His gavel was in his fist, but he wasn't using it. Dimly, I saw Atticus pushing papers from the table into his briefcase. He snapped it shut, went to the court reporter and said something, nodded to Mr. Gilmer, and then went to Tom Robinson and whispered something to him. Atticus put his hand on Tom's shoulder as he whispered. Atticus took his coat off the back of his chair and pulled it over his shoulder. Then he left the courtroom, but not by his usual exit. He must have wanted to go home the short way, because he walked quickly down the middle aisle toward the south exit. I followed the top of his head as he made his way to the door. He did not look up.

Someone was punching me, but I was reluctant to take my eyes from the people below us, and from the image of Atticus's lonely walk down the aisle.

"Miss Jean Louise?"

I looked around. They were standing. All around us and in the balcony on the opposite wall, the Negroes were getting to their feet. Reverend Sykes's voice was as distant as Judge Taylor's:

"Miss Jean Louise, stand up. Your father's passin'."

22

It was Jem's turn to cry. His face was streaked with angry tears as we made our way through the cheerful crowd. "It ain't right," he muttered, all the way to the corner of the square where we found Atticus waiting. Atticus was standing under the street light looking as though nothing had happened: his vest was buttoned, his collar and tie were neatly in place, his watch-chain glistened, he was his impassive self again.

"It ain't right, Atticus," said Jem.

"No son, it's not right."

We walked home.

Aunt Alexandra was waiting up. She was in her dressing gown, and I could have sworn she had on her corset underneath it. "I'm sorry, brother," she murmured. Having never heard her call Atticus "brother" before, I stole a glance at Jem, but he was not listening. He would look up at Atticus, then down at the floor, and I wondered if he thought Atticus somehow responsible for Tom Robinson's conviction.

"Is he all right?" Aunty asked, indicating Jem.

"He'll be so presently," said Atticus. "It was a little too strong for him." Our father sighed. "I'm going to bed," he said. "If I don't wake up in the morning, don't call me."

"I didn't think it wise in the first place to let them—"

"This is their home, sister," said Atticus. "We've made it this way for them, they might as well learn to cope with it."

"But they don't have to go to the courthouse and wallow in it—"

"It's just as much Maycomb County as missionary teas."

"Atticus—" Aunt Alexandra's eyes were anxious. "You are the last person I thought would turn bitter over this."

"I'm not bitter, just tired. I'm going to bed."

"Atticus—" said Jem bleakly.

He turned in the doorway. "What, son?"

"How could they do it, how could they?"

"I don't know, but they did it. They've done it before and they did it tonight and they'll do it again and when they do it—seems that only children weep. Good night."

But things are always better in the morning. Atticus rose at his usual ungodly hour and was in the livingroom behind the *Mobile Register* when we stumbled in. Jem's morning face posed the question his sleepy lips struggled to ask.

"It's not time to worry yet," Atticus reassured him, as we went to the diningroom. "We're not through yet. There'll be an appeal, you can count on that. Gracious alive, Cal, what's all this?" He was staring at his breakfast plate.

Calpurnia said, "Tom Robinson's daddy sent you along this chicken this morning. I fixed it."

"You tell him I'm proud to get it—bet they don't have chicken for breakfast at the White House. What are these?"

"Rolls," said Calpurnia. "Estelle down at the hotel sent 'em."

Atticus looked up at her, puzzled, and she said, "You better step out here and see what's in the kitchen, Mr. Finch."

We followed him. The kitchen table was loaded with enough food to bury the family: hunks of salt pork, tomatoes, beans, even scuppernongs. Atticus grinned when he found a jar of pickled pigs' knuckles. "Reckon Aunty'll let me eat these in the diningroom?"

Calpurnia said, "This was all 'round the back steps when I got here this morning. They—they 'preciate what you did, Mr. Finch. They—they aren't oversteppin' themselves, are they?"

Atticus's eyes filled with tears. He did not speak for a moment. "Tell them I'm very grateful," he said. "Tell them—tell them they must never do this again. Times are too hard. . . ."

He left the kitchen, went in the diningroom and excused himself to Aunt Alexandra, put on his hat and went to town.

We heard Dill's step in the hall, so Calpurnia left Atticus's uneaten breakfast on the table. Between rabbit-bites Dill told us of Miss Rachel's reaction to last night, which was: if a man like Atticus Finch wants to butt his head against a stone wall it's his head.

"I'da got her told," growled Dill, gnawing a chicken leg,

"but she didn't look much like tellin' this morning. Said she was up half the night wonderin' where I was, said she'da had the sheriff after me but he was at the hearing."

"Dill, you've got to stop goin' off without tellin' her," said Jem. "It just aggravates her."

Dill sighed patiently. "I told her till I was blue in the face where I was goin'—she's just seein' too many snakes in the closet. Bet that woman drinks a pint for breakfast every morning—know she drinks two glasses full. Seen her."

"Don't talk like that, Dill," said Aunt Alexandra. "It's not becoming to a child. It's—cynical."

"I ain't cynical, Miss Alexandra. Tellin' the truth's not cynical, is it?"

"The way you tell it, it is."

Jem's eyes flashed at her, but he said to Dill, "Let's go. You can take that runner with you."

When we went to the front porch, Miss Stephanie Crawford was busy telling it to Miss Maudie Atkinson and Mr. Avery. They looked around at us and went on talking. Jem made a feral noise in his throat. I wished for a weapon.

"I hate grown folks lookin' at you," said Dill. "Makes you feel like you've done something."

Miss Maudie yelled for Jem Finch to come there.

Jem groaned and heaved himself up from the swing. "We'll go with you," Dill said.

Miss Stephanie's nose quivered with curiosity. She wanted to know who all gave us permission to go to court—she didn't see us but it was all over town this morning that we were in the Colored balcony. Did Atticus put us up there as a sort of—? Wasn't it right close up there with all those—? Did Scout understand all the—? Didn't it make us mad to see our daddy beat?

"Hush, Stephanie." Miss Maudie's diction was deadly. "I've not got all the morning to pass on the porch—Jem Finch, I called to find out if you and your colleagues can eat some cake. Got up at five to make it, so you better say yes. Excuse us, Stephanie. Good morning, Mr. Avery."

There was a big cake and two little ones on Miss Maudie's kitchen table. There should have been three little ones. It was not like Miss Maudie to forget Dill, and we must have shown it. But we understood when she cut from the big cake and gave the slice to Jem.

As we ate, we sensed that this was Miss Maudie's way of saying that as far as she was concerned, nothing had changed. She sat quietly in a kitchen chair, watching us.

Suddenly she spoke: "Don't fret, Jem. Things are never as bad as they seem."

Indoors, when Miss Maudie wanted to say something lengthy she spread her fingers on her knees and settled her bridgework. This she did, and we waited.

"I simply want to tell you that there are some men in this world who were born to do our unpleasant jobs for us. Your father's one of them."

"Oh," said Jem. "Well."

"Don't you oh well me, sir," Miss Maudie replied, recognizing Jem's fatalistic noises, "you are not old enough to appreciate what I said."

Jem was staring at his half-eaten cake. "It's like bein' a caterpillar in a cocoon, that's what it is," he said. "Like somethin' asleep wrapped up in a warm place. I always thought Maycomb folks were the best folks in the world, least that's what they seemed like."

"We're the safest folks in the world," said Miss Maudie. "We're so rarely called on to be Christians, but when we are, we've got men like Atticus to go for us."

Jem grinned ruefully. "Wish the rest of the county thought that."

"You'd be surprised how many of us do."

"Who?" Jem's voice rose. "Who in this town did one thing to help Tom Robinson, just who?"

"His colored friends for one thing, and people like us. People like Judge Taylor. People like Mr. Heck Tate. Stop eating and start thinking, Jem. Did it ever strike you that Judge Taylor naming Atticus to defend that boy was no accident? That Judge Taylor might have had his reasons for naming him?"

This was a thought. Court-appointed defenses were usually given to Maxwell Green, Maycomb's latest addition to the bar, who needed the experience. Maxwell Green should have had Tom Robinson's case.

"You think about that," Miss Maudie was saying. "It was no accident. I was sittin' there on the porch last night, waiting. I waited and waited to see you all come down the sidewalk, and as I waited I thought, Atticus Finch won't win, he can't win, but he's the only man in these parts who can keep a jury out so long in a case like that. And I thought to myself, well, we're making a step—it's just a baby-step, but it's a step."

" 't's all right to talk like that—can't any Christian judges an' lawyers make up for heathen juries," Jem muttered. "Soon's I get grown—"

"That's something you'll have to take up with your father," Miss Maudie said.

We went down Miss Maudie's cool new steps into the sunshine and found Mr. Avery and Miss Stephanie Crawford still at it. They had moved down the sidewalk and were standing in front of Miss Stephanie's house. Miss Rachel was walking toward them.

"I think I'll be a clown when I get grown," said Dill.

Jem and I stopped in our tracks.

"Yes sir, a clown," he said. "There ain't one thing in this world I can do about folks except laugh, so I'm gonna join the circus and laugh my head off."

"You got it backwards, Dill," said Jem. "Clowns are sad, it's folks that laugh at them."

"Well I'm gonna be a new kind of clown. I'm gonna stand in the middle of the ring and laugh at the folks. Just looka yonder," he pointed. "Every one of 'em oughta be ridin' broomsticks. Aunt Rachel already does."

Miss Stephanie and Miss Rachel were waving wildly at us, in a way that did not give the lie to Dill's observation.

"Oh gosh," breathed Jem. "I reckon it'd be ugly not to see 'em."

Something was wrong. Mr. Avery was red in the face from a sneezing spell and nearly blew us off the sidewalk when we came up. Miss Stephanie was trembling with excitement, and Miss Rachel caught Dill's shoulder. "You get on in the back yard and stay there," she said. "There's danger a'-comin'."

" 's matter?" I asked.

"Ain't you heard yet? It's all over town—"

At that moment Aunt Alexandra came to the door and called us, but she was too late. It was Miss Stephanie's pleasure to tell us: this morning Mr. Bob Ewell stopped Atticus on the post office corner, spat in his face, and told him he'd get him if it took the rest of his life.

23

"I wish Bob Ewell wouldn't chew tobacco," was all Atticus said about it.

According to Miss Stephanie Crawford, however, Atticus was leaving the post office when Mr. Ewell approached him, cursed him, spat on him, and threatened to kill him. Miss Stephanie (who, by the time she had told it twice was there and had seen it all—passing by from the Jitney Jungle, she was)—Miss Stephanie said Atticus didn't bat an eye, just took out his handkerchief and wiped his face and stood there and let Mr. Ewell call him names wild horses could not bring her to repeat. Mr. Ewell was a veteran of an obscure war; that plus Atticus's peaceful reaction probably prompted him to inquire, "Too proud to fight, you nigger-lovin' bastard?" Miss Stephanie said Atticus said, "No, too old," put his hands in his pockets and strolled on. Miss Stephanie said you had to hand it to Atticus Finch, he could be right dry sometimes.

Jem and I didn't think it entertaining.

"After all, though," I said, "he was the deadest shot in the county one time. He could—"

"You know he wouldn't carry a gun, Scout. He ain't even got one—" said Jem. "You know he didn't even have one down at the jail that night. He told me havin' a gun around's an invitation to somebody to shoot you."

"This is different," I said. "We can ask him to borrow one."

We did, and he said, "Nonsense."

Dill was of the opinion that an appeal to Atticus's better nature might work: after all, we would starve if Mr. Ewell killed him, besides be raised exclusively by Aunt Alexandra, and we all knew the first thing she'd do before Atticus was under the ground good would be to fire Calpurnia. Jem said it might work if I cried and flung a fit, being young and a girl. That didn't work either.

But when he noticed us dragging around the neighborhood, not eating, taking little interest in our normal pursuits, Atticus discovered how deeply frightened we were. He tempted Jem with a new football magazine one night; when he saw Jem flip the pages and toss it aside, he said, "What's bothering you, son?"

Jem came to the point: "Mr. Ewell."

"What has happened?"

"Nothing's happened. We're scared for you, and we think you oughta do something about him."

Atticus smiled wryly. "Do what? Put him under a peace bond?"

"When a man says he's gonna get you, looks like he means it."

"He meant it when he said it," said Atticus. "Jem, see if you can stand in Bob Ewell's shoes a minute. I destroyed his last shred of credibility at that trial, if he had any to begin with. The man had to have some kind of comeback, his kind always does. So if spitting in my face and threatening me saved Mayella Ewell one extra beating, that's something I'll gladly take. He had to take it out on somebody and I'd rather it be me than that houseful of children out there. You understand?"

Jem nodded.

Aunt Alexandra entered the room as Atticus was saying, "We don't have anything to fear from Bob Ewell, he got it all out of his system that morning."

"I wouldn't be so sure of that, Atticus," she said. "His kind'd do anything to pay off a grudge. You know how those people are."

"What on earth could Ewell do to me, sister?"

"Something furtive," Aunt Alexandra said. "You may count on that."

"Nobody has much chance to be furtive in Maycomb," Atticus answered.

After that, we were not afraid. Summer was melting away,

and we made the most of it. Atticus assured us that nothing would happen to Tom Robinson until the higher court reviewed his case, and that Tom had a good chance of going free, or at least of having a new trial. He was at Enfield Prison Farm, seventy miles away in Chester County. I asked Atticus if Tom's wife and children were allowed to visit him, but Atticus said no.

"If he loses his appeal," I asked one evening, "what'll happen to him?"

"He'll go to the chair," said Atticus, "unless the Governor commutes his sentence. Not time to worry yet, Scout. We've got a good chance."

Jem was sprawled on the sofa reading *Popular Mechanics*. He looked up. "It ain't right. He didn't kill anybody even if he was guilty. He didn't take anybody's life."

"You know rape's a capital offense in Alabama," said Atticus.

"Yessir, but the jury didn't have to give him death—if they wanted to they could've gave him twenty years."

"Given," said Atticus. "Tom Robinson's a colored man, Jem. No jury in this part of the world's going to say, 'We think you're guilty, but not very,' on a charge like that. It was either a straight acquittal or nothing."

Jem was shaking his head. "I know it's not right, but I can't figure out what's wrong—maybe rape shouldn't be a capital offense. . . ."

Atticus dropped his newspaper beside his chair. He said he didn't have any quarrel with the rape statute, none whatever, but he did have deep misgivings when the state asked for and the jury gave a death penalty on purely circumstantial evidence. He glanced at me, saw I was listening, and made it easier. "—I mean, before a man is sentenced to death for murder, say, there should be one or two eye-witnesses. Someone should be able to say, 'Yes, I was there and saw him pull the trigger.'"

"But lots of folks have been hung—hanged—on circumstantial evidence," said Jem.

"I know, and lots of 'em probably deserved it, too—but in the absence of eye-witnesses there's always a doubt, sometimes only the shadow of a doubt. The law says 'reasonable doubt,' but I think a defendant's entitled to the shadow of a doubt. There's always the possibility, no matter how improbable, that he's innocent.''

"Then it all goes back to the jury, then. We oughta do away with juries." Jem was adamant.

Atticus tried hard not to smile but couldn't help it. "You're rather hard on us, son. I think maybe there might be a better way. Change the law. Change it so that only judges have the power of fixing the penalty in capital cases.''

"Then go up to Montgomery and change the law."

"You'd be surprised how hard that'd be. I won't live to see the law changed, and if you live to see it you'll be an old man.''

This was not good enough for Jem. "No sir, they oughta do away with juries. He wasn't guilty in the first place and they said he was.''

"If you had been on that jury, son, and eleven other boys like you, Tom would be a free man," said Atticus. "So far nothing in your life has interfered with your reasoning process. Those are twelve reasonable men in everyday life, Tom's jury, but you saw something come between them and reason. You saw the same thing that night in front of the jail. When that crew went away, they didn't go as reasonable men, they went because we were there. There's something in our world that makes men lose their heads—they couldn't be fair if they tried. In our courts, when it's a white man's word against a black man's, the white man always wins. They're ugly, but those are the facts of life.''

"Doesn't make it right," said Jem stolidly. He beat his fist softly on his knee. "You just can't convict a man on evidence like that—you can't.''

"You couldn't, but they could and did. The older you grow the more of it you'll see. The one place where a man ought to get a square deal is in a courtroom, be he any color of the rainbow, but people have a way of carrying their resentments right into a jury box. As you grow older, you'll see white men cheat black men every day of your life, but let me tell you something and don't you forget it—whenever a white man does that to a black man, no matter who he is, how rich he is, or how fine a family he comes from, that white man is trash.''

Atticus was speaking so quietly his last word crashed on our ears. I looked up, and his face was vehement. "There's nothing more sickening to me than a low-grade white man who'll take advantage of a Negro's ignorance. Don't fool yourselves—it's all adding up and one of these days we're going to pay the bill for it. I hope it's not in you children's time."

Jem was scratching his head. Suddenly his eyes widened. "Atticus," he said, "why don't people like us and Miss Maudie ever sit on juries? You never see anybody from Maycomb on a jury—they all come from out in the woods."

Atticus leaned back in his rocking-chair. For some reason he looked pleased with Jem. "I was wondering when that'd occur to you," he said. "There are lots of reasons. For one thing, Miss Maudie can't serve on a jury because she's a woman—"

"You mean women in Alabama can't—?" I was indignant.

"I do. I guess it's to protect our frail ladies from sordid cases like Tom's. Besides," Atticus grinned, "I doubt if we'd ever get a complete case tried—the ladies'd be interrupting to ask questions."

Jem and I laughed. Miss Maudie on a jury would be impressive. I thought of old Mrs. Dubose in her wheelchair— "Stop that rapping, John Taylor, I want to ask this man something." Perhaps our forefathers were wise.

Atticus was saying, "With people like us—that's our share of the bill. We generally get the juries we deserve. Our stout Maycomb citizens aren't interested, in the first place. In the second place, they're afraid. Then, they're—"

"Afraid, why?" asked Jem.

"Well, what if—say, Mr. Link Deas had to decide the amount of damages to award, say, Miss Maudie, when Miss Rachel ran over her with a car. Link wouldn't like the thought of losing either lady's business at his store, would he? So he tells Judge Taylor that he can't serve on the jury because he doesn't have anybody to keep store for him while he's gone So Judge Taylor excuses him. Sometimes he excuses him wrathfully."

"What'd make him think either one of 'em'd stop trading with him?" I asked.

Jem said, "Miss Rachel would, Miss Maudie wouldn't. But a jury's vote's secret, Atticus."

Our father chuckled. "You've many more miles to go, son. A jury's vote's supposed to be secret. Serving on a jury forces a man to make up his mind and declare himself about something. Men don't like to do that. Sometimes it's unpleasant."

"Tom's jury sho' made up its mind in a hurry," Jem muttered.

Atticus's fingers went to his watchpocket. "No it didn't," he said, more to himself than to us. "That was the one thing that made me think, well, this may be the shadow of a beginning. That jury took a few hours. An inevitable verdict, maybe, but usually it takes 'em just a few minutes. This time—" he broke off and looked at us. "You might like to know that there was one fellow who took considerable wearing down—in the beginning he was rarin' for an outright acquittal."

"Who?" Jem was astonished.

Atticus's eyes twinkled. "It's not for me to say, but I'll tell you this much. He was one of your Old Sarum friends . . ."

"One of the Cunninghams?" Jem yelped. "One of—I didn't recognize any of 'em . . . you're jokin'." He looked at Atticus from the corners of his eyes.

"One of their connections. On a hunch, I didn't strike him. Just on a hunch. Could've, but I didn't."

"Golly Moses," Jem said reverently. "One minute they're tryin' to kill him and the next they're tryin' to turn him loose . . . I'll never understand those folks as long as I live."

Atticus said you just had to know 'em. He said the Cunninghams hadn't taken anything from or off of anybody since they migrated to the New World. He said the other thing about them was, once you earned their respect they were for you tooth and nail. Atticus said he had a feeling, nothing more than a suspicion, that they left the jail that night with considerable respect for the Finches. Then too, he said, it took a thunderbolt plus another Cunningham to make one of them change his mind. "If we'd had two of that crowd, we'd've had a hung jury."

Jem said slowly, "You mean you actually put on the jury

a man who wanted to kill you the night before? How could you take such a risk, Atticus, how could you?"

"When you analyze it, there was little risk. There's no difference between one man who's going to convict and another man who's going to convict, is there? There's a faint difference between a man who's going to convict and a man who's a little disturbed in his mind, isn't there? He was the only uncertainty on the whole list."

"What kin was that man to Mr. Walter Cunningham?" I asked.

Atticus rose, stretched and yawned. It was not even our bedtime, but we knew he wanted a chance to read his newspaper. He picked it up, folded it, and tapped my head. "Let's see now," he droned to himself. "I've got it. Double first cousin."

"How can that be?"

"Two sisters married two brothers. That's all I'll tell you—you figure it out."

I tortured myself and decided that if I married Jem and Dill had a sister whom he married our children would be double first cousins. "Gee minetti, Jem," I said, when Atticus had gone, "they're funny folks. 'd you hear that, Aunty?"

Aunt Alexandra was hooking a rug and not watching us, but she was listening. She sat in her chair with her workbasket beside it, her rug spread across her lap. Why ladies hooked woolen rugs on boiling nights never became clear to me.

"I heard it," she said.

I remembered the distant disastrous occasion when I rushed to young Walter Cunningham's defense. Now I was glad I'd done it. "Soon's school starts I'm gonna ask Walter home to dinner," I planned, having forgotten my private resolve to beat him up the next time I saw him. "He can stay over sometimes after school, too. Atticus could drive him back to Old Sarum. Maybe he could spend the night with us sometime, okay, Jem?"

"We'll see about that," Aunt Alexandra said, a declaration that with her was always a threat, never a promise. Surprised, I turned to her. "Why not, Aunty? They're good folks."

She looked at me over her sewing glasses. "Jean Louise,

there is no doubt in my mind that they're good folks. But they're not our kind of folks.''

Jem says, ''She means they're yappy, Scout.''

''What's a yap?''

''Aw, tacky. They like fiddlin' and things like that.''

''Well I do too—''

''Don't be silly, Jean Louise,'' said Aunt Alexandra. ''The thing is, you can scrub Walter Cunningham till he shines, you can put him in shoes and a new suit, but he'll never be like Jem. Besides, there's a drinking streak in that family a mile wide. Finch women aren't interested in that sort of people.''

''Aun-ty,'' said Jem, ''she ain't nine yet.''

''She may as well learn it now.''

Aunt Alexandra had spoken. I was reminded vividly of the last time she had put her foot down. I never knew why. It was when I was absorbed with plans to visit Calpurnia's house—I was curious, interested; I wanted to be her ''company,'' to see how she lived, who her friends were. I might as well have wanted to see the other side of the moon. This time the tactics were different, but Aunt Alexandra's aim was the same. Perhaps this was why she had come to live with us—to help us choose our friends. I would hold her off as long as I could: ''If they're good folks, then why can't I be nice to Walter?''

''I didn't say not to be nice to him. You should be friendly and polite to him, you should be gracious to everybody, dear. But you don't have to invite him home.''

''What if he was kin to us, Aunty?''

''The fact is that he is not kin to us, but if he were, my answer would be the same.''

''Aunty,'' Jem spoke up, ''Atticus says you can choose your friends but you sho' can't choose your family, an' they're still kin to you no matter whether you acknowledge 'em or not, and it makes you look right silly when you don't.''

''That's your father all over again,'' said Aunt Alexandra, ''and I still say that Jean Louise will not invite Walter Cunningham to this house. If he were her double first cousin once removed he would still not be received in this house unless he comes to see Atticus on business. Now that is that.''

She had said Indeed Not, but this time she would give her

reasons: "But I want to play with Walter, Aunty, why can't I?"

She took off her glasses and stared at me. "I'll tell you why," she said. "Because—he—is—trash, that's why you can't play with him. I'll not have you around him, picking up his habits and learning Lord-knows-what. You're enough of a problem to your father as it is."

I don't know what I would have done, but Jem stopped me. He caught me by the shoulders, put his arm around me, and led me sobbing in fury to his bedroom. Atticus heard us and poked his head around the door. " 's all right, sir," Jem said gruffly, " 's not anything." Atticus went away.

"Have a chew, Scout." Jem dug into his pocket and extracted a Tootsie Roll. It took a few minutes to work the candy into a comfortable wad inside my jaw.

Jem was rearranging the objects on his dresser. His hair stuck up behind and down in front, and I wondered if it would ever look like a man's—maybe if he shaved it off and started over, his hair would grow back neatly in place. His eyebrows were becoming heavier, and I noticed a new slimness about his body. He was growing taller.

When he looked around, he must have thought I would start crying again, for he said, "Show you something if you won't tell anybody." I said what. He unbuttoned his shirt, grinning shyly.

"Well what?"

"Well can't you see it?"

"Well no."

"Well it's hair."

"Where?"

"There. Right there."

He had been a comfort to me, so I said it looked lovely, but I didn't see anything. "It's real nice, Jem."

"Under my arms, too," he said. "Goin' out for football next year. Scout, don't let Aunty aggravate you."

It seemed only yesterday that he was telling me not to aggravate Aunty.

"You know she's not used to girls," said Jem, "leastways, not girls like you. She's trying to make you a lady. Can't you take up sewin' or somethin'?"

"Hell no. She doesn't like me, that's all there is to it, and

I don't care. It was her callin' Walter Cunningham trash that got me goin', Jem, not what she said about being a problem to Atticus. We got that all straight one time, I asked him if I was a problem and he said not much of one, at most one that he could always figure out, and not to worry my head a second about botherin' him. Naw, it was Walter—that boy's not trash, Jem. He ain't like the Ewells.''

Jem kicked off his shoes and swung his feet to the bed. He propped himself against a pillow and switched on the reading light. "You know something, Scout? I've got it all figured out, now. I've thought about it a lot lately and I've got it figured out. There's four kinds of folks in the world. There's the ordinary kind like us and the neighbors, there's the kind like the Cunninghams out in the woods, the kind like the Ewells down at the dump, and the Negroes.''

"What about the Chinese, and the Cajuns down yonder in Baldwin County?''

"I mean in Maycomb County. The thing about it is, our kind of folks don't like the Cunninghams, the Cunninghams don't like the Ewells, and the Ewells hate and despise the colored folks.''

I told Jem if that was so, then why didn't Tom's jury, made up of folks like the Cunninghams, acquit Tom to spite the Ewells?

Jem waved my question away as being infantile.

"You know,'' he said, "I've seen Atticus pat his foot when there's fiddlin' on the radio, and he loves pot liquor better'n any man I ever saw—''

"Then that makes us like the Cunninghams,'' I said. "I can't see why Aunty—''

"No, lemme finish—it does, but we're still different somehow. Atticus said one time the reason Aunty's so hipped on the family is because all we've got's background and not a dime to our names.''

"Well Jem, I don't know—Atticus told me one time that most of this Old Family stuff's foolishness because everybody's family's just as old as everybody else's. I said did that include the colored folks and Englishmen and he said yes.''

"Background doesn't mean Old Family,'' said Jem. "I think it's how long your family's been readin' and writin'.

Scout, I've studied this real hard and that's the only reason I can think of. Somewhere along when the Finches were in Egypt one of 'em must have learned a hieroglyphic or two and he taught his boy." Jem laughed. "Imagine Aunty being proud her great-grandaddy could read an' write—ladies pick funny things to be proud of."

"Well I'm glad he could, or who'da taught Atticus and them, and if Atticus couldn't read, you and me'd be in a fix. I don't think that's what background is, Jem."

"Well then, how do you explain why the Cunninghams are different? Mr. Walter can hardly sign his name, I've seen him. We've just been readin' and writin' longer'n they have."

"No, everybody's gotta learn, nobody's born knowin'. That Walter's as smart as he can be, he just gets held back sometimes because he has to stay out and help his daddy. Nothin's wrong with him. Naw, Jem, I think there's just one kind of folks. Folks."

Jem turned around and punched his pillow. When he settled back his face was cloudy. He was going into one of his declines, and I grew wary. His brows came together; his mouth became a thin line. He was silent for a while.

"That's what I thought, too," he said at last, "when I was your age. If there's just one kind of folks, why can't they get along with each other? If they're all alike, why do they go out of their way to despise each other? Scout, I think I'm beginning to understand something. I think I'm beginning to understand why Boo Radley's stayed shut up in the house all this time . . . it's because he *wants* to stay inside."

24

Calpurnia wore her stiffest starched apron. She carried a tray of charlotte. She backed up to the swinging door and pressed gently. I admired the ease and grace with which she handled heavy loads of dainty things. So did Aunt Alexandra, I guess, because she had let Calpurnia serve today.

August was on the brink of September. Dill would be leaving for Meridian tomorrow; today he was off with Jem at Barker's Eddy. Jem had discovered with angry amazement that nobody had ever bothered to teach Dill how to swim, a skill Jem considered necessary as walking. They had spent two afternoons at the creek, they said they were going in naked and I couldn't come, so I divided the lonely hours between Calpurnia and Miss Maudie.

Today Aunt Alexandra and her missionary circle were fighting the good fight all over the house. From the kitchen, I heard Mrs. Grace Merriweather giving a report in the livingroom on the squalid lives of the Mrunas, it sounded like to me. They put the women out in huts when their time came, whatever that was; they had no sense of family——I knew that'd distress Aunty——they subjected children to terrible ordeals when they were thirteen; they were crawling with yaws and earworms, they chewed up and spat out the bark of a tree into a communal pot and then got drunk on it.

Immediately thereafter, the ladies adjourned for refreshments.

I didn't know whether to go into the diningroom or stay out. Aunt Alexandra told me to join them for refreshments; it was not necessary that I attend the business part of the meeting, she said it'd bore me. I was wearing my pink Sunday dress, shoes, and a petticoat, and reflected that if I spilled anything Calpurnia would have to wash my dress again for tomorrow. This had been a busy day for her. I decided to stay out.

"Can I help you, Cal?" I asked, wishing to be of some service.

Calpurnia paused in the doorway. "You be still as a mouse in that corner," she said, "an' you can help me load up the trays when I come back."

The gentle hum of ladies' voices grew louder as she opened the door: "Why, Alexandra, I never saw such charlotte . . . just lovely . . . I never can get my crust like this, never can . . . who'd've thought of little dewberry tarts . . . Calpurnia? . . . who'da thought it . . . anybody tell you that the preacher's wife's . . . nooo, well she is, and that other one not walkin' yet . . ."

They became quiet, and I knew they had all been served.

Calpurnia returned and put my mother's heavy silver pitcher on a tray. "This coffee pitcher's a curiosity," she murmured, "they don't make 'em these days."

"Can I carry it in?"

"If you be careful and don't drop it. Set it down at the end of the table by Miss Alexandra. Down there by the cups'n things. She's gonna pour."

I tried pressing my behind against the door as Calpurnia had done, but the door didn't budge. Grinning, she held it open for me. "Careful now, it's heavy. Don't look at it and you won't spill it."

My journey was successful: Aunt Alexandra smiled brilliantly. "Stay with us, Jean Louise," she said. This was a part of her campaign to teach me to be a lady.

It was customary for every circle hostess to invite her neighbors in for refreshments, be they Baptists or Presbyterians, which accounted for the presence of Miss Rachel (sober as a judge), Miss Maudie and Miss Stephanie Crawford. Rather nervous, I took a seat beside Miss Maudie and wondered why ladies put on their hats to go across the street. Ladies in bunches always filled me with vague apprehension and a firm desire to be elsewhere, but this feeling was what Aunt Alexandra called being "spoiled."

The ladies were cool in fragile pastel prints: most of them were heavily powdered but unrouged; the only lipstick in the room was Tangee Natural. Cutex Natural sparkled on their fingernails, but some of the younger ladies wore Rose. They smelled heavenly. I sat quietly, having conquered my hands by tightly gripping the arms of the chair, and waited for someone to speak to me.

Miss Maudie's gold bridgework twinkled. "You're mighty dressed up, Miss Jean Louise," she said. "Where are your britches today?"

"Under my dress."

I hadn't meant to be funny, but the ladies laughed. My cheeks grew hot as I realized my mistake, but Miss Maudie looked gravely down at me. She never laughed at me unless I meant to be funny.

In the sudden silence that followed, Miss Stephanie Crawford called from across the room, "Whatcha going to be when you grow up, Jean Louise? A lawyer?"

"Nome, I hadn't thought about it . . ." I answered, grateful that Miss Stephanie was kind enough to change the subject. Hurriedly I began choosing my vocation. Nurse? Aviator? "Well . . ."

"Why shoot, I thought you wanted to be a lawyer, you've already commenced going to court."

The ladies laughed again. "That Stephanie's a card," somebody said. Miss Stephanie was encouraged to pursue the subject: "Don't you want to grow up to be a lawyer?"

Miss Maudie's hand touched mine and I answered mildly enough, "Nome, just a lady."

Miss Stephanie eyed me suspiciously, decided that I meant no impertinence, and contented herself with, "Well, you won't get very far until you start wearing dresses more often."

Miss Maudie's hand closed tightly on mine, and I said nothing. Its warmth was enough.

Mrs. Grace Merriweather sat on my left, and I felt it would be polite to talk to her. Mr. Merriweather, a faithful Methodist under duress, apparently saw nothing personal in singing, "Amazing Grace, how sweet the sound, that saved a wretch like me . . ." It was the general opinion of Maycomb, however, that Mrs. Merriweather had sobered him up and made a reasonably useful citizen of him. For certainly Mrs. Merriweather was the most devout lady in Maycomb. I searched for a topic of interest to her. "What did you all study this afternoon?" I asked.

"Oh child, those poor Mrunas," she said, and was off. Few other questions would be necessary.

Mrs. Merriweather's large brown eyes always filled with tears when she considered the oppressed. "Living in that jungle with nobody but J. Grimes Everett," she said. "Not a white person'll go near 'em but that saintly J. Grimes Everett."

Mrs. Merriweather played her voice like an organ; every word she said received its full measure: "The poverty . . . the darkness . . . the immorality—nobody but J. Grimes Everett knows. You know, when the church gave me that trip to the camp grounds J. Grimes Everett said to me—"

"Was he there, ma'am? I thought—"

"Home on leave. J. Grimes Everett said to me, he said,

'Mrs. Merriweather, you have no conception, no *conception* of what we are fighting over there.' That's what he said to me.''

"Yes ma'am."

"I said to him, 'Mr. Everett,' I said, 'the ladies of the Maycomb Alabama Methodist Episcopal Church South are behind you one hundred percent.' That's what I said to him. And you know, right then and there I made a pledge in my heart. I said to myself, when I go home I'm going to give a course on the Mrunas and bring J. Grimes Everett's message to Maycomb and that's just what I'm doing.''

"Yes ma'am."

When Mrs. Merriweather shook her head, her black curls jiggled. "Jean Louise," she said, "you are a fortunate girl. You live in a Christian home with Christian folks in a Christian town. Out there in J. Grimes Everett's land there's nothing but sin and squalor."

"Yes ma'am."

"Sin and squalor—what was that, Gertrude?" Mrs. Merriweather turned on her chimes for the lady sitting beside her. "Oh that. Well, I always say forgive and forget, forgive and forget. Thing that church ought to do is help her lead a Christian life for those children from here on out. Some of the men ought to go out there and tell that preacher to encourage her."

"Excuse me, Mrs. Merriweather," I interrupted, "are you all talking about Mayella Ewell?"

"May—? No, child. That darky's wife. Tom's wife, Tom—"

"Robinson, ma'am."

Mrs. Merriweather turned back to her neighbor. "There's one thing I truly believe, Gertrude," she continued, "but some people just don't see it my way. If we just let them know we forgive 'em, that we've forgotten it, then this whole thing'll blow over."

"Ah—Mrs. Merriweather," I interrupted once more, "what'll blow over?"

Again, she turned to me. Mrs. Merriweather was one of those childless adults who find it necessary to assume a different tone of voice when speaking to children. "Nothing,

Jean Louise," she said, in stately largo, "the cooks and field hands are just dissatisfied, but they're settling down now—they grumbled all next day after that trial."

Mrs. Merriweather faced Mrs. Farrow: "Gertrude, I tell you there's nothing more distracting than a sulky darky. Their mouths go down to here. Just ruins your day to have one of 'em in the kitchen. You know what I said to my Sophy, Gertrude? I said, 'Sophy,' I said, 'you simply are not being a Christian today. Jesus Christ never went around grumbling and complaining,' and you know, it did her good. She took her eyes off that floor and said, 'Nome, Miz Merriweather, Jesus never went around grumblin'.' I tell you, Gertrude, you never ought to let an opportunity go by to witness for the Lord."

I was reminded of the ancient little organ in the chapel at Finch's Landing. When I was very small, and if I had been very good during the day, Atticus would let me pump its bellows while he picked out a tune with one finger. The last note would linger as long as there was air to sustain it. Mrs. Merriweather had run out of air, I judged, and was replenishing her supply while Mrs. Farrow composed herself to speak.

Mrs. Farrow was a splendidly built woman with pale eyes and narrow feet. She had a fresh permanent wave, and her hair was a mass of tight gray ringlets. She was the second most devout lady in Maycomb. She had a curious habit of prefacing everything she said with a soft sibilant sound.

"S-s-s Grace," she said, "it's just like I was telling Brother Hutson the other day. 'S-s-s Brother Hutson,' I said, 'looks like we're fighting a losing battle, a losing battle.' I said, 'S-s-s it doesn't matter to 'em one bit. We can educate 'em till we're blue in the face, we can try till we drop to make Christians out of 'em, but there's no lady safe in her bed these nights.' He said to me, 'Mrs. Farrow, I don't know what we're coming to down here.' S-s-s I told him that was certainly a fact."

Mrs. Merriweather nodded wisely. Her voice soared over the clink of coffee cups and the soft bovine sounds of the ladies munching their dainties. "Gertrude," she said, "I tell you there are some good but misguided people in this town. Good, but misguided. Folks in this town who think they're doing right, I mean. Now far be it from me to say who, but some of 'em in this town thought they were doing the right thing a while back, but all they did was stir 'em up. That's all they did. Might've looked like the right thing to do at the time, I'm sure I don't know, I'm not read in that field, but sulky . . . dissatisfied . . . I tell you if my Sophy'd kept it up another day I'd have let her go. It's never entered that wool of hers that the only reason I keep her is because this depression's on and she needs her dollar and a quarter every week she can get it."

"His food doesn't stick going down, does it?"

Miss Maudie said it. Two tight lines had appeared at the corners of her mouth. She had been sitting silently beside me, her coffee cup balanced on one knee. I had lost the thread of conversation long ago, when they quit talking about Tom Robinson's wife, and had contented myself with thinking of Finch's Landing and the river. Aunt Alexandra had got it backwards: the business part of the meeting was blood-curdling, the social hour was dreary.

"Maudie, I'm sure I don't know what you mean," said Mrs. Merriweather.

"I'm sure you do," Miss Maudie said shortly.

She said no more. When Miss Maudie was angry her brevity was icy. Something had made her deeply angry, and her gray eyes were as cold as her voice. Mrs. Merriweather reddened, glanced at me, and looked away. I could not see Mrs. Farrow.

Aunt Alexandra got up from the table and swiftly passed more refreshments, neatly engaging Mrs. Merriweather and Mrs. Gates in brisk conversation. When she had them well on the road with Mrs. Perkins, Aunt Alexandra stepped back. She gave Miss Maudie a look of pure gratitude, and I wondered at the world of women. Miss Maudie and Aunt Alexandra had never been especially close, and here was Aunty silently thanking her for something. For what, I knew not. I was content to learn that Aunt Alexandra could be pierced sufficiently to feel gratitude for help given. There was no doubt about it, I must soon enter this world, where on its surface fragrant ladies rocked slowly, fanned gently, and drank cool water.

But I was more at home in my father's world. People like

Mr. Heck Tate did not trap you with innocent questions to make fun of you; even Jem was not highly critical unless you said something stupid. Ladies seemed to live in faint horror of men, seemed unwilling to approve wholeheartedly of them. But I liked them. There was something about them, no matter how much they cussed and drank and gambled and chewed; no matter how undelectable they were, there was something about them that I instinctively liked . . . they weren't—

"Hypocrites, Mrs. Perkins, born hypocrites," Mrs. Merriweather was saying. "At least we don't have that sin on our shoulders down here. People up there set 'em free, but you don't see 'em settin' at the table with 'em. At least we don't have the deceit to say to 'em yes you're as good as we are but stay away from us. Down here we just say you live your way and we'll live ours. I think that woman, that Mrs. Roosevelt's lost her mind—just plain lost her mind coming down to Birmingham and tryin' to sit with 'em. If I was the Mayor of Birmingham I'd—"

Well, neither of us was the Mayor of Birmingham, but I wished I was the Governor of Alabama for one day: I'd let Tom Robinson go so quick the Missionary Society wouldn't have time to catch its breath. Calpurnia was telling Miss Rachel's cook the other day how bad Tom was taking things and she didn't stop talking when I came into the kitchen. She said there wasn't a thing Atticus could do to make being shut up easier for him, that the last thing he said to Atticus before they took him down to the prison camp was, "Good-bye, Mr. Finch, there ain't nothin' you can do now, so there ain't no use tryin'." Calpurnia said Atticus told her that the day they took Tom to prison he just gave up hope. She said Atticus tried to explain things to him, and that he must do his best not to lose hope because Atticus was doing his best to get him free. Miss Rachel's cook asked Calpurnia why didn't Atticus just say yes, you'll go free, and leave it at that—seemed like that'd be a big comfort to Tom. Calpurnia said, "Because you ain't familiar with the law. First thing you learn when you're in a lawin' family is that there ain't any definite answers to anything. Mr. Finch couldn't say somethin's so when he doesn't know for sure it's so."

The front door slammed and I heard Atticus's footsteps in the hall. Automatically I wondered what time it was. Not nearly time for him to be home, and on Missionary Society days he usually stayed downtown until black dark.

He stopped in the doorway. His hat was in his hand, and his face was white.

"Excuse me, ladies," he said. "Go right ahead with your meeting, don't let me disturb you. Alexandra, could you come to the kitchen a minute? I want to borrow Calpurnia for a while."

He didn't go through the diningroom, but went down the back hallway and entered the kitchen from the rear door. Aunt Alexandra and I met him. The diningroom door opened again and Miss Maudie joined us. Calpurnia had half risen from her chair.

"Cal," Atticus said, "I want you to go with me out to Helen Robinson's house—"

"What's the matter?" Aunt Alexandra asked, alarmed by the look on my father's face.

"Tom's dead."

Aunt Alexandra put her hands to her mouth.

"They shot him," said Atticus. "He was running. It was during their exercise period. They said he just broke into a blind raving charge at the fence and started climbing over. Right in front of them—"

"Didn't they try to stop him? Didn't they give him any warning?" Aunt Alexandra's voice shook.

"Oh yes, the guards called to him to stop. They fired a few shots in the air, then to kill. They got him just as he went over the fence They said if he'd had two good arms he'd have made it, he was moving that fast. Seventeen bullet holes in him. They didn't have to shoot him that much. Cal, I want you to come out with me and help me tell Helen."

"Yes sir," she murmured, fumbling at her apron. Miss Maudie went to Calpurnia and untied it.

"This is the last straw, Atticus," Aunt Alexandra said.

"Depends on how you look at it," he said. "What was one Negro, more or less, among two hundred of 'em? He wasn't Tom to them, he was an escaping prisoner."

Atticus leaned against the refrigerator, pushed up his glasses, and rubbed his eyes. "We had such a good chance," he said. "I told him what I thought, but I couldn't in truth say that we had more than a good chance. I guess Tom was tired of white men's chances and preferred to take his own. Ready, Cal?"

"Yessir, Mr. Finch."

"Then let's go."

Aunt Alexandra sat down in Calpurnia's chair and put her hands to her face. She sat quite still; she was so quiet I wondered if she would faint. I heard Miss Maudie breathing as if she had just climbed the steps, and in the diningroom the ladies chattered happily.

I thought Aunt Alexandra was crying, but when she took her hands away from her face, she was not. She looked weary. She spoke, and her voice was flat.

"I can't say I approve of everything he does, Maudie, but he's my brother, and I just want to know when this will ever end." Her voice rose: "It tears him to pieces. He doesn't show it much, but it tears him to pieces. I've seen him when—what else do they want from him, Maudie, what else?"

"What does who want, Alexandra?" Miss Maudie asked.

"I mean this town. They're perfectly willing to let him do what they're too afraid to do themselves—it might lose 'em a nickel. They're perfectly willing to let him wreck his health doing what they're afraid to do, they're—"

"Be quiet, they'll hear you," said Miss Maudie. "Have you ever thought of it this way, Alexandra? Whether Maycomb knows it or not, we're paying the highest tribute we can pay a man. We trust him to do right. It's that simple."

"Who?" Aunt Alexandra never knew she was echoing her twelve-year-old nephew.

"The handful of people in this town who say that fair play is not marked White Only; the handful of people who say a fair trial is for everybody, not just us; the handful of people with enough humility to think, when they look at a Negro, there but for the Lord's kindness am I." Miss Maudie's old crispness was returning: "The handful of people in this town with background, that's who they are."

Had I been attentive, I would have had another scrap to add to Jem's definition of background, but I found myself shaking and couldn't stop. I had seen Enfield Prison Farm, and Atticus had pointed out the exercise yard to me. It was the size of a football field.

"Stop that shaking," commanded Miss Maudie, and I stopped. "Get up, Alexandra, we've left 'em long enough."

Aunt Alexandra rose and smoothed the various whalebone ridges along her hips. She took her handkerchief from her belt and wiped her nose. She patted her hair and said, "Do I show it?"

"Not a sign," said Miss Maudie. "Are you together again, Jean Louise?"

"Yes ma'am."

"Then let's join the ladies," she said grimly.

Their voices swelled when Miss Maudie opened the door to the diningroom. Aunt Alexandra was ahead of me, and I saw her head go up as she went through the door.

"Oh, Mrs. Perkins," she said, "you need some more coffee. Let me get it."

"Calpurnia's on an errand for a few minutes, Grace," said Miss Maudie. "Let me pass you some more of those dewberry tarts. 'dyou hear what that cousin of mine did the other day, the one who likes to go fishing? . . ."

And so they went, down the row of laughing women, around the diningroom, refilling coffee cups, dishing out goodies as though their only regret was the temporary domestic disaster of losing Calpurnia.

The gentle hum began again. "Yes sir, Mrs. Perkins, that J. Grimes Everett is a martyred saint, he . . . needed to get married so they ran . . . to the beauty parlor every Saturday afternoon . . . soon as the sun goes down. He goes to bed with the . . . chickens, a crate full of sick chickens, Fred says that's what started it all. Fred says. . . ."

Aunt Alexandra looked across the room at me and smiled. She looked at a tray of cookies on the table and nodded at them. I carefully picked up the tray and watched myself walk to Mrs. Merriweather. With my best company manners, I asked her if she would have some.

After all, if Aunty could be a lady at a time like this, so could I.

25

"Don't do that, Scout. Set him out on the back steps."

"Jem, are you crazy? . . . ."

"I said set him out on the back steps."

Sighing, I scooped up the small creature, placed him on the bottom step and went back to my cot. September had come, but not a trace of cool weather with it, and we were still sleeping on the back screen porch. Lightning bugs were still about, the night crawlers and flying insects that beat against the screen the summer long had not gone wherever they go when autumn comes.

A roly-poly had found his way inside the house; I reasoned that the tiny varmint had crawled up the steps and under the door. I was putting my book on the floor beside my cot when I saw him. The creatures are no more than an inch long, and when you touch them they roll themselves into a tight gray ball.

I lay on my stomach, reached down and poked him. He rolled up. Then, feeling safe, I suppose, he slowly unrolled. He traveled a few inches on his hundred legs and I touched him again. He rolled up. Feeling sleepy, I decided to end things. My hand was going down on him when Jem spoke.

Jem was scowling. It was probably a part of the stage he was going through, and I wished he would hurry up and get through it. He was certainly never cruel to animals, but I had never known his charity to embrace the insect world.

"Why couldn't I mash him?" I asked.

"Because they don't bother you," Jem answered in the darkness. He had turned out his reading light.

"Reckon you're at the stage now where you don't kill flies and mosquitoes now, I reckon," I said. "Lemme know when you change your mind. Tell you one thing, though, I ain't gonna sit around and not scratch a redbug."

"Aw dry up," he answered drowsily.

Jem was the one who was getting more like a girl every day, not I. Comfortable, I lay on my back and waited for sleep, and while waiting I thought of Dill. He had left us the first of the month with firm assurances that he would return the minute school was out—he guessed his folks had got the general idea that he liked to spend his summers in Maycomb. Miss Rachel took us with them in the taxi to Maycomb Junction, and Dill waved to us from the train window until he was out of sight. He was not out of mind: I missed him. The last two days of his time with us, Jem had taught him to swim—

Taught him to swim. I was wide awake, remembering what Dill had told me.

Barker's Eddy is at the end of a dirt road off the Meridian highway about a mile from town. It is easy to catch a ride down the highway on a cotton wagon or from a passing motorist, and the short walk to the creek is easy, but the prospect of walking all the way back home at dusk, when the traffic is light, is tiresome, and swimmers are careful not to stay too late.

According to Dill, he and Jem had just come to the highway when they saw Atticus driving toward them. He looked like he had not seen them, so they both waved. Atticus finally slowed down; when they caught up with him he said, "You'd better catch a ride back. I won't be going home for a while." Calpurnia was in the back seat.

Jem protested, then pleaded, and Atticus said, "All right, you can come with us if you stay in the car."

On the way to Tom Robinson's, Atticus told them what had happened.

They turned off the highway, rode slowly by the dump and past the Ewell residence, down the narrow lane to the Negro cabins. Dill said a crowd of black children were playing marbles in Tom's front yard. Atticus parked the car and got out. Calpurnia followed him through the front gate.

Dill heard him ask one of the children, "Where's your mother, Sam?" and heard Sam say, "She down at Sis Stevens's, Mr. Finch. Want me run fetch her?"

Dill said Atticus looked uncertain, then he said yes, and Sam scampered off. "Go on with your game, boys," Atticus said to the children.

A little girl came to the cabin door and stood looking at Atticus. Dill said her hair was a wad of tiny stiff pigtails, each ending in a bright bow. She grinned from ear to ear and walked toward our father, but she was too small to navigate the steps. Dill said Atticus went to her, took off his hat, and offered her his finger. She grabbed it and he eased her down the steps. Then he gave her to Calpurnia.

Sam was trotting behind his mother when they came up. Dill said Helen said, " 'evenin', Mr. Finch, won't you have a seat?" But she didn't say any more. Neither did Atticus.

"Scout," said Dill, "she just fell down in the dirt. Just fell down in the dirt, like a giant with a big foot just came along and stepped on her. Just ump—" Dill's fat foot hit the ground. "Like you'd step on an ant."

Dill said Calpurnia and Atticus lifted Helen to her feet and half carried, half walked her to the cabin. They stayed inside a long time, and Atticus came out alone. When they drove back by the dump, some of the Ewells hollered at them, but Dill didn't catch what they said.

Maycomb was interested by the news of Tom's death for perhaps two days; two days was enough for the information to spread through the county. "Did you hear about? . . . . No? Well, they say he was runnin' fit to beat lightnin' . . ." To Maycomb, Tom's death was typical. Typical of a nigger to cut and run. Typical of a nigger's mentality to have no plan, no thought for the future, just run blind first chance he saw. Funny thing, Atticus Finch might've got him off scot free, but wait—? Hell no. You know how they are. Easy come, easy go. Just shows you, that Robinson boy was legally married, they say he kept himself clean, went to church and all that, but when it comes down to the line the veneer's mighty thin. Nigger always comes out in 'em.

A few more details, enabling the listener to repeat his version in turn, then nothing to talk about until *The Maycomb Tribune* appeared the following Thursday. There was a brief obituary in the Colored News, but there was also an editorial.

Mr. B. B. Underwood was at his most bitter, and he couldn't have cared less who canceled advertising and subscriptions. (But Maycomb didn't play that way: Mr. Underwood could holler till he sweated and write whatever he wanted to, he'd still get his advertising and subscriptions. If he wanted to make a fool of himself in his paper that was his business.) Mr. Underwood didn't talk about miscarriages of justice, he was writing so children could understand. Mr. Underwood simply figured it was a sin to kill cripples, be they standing, sitting, or escaping. He likened Tom's death to the senseless slaughter of songbirds by hunters and children, and Maycomb thought he was trying to write an editorial poetical enough to be reprinted in *The Montgomery Advertiser*.

How could this be so, I wondered, as I read Mr. Underwood's editorial. Senseless killing—Tom had been given due process of law to the day of his death; he had been tried openly and convicted by twelve good men and true; my father had fought for him all the way. Then Mr. Underwood's meaning became clear: Atticus had used every tool available to free men to save Tom Robinson, but in the secret courts of men's hearts Atticus had no case. Tom was a dead man the minute Mayella Ewell opened her mouth and screamed.

The name Ewell gave me a queasy feeling. Maycomb had lost no time in getting Mr. Ewell's views on Tom's demise and passing them along through that English Channel of gossip, Miss Stephanie Crawford. Miss Stephanie told Aunt Alexandra in Jem's presence ("Oh foot, he's old enough to listen.") that Mr. Ewell said it made one down and about two more to go. Jem told me not to be afraid, Mr. Ewell was more hot gas than anything. Jem also told me that if I breathed a word to Atticus, if in any way I let Atticus know I knew, Jem would personally never speak to me again.

26

School started, and so did our daily trips past the Radley Place. Jem was in the seventh grade and went to high school, beyond the grammar-school building; I was now in the third grade, and our routines were so different I only walked to school with Jem in the mornings and saw him at mealtimes.

He went out for football, but was too slender and too young yet to do anything but carry the team water buckets. This he did with enthusiasm; most afternoons he was seldom home before dark.

The Radley Place had ceased to terrify me, but it was no less gloomy, no less chilly under its great oaks, and no less uninviting. Mr. Nathan Radley could still be seen on a clear day, walking to and from town; we knew Boo was there, for the same old reason—nobody'd seen him carried out yet. I sometimes felt a twinge of remorse, when passing by the old place, at ever having taken part in what must have been sheer torment to Arthur Radley—what reasonable recluse wants children peeping through his shutters, delivering greetings on the end of a fishing-pole, wandering in his collards at night?

And yet I remembered. Two Indian-head pennies, chewing gum, soap dolls, a rusty medal, a broken watch and chain. Jem must have put them away somewhere. I stopped and looked at the tree one afternoon: the trunk was swelling around its cement patch. The patch itself was turning yellow.

We had almost seen him a couple of times, a good enough score for anybody.

But I still looked for him each time I went by. Maybe someday we would see him. I imagined how it would be: when it happened, he'd just be sitting in the swing when I came along. "Hidy do, Mr. Arthur," I would say, as if I had said it every afternoon of my life. "Evening, Jean Louise," he would say, as if he had said it every afternoon of my life, "right pretty spell we're having, isn't it?" "Yes sir, right pretty," I would say, and go on.

It was only a fantasy. We would never see him. He probably did go out when the moon was down and gaze upon Miss Stephanie Crawford. I'd have picked somebody else to look at, but that was his business. He would never gaze at us.

"You aren't starting that again, are you?" said Atticus one night, when I expressed a stray desire just to have one good look at Boo Radley before I died. "If you are, I'll tell you right now: stop it. I'm too old to go chasing you off the Radley property. Besides, it's dangerous. You might get shot. You know Mr. Nathan shoots at every shadow he sees, even shadows that leave size-four bare footprints. You were lucky not to be killed.''

I hushed then and there. At the same time I marveled at Atticus. This was the first he had let us know he knew a lot more about something than we thought he knew. And it had happened years ago. No, only last summer—no, summer before last, when . . . time was playing tricks on me. I must remember to ask Jem.

So many things had happened to us, Boo Radley was the least of our fears. Atticus said he didn't see how anything else could happen, that things had a way of settling down, and after enough time passed people would forget that Tom Robinson's existence was ever brought to their attention.

Perhaps Atticus was right, but the events of the summer hung over us like smoke in a closed room. The adults in Maycomb never discussed the case with Jem and me; it seemed that they discussed it with their children, and their attitude must have been that neither of us could help having Atticus for a parent, so their children must be nice to us in spite of him. The children would never have thought that up for themselves: had our classmates been left to their own devices, Jem and I would have had several swift, satisfying fist-fights apiece and ended the matter for good. As it was, we were compelled to hold our heads high and be, respectively, a gentleman and a lady. In a way, it was like the era of Mrs. Henry Lafayette Dubose, without all her yelling. There was one odd thing, though, that I never understood: in spite of Atticus's shortcomings as a parent, people were content to re-elect him to the state legislature that year, as usual, without opposition. I came to the conclusion that people were just peculiar, I withdrew from them, and never thought about them until I was forced to.

I was forced to one day in school. Once a week, we had a Current Events period. Each child was supposed to clip an item from a newspaper, absorb its contents, and reveal them to the class. This practice allegedly overcame a variety of evils: standing in front of his fellows encouraged good posture and gave a child poise; delivering a short talk made him word-conscious; learning his current event strengthened his memory; being singled out made him more than ever anxious to return to the Group.

The idea was profound, but as usual, in Maycomb it didn't work very well. In the first place, few rural children had access to newspapers, so the burden of Current Events was borne by the town children, convincing the bus children more deeply that the town children got all the attention anyway. The rural children who could, usually brought clippings from what they called The Grit Paper, a publication spurious in the eyes of Miss Gates, our teacher. Why she frowned when a child recited from The Grit Paper I never knew, but in some way it was associated with liking fiddling, eating syrupy biscuits for lunch, being a holy-roller, singing *Sweetly Sings the Donkey* and pronouncing it dunkey, all of which the state paid teachers to discourage.

Even so, not many of the children knew what a Current Event was. Little Chuck Little, a hundred years old in his knowledge of cows and their habits, was halfway through an Uncle Natchell story when Miss Gates stopped him: "Charles, that is not a current event. That is an advertisement."

Cecil Jacobs knew what one was, though. When his turn came, he went to the front of the room and began, "Old Hitler—"

"Adolf Hitler, Cecil," said Miss Gates. "One never begins with Old anybody."

"Yes ma'am," he said. "Old Adolf Hitler has been prosecutin' the—"

"Persecuting Cecil. . . ."

"Nome, Miss Gates, it says here—well anyway, old Adolf Hitler has been after the Jews and he's puttin' 'em in prisons and he's taking away all their property and he won't let any of 'em out of the country and he's washin' all the feeble-minded and—"

"Washing the feeble-minded?"

"Yes ma'am, Miss Gates, I reckon they don't have sense enough to wash themselves, I don't reckon an idiot could keep hisself clean. Well anyway, Hitler's started a program to round up all the half-Jews too and he wants to register 'em in case they might wanta cause him any trouble and I think this is a bad thing and that's my current event."

"Very good, Cecil," said Miss Gates. Puffing, Cecil returned to his seat.

A hand went up in the back of the room. "How can he do that?"

"Who do what?" asked Miss Gates patiently.

"I mean how can Hitler just put a lot of folks in a pen like that, looks like the govamint'd stop him," said the owner of the hand.

"Hitler is the government," said Miss Gates, and seizing an opportunity to make education dynamic, she went to the blackboard. She printed DEMOCRACY in large letters. "Democracy," she said. "Does anybody have a definition?"

"Us," somebody said.

I raised my hand, remembering an old campaign slogan Atticus had once told me about.

"What do you think it means, Jean Louise?"

" 'Equal rights for all, special privileges for none,' " I quoted.

"Very good, Jean Louise, very good," Miss Gates smiled. In front of DEMOCRACY, she printed WE ARE A. "Now class, say it all together, 'We are a democracy.' "

We said it. Then Miss Gates said, "That's the difference between America and Germany. We are a democracy and Germany is a dictatorship. Dictator-ship," she said. "Over here we don't believe in persecuting anybody. Persecution comes from people who are prejudiced. Prejudice," she enunciated carefully. "There are no better people in the world than the Jews, and why Hitler doesn't think so is a mystery to me."

An inquiring soul in the middle of the room said, "Why don't they like the Jews, you reckon, Miss Gates?"

"I don't know, Henry. They contribute to every society they live in, and most of all, they are a deeply religious people. Hitler's trying to do away with religion, so maybe he doesn't like them for that reason."

Cecil spoke up. "Well I don't know for certain," he said, "they're supposed to change money or somethin', but that ain't no cause to persecute 'em. They're white, ain't they?"

Miss Gates said, "When you get to high school, Cecil, you'll learn that the Jews have been persecuted since the beginning of history, even driven out of their own country. It's one of the most terrible stories in history. Time for arithmetic, children."

As I had never liked arithmetic, I spent the period looking out the window. The only time I ever saw Atticus scowl was when Elmer Davis would give us the latest on Hitler. Atticus would snap off the radio and say, "Hmp!" I asked him once why he was impatient with Hitler and Atticus said, "Because he's a maniac."

This would not do, I mused, as the class proceeded with its sums. One maniac and millions of German folks. Looked to me like they'd shut Hitler in a pen instead of letting him shut them up. There was something else wrong—I would ask my father about it.

I did, and he said he could not possibly answer my question because he didn't know the answer.

"But it's okay to hate Hitler?"

"It is not," he said. "It's not okay to hate anybody."

"Atticus," I said, "there's somethin' I don't understand. Miss Gates said it was awful, Hitler doin' like he does, she got real red in the face about it—"

"I should think she would."

"But—"

"Yes?"

"Nothing, sir." I went away, not sure that I could explain to Atticus what was on my mind, not sure that I could clarify what was only a feeling. Perhaps Jem could provide the answer. Jem understood school things better than Atticus.

Jem was worn out from a day's water-carrying. There were at least twelve banana peels on the floor by his bed, surrounding an empty milk bottle. "Whatcha stuffin' for?" I asked.

"Coach says if I can gain twenty-five pounds by year after next I can play," he said. "This is the quickest way."

"If you don't throw it all up. Jem," I said, "I wanta ask you somethin'."

"Shoot." He put down his book and stretched his legs.

"Miss Gates is a nice lady, ain't she?"

"Why sure," said Jem. "I liked her when I was in her room."

"She hates Hitler a lot . . ."

"What's wrong with that?"

"Well, she went on today about how bad it was him treatin'

the Jews like that. Jem, it's not right to persecute anybody, is it? I mean have mean thoughts about anybody, even, is it?"

"Gracious no, Scout. What's eatin' you?"

"Well, coming out of the courthouse that night Miss Gates was—she was goin' down the steps in front of us, you musta not seen her—she was talking with Miss Stephanie Crawford. I heard her say it's time somebody taught 'em a lesson, they were gettin' way above themselves, an' the next thing they think they can do is marry us. Jem, how can you hate Hitler so bad an' then turn around and be ugly about folks right at home—"

Jem was suddenly furious. He leaped off the bed, grabbed me by the collar and shook me. "I never wanta hear about that courthouse again, ever, ever, you hear me? You hear me? Don't you ever say one word to me about it again, you hear? Now go on!"

I was too surprised to cry. I crept from Jem's room and shut the door softly, lest undue noise set him off again. Suddenly tired, I wanted Atticus. He was in the livingroom, and I went to him and tried to get in his lap.

Atticus smiled. "You're getting so big now, I'll just have to hold a part of you." He held me close. "Scout," he said softly, "don't let Jem get you down. He's having a rough time these days. I heard you back there."

Atticus said that Jem was trying hard to forget something, but what he was really doing was storing it away for a while, until enough time passed. Then he would be able to think about it and sort things out. When he was able to think about it, Jem would be himself again.

27

Things did settle down, after a fashion, as Atticus said they would. By the middle of October, only two small things out of the ordinary happened to two Maycomb citizens. No, there were three things, and they did not directly concern us—the Finches—but in a way they did.

The first thing was that Mr. Bob Ewell acquired and lost a job in a matter of days and probably made himself unique in the annals of the nineteen-thirties: he was the only man I ever heard of who was fired from the WPA for laziness. I suppose his brief burst of fame brought on a briefer burst of industry, but his job lasted only as long as his notoriety: Mr. Ewell found himself as forgotten as Tom Robinson. Thereafter, he resumed his regular weekly appearances at the welfare office for his check, and received it with no grace amid obscure mutterings that the bastards who thought they ran this town wouldn't permit an honest man to make a living. Ruth Jones, the welfare lady, said Mr. Ewell openly accused Atticus of getting his job. She was upset enough to walk down to Atticus's office and tell him about it. Atticus told Miss Ruth not to fret, that if Bob Ewell wanted to discuss Atticus's "getting" his job, he knew the way to the office.

The second thing happened to Judge Taylor. Judge Taylor was not a Sunday-night churchgoer: Mrs. Taylor was. Judge Taylor savored his Sunday night hour alone in his big house, and churchtime found him holed up in his study reading the writings of Bob Taylor (no kin, but the judge would have been proud to claim it). One Sunday night, lost in fruity metaphors and florid diction, Judge Taylor's attention was wrenched from the page by an irritating scratching noise. "Hush," he said to Ann Taylor, his fat nondescript dog. Then he realized he was speaking to an empty room; the scratching noise was coming from the rear of the house. Judge Taylor clumped to the back porch to let Ann out and found the screen door swinging open. A shadow on the corner of the house caught his eye, and that was all he saw of his visitor. Mrs. Taylor came home from church to find her husband in his chair, lost in the writings of Bob Taylor, with a shotgun across his lap.

The third thing happened to Helen Robinson, Tom's widow. If Mr. Ewell was as forgotten as Tom Robinson, Tom Robinson was as forgotten as Boo Radley. But Tom was not forgotten by his employer, Mr. Link Deas. Mr. Link Deas made a job for Helen. He didn't really need her, but he said he felt right bad about the way things turned out. I never knew who took care of her children while Helen was away. Calpurnia said it was hard on Helen, because she had to walk nearly a mile out of her way to avoid the Ewells, who, according to Helen, "chunked at her" the first time she tried to use the public road. Mr. Link Deas eventually received the impression that Helen was coming to work each morning from the wrong direction, and dragged the reason out of her. "Just let it be, Mr. Link, please suh," Helen begged. "The hell I will," said Mr. Link. He told her to come by his store that afternoon before she left. She did, and Mr. Link closed his store, put his hat firmly on his head, and walked Helen home. He walked her the short way, by the Ewells'. On his way back, Mr. Link stopped at the crazy gate.

"Ewell?" he called. "I say Ewell!"

The windows, normally packed with children, were empty.

"I know every last one of you's in there a-layin' on the floor! Now hear me, Bob Ewell: if I hear one more peep outa my girl Helen about not bein' able to walk this road I'll have you in jail before sundown!" Mr. Link spat in the dust and walked home.

Helen went to work next morning and used the public road. Nobody chunked at her, but when she was a few yards beyond the Ewell house, she looked around and saw Mr. Ewell walking behind her. She turned and walked on, and Mr. Ewell kept the same distance behind her until she reached Mr. Link Deas's house. All the way to the house, Helen said, she heard a soft voice behind her, crooning foul words. Thoroughly frightened, she telephoned Mr. Link at his store, which was not too far from his house. As Mr. Link came out of his store he saw Mr. Ewell leaning on the fence. Mr. Ewell said, "Don't you look at me, Link Deas, like I was dirt. I ain't jumped your—"

"First thing you can do, Ewell, is get your stinkin' carcass off my property. You're leanin' on it an' I can't afford fresh paint for it. Second thing you can do is stay away from my cook or I'll have you up for assault—"

"I ain't touched her, Link Deas, and ain't about to go with no nigger!"

"You don't have to touch her, all you have to do is make her afraid, an' if assault ain't enough to keep you locked up awhile, I'll get you in on the Ladies' Law, so get outa my sight! If you don't think I mean it, just bother that girl again!''

Mr. Ewell evidently thought he meant it, for Helen reported no further trouble.

"I don't like it, Atticus, I don't like it at all," was Aunt Alexandra's assessment of these events. "That man seems to have a permanent running grudge against everybody connected with that case. I know how that kind are about paying off grudges, but I don't understand why he should harbor one—he had his way in court, didn't he?"

"I think I understand," said Atticus. "It might be because he knows in his heart that very few people in Maycomb really believed his and Mayella's yarns. He thought he'd be a hero, but all he got for his pain was . . . was, okay, we'll convict this Negro but get back to your dump. He's had his fling with about everybody now, so he ought to be satisfied. He'll settle down when the weather changes."

"But why should he try to burgle John Taylor's house? He obviously didn't know John was home or he wouldn't've tried. Only lights John shows on Sunday nights are on the front porch and back in his den . . ."

"You don't know if Bob Ewell cut that screen, you don't know who did it," said Atticus. "But I can guess. I proved him a liar but John made him look like a fool. All the time Ewell was on the stand I couldn't dare look at John and keep a straight face. John looked at him as if he were a three-legged chicken or a square egg. Don't tell me judges don't try to prejudice juries," Atticus chuckled.

By the end of October, our lives had become the familiar routine of school, play, study. Jem seemed to have put out of his mind whatever it was he wanted to forget, and our classmates mercifully let us forget our father's eccentricities. Cecil Jacobs asked me one time if Atticus was a Radical. When I asked Atticus, Atticus was so amused I was rather annoyed, but he said he wasn't laughing at me. He said, "You tell Cecil I'm about as radical as Cotton Tom Heflin."

Aunt Alexandra was thriving. Miss Maudie must have silenced the whole missionary society at one blow, for Aunty again ruled that roost. Her refreshments grew even more delicious. I learned more about the poor Mrunas' social life from listening to Mrs. Merriweather: they had so little sense of family that the whole tribe was one big family. A child had as many fathers as there were men in the community, as many mothers as there were women. J. Grimes Everett was doing his utmost to change this state of affairs, and desperately needed our prayers.

Maycomb was itself again. Precisely the same as last year and the year before that, with only two minor changes. Firstly, people had removed from their store windows and automobiles the stickers that said NRA—WE DO OUR PART. I asked Atticus why, and he said it was because the National Recovery Act was dead. I asked who killed it: he said nine old men.

The second change in Maycomb since last year was not one of national significance. Until then, Halloween in Maycomb was a completely unorganized affair. Each child did what he wanted to do, with assistance from other children if there was anything to be moved, such as placing a light buggy on top of the livery stable. But parents thought things went too far last year, when the peace of Miss Tutti and Miss Frutti was shattered.

Misses Tutti and Frutti Barber were maiden ladies, sisters, who lived together in the only Maycomb residence boasting a cellar. The Barber ladies were rumored to be Republicans, having migrated from Clanton, Alabama, in 1911. Their ways were strange to us, and why they wanted a cellar nobody knew, but they wanted one and they dug one, and they spent the rest of their lives chasing generations of children out of it.

Misses Tutti and Frutti (their names were Sarah and Frances), aside from their Yankee ways, were both deaf. Miss Tutti denied it and lived in a world of silence, but Miss Frutti, not about to miss anything, employed an ear trumpet so enormous that Jem declared it was a loudspeaker from one of those dog Victrolas.

With these facts in mind and Halloween at hand, some wicked children had waited until the Misses Barber were thoroughly asleep, slipped into their livingroom (nobody but the Radleys locked up at night), stealthily made away with every stick of furniture therein, and hid it in the cellar. I deny having taken part in such a thing.

"I heard 'em!" was the cry that awoke the Misses Barber's

neighbors at dawn next morning. "Heard 'em drive a truck up to the door! Stomped around like horses. They're in New Orleans by now!"

Miss Tutti was sure those traveling fur sellers who came through town two days ago had purloined their furniture. "Da-rk they were," she said. "Syrians."

Mr. Heck Tate was summoned. He surveyed the area and said he thought it was a local job. Miss Frutti said she'd know a Maycomb voice anywhere, and there were no Maycomb voices in that parlor last night—rolling their r's all over her premises, they were. Nothing less than the bloodhounds must be used to locate their furniture, Miss Tutti insisted, so Mr. Tate was obliged to go ten miles out the road, round up the county hounds, and put them on the trail.

Mr. Tate started them off at the Misses Barber's front steps, but all they did was run around to the back of the house and howl at the cellar door. When Mr. Tate set them in motion three times, he finally guessed the truth. By noontime that day, there was not a barefooted child to be seen in Maycomb and nobody took off his shoes until the hounds were returned.

So the Maycomb ladies said things would be different this year. The high-school auditorium would be open, there would be a pageant for the grown-ups; apple-bobbing, taffy-pulling, pinning the tail on the donkey for the children. There would also be a prize of twenty-five cents for the best Halloween costume, created by the wearer.

Jem and I both groaned. Not that we'd ever done anything, it was the principle of the thing. Jem considered himself too old for Halloween anyway; he said he wouldn't be caught anywhere near the high school at something like that. Oh well, I thought, Atticus would take me.

I soon learned, however, that my services would be required on stage that evening. Mrs. Grace Merriweather had composed an original pageant entitled *Maycomb County: Ad Astra Per Aspera*, and I was to be a ham. She thought it would be adorable if some of the children were costumed to represent the county's agricultural products: Cecil Jacobs would be dressed up to look like a cow; Agnes Boone would make a lovely butterbean, another child would be a peanut, and on down the line until Mrs. Merriweather's imagination and the supply of children were exhausted.

Our only duties, as far as I could gather from our two rehearsals, were to enter from stage left as Mrs. Merriweather (not only the author, but the narrator) identified us. When she called out, "Pork," that was my cue. Then the assembled company would sing, "Maycomb County, Maycomb County, we will aye be true to thee," as the grand finale, and Mrs. Merriweather would mount the stage with the state flag.

My costume was not much of a problem. Mrs. Crenshaw, the local seamstress, had as much imagination as Mrs. Merriweather. Mrs. Crenshaw took some chicken wire and bent it into the shape of a cured ham. This she covered with brown cloth, and painted it to resemble the original. I could duck under and someone would pull the contraption down over my head. It came almost to my knees. Mrs. Crenshaw thoughtfully left two peepholes for me. She did a fine job. Jem said I looked exactly like a ham with legs. There were several discomforts, though: it was hot, it was a close fit; if my nose itched I couldn't scratch, and once inside I could not get out of it alone.

When Halloween came, I assumed that the whole family would be present to watch me perform, but I was disappointed. Atticus said as tactfully as he could that he just didn't think he could stand a pageant tonight, he was all in. He had been in Montgomery for a week and had come home late that afternoon. He thought Jem might escort me if I asked him.

Aunt Alexandra said she just had to get to bed early, she'd been decorating the stage all afternoon and was worn out— she stopped short in the middle of her sentence. She closed her mouth, then opened it to say something, but no words came.

" 's matter, Aunty?" I asked.

"Oh nothing, nothing," she said, "somebody just walked over my grave." She put away from her whatever it was that gave her a pinprick of apprehension, and suggested that I give the family a preview in the livingroom. So Jem squeezed me into my costume, stood at the livingroom door, called out "Po-ork," exactly as Mrs. Merriweather would have done, and I marched in. Atticus and Aunt Alexandra were delighted.

I repeated my part for Calpurnia in the kitchen and she said I was wonderful. I wanted to go across the street to show

Miss Maudie, but Jem said she'd probably be at the pageant anyway.

After that, it didn't matter whether they went or not. Jem said he would take me. Thus began our longest journey together.

28

The weather was unusually warm for the last day of October. We didn't even need jackets. The wind was growing stronger, and Jem said it might be raining before we got home. There was no moon.

The street light on the corner cast sharp shadows on the Radley house. I heard Jem laugh softly. "Bet nobody bothers them tonight," he said. Jem was carrying my ham costume, rather awkwardly, as it was hard to hold. I thought it gallant of him to do so.

"It is a scary place though, ain't it?" I said. "Boo doesn't mean anybody any harm, but I'm right glad you're along."

"You know Atticus wouldn't let you go to the schoolhouse by yourself," Jem said.

"Don't see why, it's just around the corner and across the yard."

"That yard's a mighty long place for little girls to cross at night," Jem teased. "Ain't you scared of haints?"

We laughed. Haints, Hot Steams, incantations, secret signs, had vanished with our years as mist with sunrise. "What was that old thing," Jem said, "Angel bright, life-in-death; get off the road, don't suck my breath."

"Cut it out, now," I said. We were in front of the Radley Place.

Jem said, "Boo must not be at home. Listen."

High above us in the darkness a solitary mocker poured out his repertoire in blissful unawareness of whose tree he sat in, plunging from the shrill kee, kee of the sunflower bird to the irascible qua-ack of a bluejay, to the sad lament of Poor Will, Poor Will, Poor Will.

We turned the corner and I tripped on a root growing in the road. Jem tried to help me, but all he did was drop my costume in the dust. I didn't fall, though, and soon we were on our way again.

We turned off the road and entered the schoolyard. It was pitch black.

"How do you know where we're at, Jem?" I asked, when we had gone a few steps.

"I can tell we're under the big oak because we're passin' through a cool spot. Careful now, and don't fall again."

We had slowed to a cautious gait, and were feeling our way forward so as not to bump into the tree. The tree was a single and ancient oak; two children could not reach around its trunk and touch hands. It was far away from teachers, their spies, and curious neighbors: it was near the Radley lot, but the Radleys were not curious. A small patch of earth beneath its branches was packed hard from many fights and furtive crap games.

The lights in the high school auditorium were blazing in the distance, but they blinded us, if anything. "Don't look ahead, Scout," Jem said. "Look at the ground and you won't fall."

"You should have brought the flashlight, Jem."

"Didn't know it was this dark. Didn't look like it'd be this dark earlier in the evening. So cloudy, that's why. It'll hold off a while, though."

Someone leaped at us.

"God almighty!" Jem yelled.

A circle of light burst in our faces, and Cecil Jacobs jumped in glee behind it. "Ha-a-a, gotcha!" he shrieked. "Thought you'd be comin' along this way!"

"What are you doin' way out here by yourself, boy? Ain't you scared of Boo Radley?"

Cecil had ridden safely to the auditorium with his parents, hadn't seen us, then had ventured down this far because he knew good and well we'd be coming along. He thought Mr. Finch'd be with us, though.

"Shucks, ain't much but around the corner," said Jem.

"Who's scared to go around the corner?" We had to admit that Cecil was pretty good, though. He *had* given us a fright, and he could tell it all over the schoolhouse, that was his privilege.

"Say," I said, "ain't you a cow tonight? Where's your costume?"

"It's up behind the stage," he said. "Mrs. Merriweather says the pageant ain't comin' on for a while. You can put yours back of the stage by mine, Scout, and we can go with the rest of 'em."

This was an excellent idea, Jem thought. He also thought it a good thing that Cecil and I would be together. This way, Jem would be left to go with people his own age.

When we reached the auditorium, the whole town was there except Atticus and the ladies worn out from decorating, and the usual outcasts and shut-ins. Most of the county, it seemed, was there: the hall was teeming with slicked-up country people. The high school building had a wide downstairs hallway; people milled around booths that had been installed along each side.

"Oh Jem. I forgot my money," I sighed, when I saw them.

"Atticus didn't," Jem said. "Here's thirty cents, you can do six things. See you later on."

"Okay," I said, quite content with thirty cents and Cecil. I went with Cecil down to the front of the auditorium, through a door on one side, and backstage. I got rid of my ham costume and departed in a hurry, for Mrs. Merriweather was standing at a lectern in front of the first row of seats making last-minute, frenzied changes in the script.

"How much money you got?" I asked Cecil. Cecil had thirty cents, too, which made us even. We squandered our first nickels on the House of Horrors, which scared us not at all; we entered the black seventh-grade room and were led around by the temporary ghoul in residence and were made to touch several objects alleged to be component parts of a human being. "Here's his eyes," we were told when we touched two peeled grapes on a saucer. "Here's his heart," which felt like raw liver. "These are his innards," and our hands were thrust into a plate of cold spaghetti.

Cecil and I visited several booths. We each bought a sack

of Mrs. Judge Taylor's homemade divinity. I wanted to bob for apples, but Cecil said it wasn't sanitary. His mother said he might catch something from everybody's heads having been in the same tub. "Ain't anything around town now to catch," I protested. But Cecil said his mother said it was unsanitary to eat after folks. I later asked Aunt Alexandra about this, and she said people who held such views were usually climbers.

We were about to purchase a blob of taffy when Mrs. Merriweather's runners appeared and told us to go backstage, it was time to get ready. The auditorium was filling with people; the Maycomb County High School band had assembled in front below the stage; the stage footlights were on and the red velvet curtain rippled and billowed from the scurrying going on behind it.

Backstage, Cecil and I found the narrow hallway teeming with people: adults in homemade three-corner hats, Confederate caps, Spanish-American War hats, and World War helmets. Children dressed as various agricultural enterprises crowded around the one small window.

"Somebody's mashed my costume," I wailed in dismay. Mrs. Merriweather galloped to me, reshaped the chicken wire, and thrust me inside.

"You all right in there, Scout?" asked Cecil. "You sound so far off, like you was on the other side of a hill."

"You don't sound any nearer," I said.

The band played the national anthem, and we heard the audience rise. Then the bass drum sounded. Mrs. Merriweather, stationed behind her lectern beside the band, said: "Maycomb County Ad Astra Per Aspera." The bass drum boomed again. "That means," said Mrs. Merriweather, translating for the rustic elements, "from the mud to the stars." She added, unnecessarily, it seemed to me, "A pageant."

"Reckon they wouldn't know what it was if she didn't tell 'em," whispered Cecil, who was immediately shushed.

"The whole town knows it," I breathed.

"But the country folks've come in," Cecil said.

"Be quiet back there," a man's voice ordered, and we were silent.

The bass drum went boom with every sentence Mrs. Merriweather uttered. She chanted mournfully about Maycomb County being older than the state, that it was a part of the Mississippi and Alabama Territories, that the first white man to set foot in the virgin forests was the Probate Judge's great-grandfather five times removed, who was never heard of again. Then came the fearless Colonel Maycomb, for whom the county was named.

Andrew Jackson appointed him to a position of authority, and Colonel Maycomb's misplaced self-confidence and slender sense of direction brought disaster to all who rode with him in the Creek Indian Wars. Colonel Maycomb persevered in his efforts to make the region safe for democracy, but his first campaign was his last. His orders, relayed to him by a friendly Indian runner, were to move south. After consulting a tree to ascertain from its lichen which way was south, and taking no lip from the subordinates who ventured to correct him, Colonel Maycomb set out on a purposeful journey to rout the enemy and entangled his troops so far northwest in the forest primeval that they were eventually rescued by settlers moving inland.

Mrs. Merriweather gave a thirty-minute description of Colonel Maycomb's exploits. I discovered that if I bent my knees I could tuck them under my costume and more or less sit. I sat down, listened to Mrs. Merriweather's drone and the bass drum's boom and was soon fast asleep.

They said later that Mrs. Merriweather was putting her all into the grand finale, that she had crooned, "Po-ork," with a confidence born of pine trees and butterbeans entering on cue. She waited a few seconds, then called, "Po-ork?" When nothing materialized, she yelled, "Pork!"

I must have heard her in my sleep, or the band playing *Dixie* woke me, but it was when Mrs. Merriweather triumphantly mounted the stage with the state flag that I chose to make my entrance. Chose is incorrect: I thought I'd better catch up with the rest of them.

They told me later that Judge Taylor went out behind the auditorium and stood there slapping his knees so hard Mrs. Taylor brought him a glass of water and one of his pills.

Mrs. Merriweather seemed to have a hit, everybody was cheering so, but she caught me backstage and told me I had ruined her pageant. She made me feel awful, but when Jem came to fetch me he was sympathetic. He said he couldn't see my costume much from where he was sitting. How he could tell I was feeling bad under my costume I don't know, but he said I did all right, I just came in a little late, that was all. Jem was becoming almost as good as Atticus at making you feel right when things went wrong. Almost—not even Jem could make me go through that crowd, and he consented to wait backstage with me until the audience left.

"You wanta take it off, Scout?" he asked.

"Naw, I'll just keep it on," I said. I could hide my mortification under it.

"You all want a ride home?" someone asked.

"No sir, thank you," I heard Jem say. "It's just a little walk."

"Be careful of haints," the voice said. "Better still, tell the haints to be careful of Scout."

"There aren't many folks left now," Jem told me. "Let's go."

We went through the auditorium to the hallway, then down the steps. It was still black dark. The remaining cars were parked on the other side of the building, and their headlights were little help. "If some of 'em were goin' in our direction we could see better," said Jem. "Here Scout, let me hold onto your—hock. You might lose your balance."

"I can see all right."

"Yeah, but you might lose your balance." I felt a slight pressure on my head, and assumed that Jem had grabbed that end of the ham. "You got me?"

"Uh huh."

We began crossing the black schoolyard, straining to see our feet. "Jem," I said, "I forgot my shoes, they're back behind the stage."

"Well let's go get 'em." But as we turned around the auditorium lights went off. "You can get 'em tomorrow," he said.

"But tomorrow's Sunday," I protested, as Jem turned me homeward.

"You can get the Janitor to let you in . . . Scout?"

"Hm?"

"Nothing."

Jem hadn't started that in a long time. I wondered what

he was thinking. He'd tell me when he wanted to, probably when we got home. I felt his fingers press the top of my costume, too hard, it seemed. I shook my head. "Jem, you don't hafta—"

"Hush a minute, Scout," he said, pinching me.

We walked along silently. "Minute's up," I said. "Whatcha thinkin' about?" I turned to look at him, but his outline was barely visible.

"Thought I heard something," he said. "Stop a minute."

We stopped.

"Hear anything?" he asked.

"No."

We had not gone five paces before he made me stop again.

"Jem, are you tryin' to scare me? You know I'm too old—"

"Be quiet," he said, and I knew he was not joking.

The night was still. I could hear his breath coming easily beside me. Occasionally there was a sudden breeze that hit my bare legs, but it was all that remained of a promised windy night. This was the stillness before a thunderstorm. We listened.

"Heard an old dog just then," I said.

"It's not that," Jem answered. "I hear it when we're walkin' along, but when we stop I don't hear it."

"You hear my costume rustlin'. Aw, it's just Halloween got you. . . ."

I said it more to convince myself than Jem, for sure enough, as we began walking, I heard what he was talking about. It was not my costume.

"It's just old Cecil," said Jem presently. "He won't get us again. Let's don't let him think we're hurrying."

We slowed to a crawl. I asked Jem how Cecil could follow us in this dark, looked to me like he'd bump into us from behind.

"I can see you, Scout," Jem said.

"How? I can't see you."

"Your fat streaks are showin'. Mrs. Crenshaw painted 'em with some of that shiny stuff so they'd show up under the footlights. I can see you pretty well, an' I expect Cecil can see you well enough to keep his distance."

I would show Cecil that we knew he was behind us and

we were ready for him. "Cecil Jacobs is a big wet he-en!" I yelled suddenly, turning around.

We stopped. There was no acknowledgement save he-en bouncing off the distant schoolhouse wall.

"I'll get him," said Jem. *"He-y!"*

Hay-e-hay-e-hay-ey, answered the schoolhouse wall. It was unlike Cecil to hold out for so long; once he pulled a joke he'd repeat it time and again. We should have been leapt at already. Jem signaled for me to stop again.

He said softly, "Scout, can you take that thing off?"

"I think so, but I ain't got anything on under it much."

"I've got your dress here."

"I can't get it on in the dark."

"Okay," he said, "never mind."

"Jem, are you afraid?"

"No. Think we're almost to the tree now. Few yards from that, an' we'll be to the road. We can see the street light then." Jem was talking in an unhurried, flat toneless voice. I wondered how long he would try to keep the Cecil myth going.

"You reckon we oughta sing, Jem?"

"No. Be real quiet again, Scout."

We had not increased our pace. Jem knew as well as I that it was difficult to walk fast without stumping a toe, tripping on stones, and other inconveniences, and I was barefooted. Maybe it was the wind rustling the trees. But there wasn't any wind and there weren't any trees except the big oak.

Our company shuffled and dragged his feet, as if wearing heavy shoes. Whoever it was wore thick cotton pants; what I thought were trees rustling was the soft swish of cotton on cotton, wheek, wheek, with every step.

I felt the sand go cold under my feet and I knew we were near the big oak. Jem pressed my head. We stopped and listened.

Shuffle-foot had not stopped with us this time. His trousers swished softly and steadily. Then they stopped. He was running, running toward us with no child's steps.

"Run, Scout! Run! Run!" Jem screamed.

I took one giant step and found myself reeling: my arms useless, in the dark, I could not keep my balance.

"Jem, Jem, help me, Jem!"

Something crushed the chicken wire around me. Metal ripped on metal and I fell to the ground and rolled as far as I could, floundering to escape my wire prison. From somewhere near by came scuffling, kicking sounds, sounds of shoes and flesh scraping dirt and roots. Someone rolled against me and I felt Jem. He was up like lightning and pulling me with him but, though my head and shoulders were free, I was so entangled we didn't get very far.

We were nearly to the road when I felt Jem's hand leave me, felt him jerk backwards to the ground. More scuffling, and there came a dull crunching sound and Jem screamed.

I ran in the direction of Jem's scream and sank into a flabby male stomach. Its owner said, "Uff!" and tried to catch my arms, but they were tightly pinioned. His stomach was soft but his arms were like steel. He slowly squeezed the breath out of me. I could not move. Suddenly he was jerked backwards and flung on the ground, almost carrying me with him. I thought, Jem's up.

One's mind works very slowly at times. Stunned, I stood there dumbly. The scuffling noises were dying; someone wheezed and the night was still again.

Still but for a man breathing heavily, breathing heavily and staggering. I thought he went to the tree and leaned against it. He coughed violently, a sobbing, bone-shaking cough.

"Jem?"

There was no answer but the man's heavy breathing.

"Jem?"

Jem didn't answer.

The man began moving around, as if searching for something. I heard him groan and pull something heavy along the ground. It was slowly coming to me that there were now four people under the tree.

"Atticus . . . ?"

The man was walking heavily and unsteadily toward the road.

I went to where I thought he had been and felt frantically along the ground, reaching out with my toes. Presently I touched someone.

"Jem?"

My toes touched trousers, a belt buckle, buttons, something I could not identify, a collar, and a face. A prickly stubble on the face told me it was not Jem's. I smelled stale whiskey.

I made my way along in what I thought was the direction of the road. I was not sure, because I had been turned around so many times. But I found it and looked down to the street light. A man was passing under it. The man was walking with the staccato steps of someone carrying a load too heavy for him. He was going around the corner. He was carrying Jem. Jem's arm was dangling crazily in front of him.

By the time I reached the corner the man was crossing our front yard. Light from our front door framed Atticus for an instant; he ran down the steps, and together, he and the man took Jem inside.

I was at the front door when they were going down the hall. Aunt Alexandra was running to meet me. "Call Dr. Reynolds!" Atticus's voice came sharply from Jem's room. "Where's Scout?"

"Here she is," Aunt Alexandra called, pulling me along with her to the telephone. She tugged at me anxiously. "I'm all right, Aunty," I said, "you better call."

She pulled the receiver from the hook and said, "Eula May, get Dr. Reynolds, quick!"

"Agnes, is your father home? Oh God, where is he? Please tell him to come over here as soon as he comes in. Please, it's urgent!"

There was no need for Aunt Alexandra to identify herself; people in Maycomb knew each other's voices.

Atticus came out of Jem's room. The moment Aunt Alexandra broke the connection, Atticus took the receiver from her. He rattled the hook, then said, "Eula May, get me the sheriff, please."

"Heck? Atticus Finch. Someone's been after my children. Jem's hurt. Between here and the schoolhouse. I can't leave my boy. Run out there for me, please, and see if he's still around. Doubt if you'll find him now, but I'd like to see him if you do. Got to go now. Thanks, Heck."

"Atticus, is Jem dead?"

"No, Scout. Look after her, sister," he called, as he went down the hall.

Aunt Alexandra's fingers trembled as she unwound the crushed fabric and wire from around me. "Are you all right, darling?" she asked over and over as she worked me free.

It was a relief to be out. My arms were beginning to tingle, and they were red with small hexagonal marks. I rubbed them, and they felt better.

"Aunty, is Jem dead?"

"No—no, darling, he's unconscious. We won't know how badly he's hurt until Dr. Reynolds gets here. Jean Louise, what happened?"

"I don't know."

She left it at that. She brought me something to put on, and had I thought about it then, I would have never let her forget it: in her distraction, Aunty brought me my overalls. "Put these on, darling," she said, handing me the garments she most despised.

She rushed back to Jem's room, then came to me in the hall. She patted me vaguely, and went back to Jem's room.

A car stopped in front of the house. I knew Dr. Reynolds's step almost as well as my father's. He had brought Jem and me into the world, had led us through every childhood disease known to man including the time Jem fell out of the treehouse, and he had never lost our friendship. Dr. Reynolds said if we had been boil-prone things would have been different, but we doubted it.

He came in the door and said, "Good Lord." He walked toward me, said, "You're still standing," and changed his course. He knew every room in the house. He also knew that if I was in bad shape, so was Jem.

After ten forevers Dr. Reynolds returned. "Is Jem dead?" I asked.

"Far from it," he said, squatting down to me. "He's got a bump on the head just like yours, and a broken arm. Scout, look that way—no, don't turn your head, roll your eyes. Now look over yonder. He's got a bad break, so far as I can tell now it's in the elbow. Like somebody tried to wring his arm off . . . Now look at me."

"Then he's not dead?"

"No-o!" Dr. Reynolds got to his feet. "We can't do much tonight," he said, "except try to make him as comfortable as we can. We'll have to X-ray his arm—looks like he'll be wearing his arm 'way out by his side for a while. Don't worry, though, he'll be as good as new. Boys his age bounce.''

While he was talking, Dr. Reynolds had been looking keenly at me, lightly fingering the bump that was coming on my forehead. "You don't feel broke anywhere, do you?''

Dr. Reynolds's small joke made me smile. "Then you don't think he's dead, then?''

He put on his hat. "Now I may be wrong, of course, but I think he's very alive. Shows all the symptoms of it. Go have a look at him, and when I come back we'll get together and decide.''

Dr. Reynolds's step was young and brisk. Mr. Heck Tate's was not. His heavy boots punished the porch and he opened the door awkwardly, but he said the same thing Dr. Reynolds said when he came in. "You all right, Scout?'' he added.

"Yes sir, I'm goin' in to see Jem. Atticus'n'them's in there.''

"I'll go with you,'' said Mr. Tate.

Aunt Alexandra had shaded Jem's reading light with a towel, and his room was dim. Jem was lying on his back. There was an ugly mark along one side of his face. His left arm lay out from his body; his elbow was bent slightly, but in the wrong direction. Jem was frowning.

"Jem . . . ?''

Atticus spoke. "He can't hear you, Scout, he's out like a light. He was coming around, but Dr. Reynolds put him out again.''

"Yes sir.'' I retreated. Jem's room was large and square. Aunt Alexandra was sitting in a rocking-chair by the fireplace. The man who brought Jem in was standing in a corner, leaning against the wall. He was some countryman I did not know. He had probably been at the pageant, and was in the vicinity when it happened. He must have heard our screams and come running.

Atticus was standing by Jem's bed.

Mr. Heck Tate stood in the doorway. His hat was in his hand, and a flashlight bulged from his pants pocket. He was in his working clothes.

"Come in, Heck," said Atticus. "Did you find anything? I can't conceive of anyone low-down enough to do a thing like this, but I hope you found him."

Mr. Tate sniffed. He glanced sharply at the man in the corner, nodded to him, then looked around the room—at Jem, at Aunt Alexandra, then at Atticus.

"Sit down, Mr. Finch," he said pleasantly.

Atticus said, "Let's all sit down. Have that chair, Heck. I'll get another one from the livingroom."

Mr. Tate sat in Jem's desk chair. He waited until Atticus returned and settled himself. I wondered why Atticus had not brought a chair for the man in the corner, but Atticus knew the ways of country people far better than I. Some of his rural clients would park their long-eared steeds under the chinaberry trees in the back yard, and Atticus would often keep appointments on the back steps. This one was probably more comfortable where he was.

"Mr. Finch," said Mr. Tate, "tell you what I found. I found a little girl's dress—it's out there in my car. That your dress, Scout?"

"Yes sir, if it's a pink one with smockin'," I said. Mr. Tate was behaving as if he were on the witness stand. He liked to tell things his own way, untrammeled by state or defense, and sometimes it took him a while.

"I found some funny-looking pieces of muddy-colored cloth—"

"That's m'costume, Mr. Tate."

Mr. Tate ran his hands down his thighs. He rubbed his left arm and investigated Jem's mantelpiece, then he seemed to be interested in the fireplace. His fingers sought his long nose.

"What is it, Heck?" said Atticus.

Mr. Tate found his neck and rubbed it. "Bob Ewell's lyin' on the ground under that tree down yonder with a kitchen knife stuck up under his ribs. He's dead, Mr. Finch."

29

Aunt Alexandra got up and reached for the mantelpiece. Mr. Tate rose, but she declined assistance. For once in his life, Atticus's instinctive courtesy failed him: he sat where he was.

Somehow, I could think of nothing but Mr. Bob Ewell saying he'd get Atticus if it took him the rest of his life. Mr. Ewell almost got him, and it was the last thing he did.

"Are you sure?" Atticus said bleakly.

"He's dead all right," said Mr. Tate. "He's good and dead. He won't hurt these children again."

"I didn't mean that." Atticus seemed to be talking in his sleep. His age was beginning to show, his one sign of inner turmoil, the strong line of his jaw melted a little, one became aware of telltale creases forming under his ears, one noticed not his jet-black hair but the gray patches growing at his temples.

"Hadn't we better go to the livingroom?" Aunt Alexandra said at last.

"If you don't mind," said Mr. Tate, "I'd rather us stay in here if it won't hurt Jem any. I want to have a look at his injuries while Scout . . . tells us about it."

"Is it all right if I leave?" she asked. "I'm just one person too many in here. I'll be in my room if you want me, Atticus." Aunt Alexandra went to the door, but she stopped and turned. "Atticus, I had a feeling about this tonight—I—this is my fault," she began. "I should have—"

Mr. Tate held up his hand. "You go ahead, Miss Alexandra, I know it's been a shock to you. And don't you fret yourself about anything—why, if we followed our feelings all the time we'd be like cats chasin' their tails. Miss Scout, see if you can tell us what happened, while it's still fresh in your mind. You think you can? Did you see him following you?"

I went to Atticus and felt his arms go around me. I buried my head in his lap. "We started home. I said Jem, I've forgot m'shoes. Soon's we started back for 'em the lights went out. Jem said I could get 'em tomorrow. . . ."

"Scout, raise up so Mr. Tate can hear you," Atticus said. I crawled into his lap.

"Then Jem said hush a minute. I thought he was thinkin'—he always wants you to hush so he can think—then he said he heard somethin'. We thought it was Cecil."

"Cecil?"

"Cecil Jacobs. He scared us once tonight, an' we thought it was him again. He had on a sheet. They gave a quarter for the best costume, I don't know who won it—"

"Where were you when you thought it was Cecil?"

"Just a little piece from the schoolhouse. I yelled somethin' at him—"

"You yelled, what?"

"Cecil Jacobs is a big fat hen, I think. We didn't hear nothin'—then Jem yelled hello or somethin' loud enough to wake the dead—"

"Just a minute, Scout," said Mr. Tate. "Mr. Finch, did you hear them?"

Atticus said he didn't. He had the radio on. Aunt Alexandra had hers going in her bedroom. He remembered because she told him to turn his down a bit so she could hear hers. Atticus smiled. "I always play a radio too loud."

"I wonder if the neighbors heard anything. . . ." said Mr. Tate.

"I doubt it, Heck. Most of them listen to their radios or go to bed with the chickens. Maudie Atkinson may have been up, but I doubt it."

"Go ahead, Scout," Mr. Tate said.

"Well, after Jem yelled we walked on. Mr. Tate, I was shut up in my costume but I could hear it myself, then. Footsteps, I mean. They walked when we walked and stopped when we stopped. Jem said he could see me because Mrs. Crenshaw put some kind of shiny paint on my costume. I was a ham."

"How's that?" asked Mr. Tate, startled.

Atticus described my role to Mr. Tate, plus the construction of my garment. "You should have seen her when she came in," he said, "it was crushed to a pulp."

Mr. Tate rubbed his chin. "I wondered why he had those marks on him. His sleeves were perforated with little holes. There were one or two little puncture marks on his arms to match the holes. Let me see that thing if you will, sir."

Atticus fetched the remains of my costume. Mr. Tate turned it over and bent it around to get an idea of its former shape. "This thing probably saved her life," he said. "Look."

He pointed with a long forefinger. A shiny clean line stood out on the dull wire. "Bob Ewell meant business," Mr. Tate muttered.

"He was out of his mind," said Atticus.

"Don't like to contradict you, Mr. Finch—wasn't crazy, mean as hell. Low-down skunk with enough liquor in him to make him brave enough to kill children. He'd never have met you face to face."

Atticus shook his head. "I can't conceive of a man who'd—"

"Mr. Finch, there's just some kind of men you have to shoot before you can say hidy to 'em. Even then, they ain't worth the bullet it takes to shoot 'em. Ewell 'as one of 'em."

Atticus said, "I thought he got it all out of him the day he threatened me. Even if he hadn't, I thought he'd come after me."

"He had guts enough to pester a poor colored woman, he had guts enough to pester Judge Taylor when he thought the house was empty, so do you think he'da met you to your face in daylight?" Mr. Tate sighed. "We'd better get on. Scout, you heard him behind you—"

"Yes sir. When we got under the tree—"

"How'd you know you were under the tree, you couldn't see thunder out there."

"I was barefooted, and Jem says the ground's always cooler under a tree."

"We'll have to make him a deputy, go ahead."

"Then all of a sudden somethin' grabbed me an' mashed my costume . . . think I ducked on the ground . . . heard a tusslin' under the tree sort of . . . they were bammin' against the trunk, sounded like. Jem found me and started pullin' me toward the road. Some—Mr. Ewell yanked him down, I reckon. They tussled some more and then there was this funny noise—Jem hollered . . .'' I stopped. That was Jem's arm.

"Anyway, Jem hollered and I didn't hear him any more an' the next thing—Mr. Ewell was tryin' to squeeze me to death, I reckon . . . then somebody yanked Mr. Ewell down. Jem must have got up, I guess. That's all I know . . .''

"And then?" Mr. Tate was looking at me sharply.

"Somebody was staggerin' around and pantin' and—coughing fit to die. I thought it was Jem at first, but it didn't sound like him, so I went lookin' for Jem on the ground. I thought Atticus had come to help us and had got wore out—''

"Who was it?"

"Why there he is, Mr. Tate, he can tell you his name."

As I said it, I half pointed to the man in the corner, but brought my arm down quickly lest Atticus reprimand me for pointing. It was impolite to point.

He was still leaning against the wall. He had been leaning against the wall when I came into the room, his arms folded across his chest. As I pointed he brought his arms down and pressed the palms of his hands against the wall. They were white hands, sickly white hands that had never seen the sun, so white they stood out garishly against the dull cream wall in the dim light of Jem's room.

I looked from his hands to his sand-stained khaki pants; my eyes traveled up his thin frame to his torn denim shirt. His face was as white as his hands, but for a shadow on his jutting chin. His cheeks were thin to hollowness; his mouth was wide; there were shallow, almost delicate indentations at his temples, and his gray eyes were so colorless I thought he was blind. His hair was dead and thin, almost feathery on top of his head.

When I pointed to him his palms slipped slightly, leaving greasy sweat streaks on the wall, and he hooked his thumbs in his belt. A strange small spasm shook him, as if he heard fingernails scrape slate, but as I gazed at him in wonder the tension slowly drained from his face. His lips parted into a timid smile, and our neighbor's image blurred with my sudden tears.

"Hey, Boo," I said.

30

"Mr. Arthur, honey," said Atticus, gently correcting me. "Jean Louise, this is Mr. Arthur Radley. I believe he already knows you."

If Atticus could blandly introduce me to Boo Radley at a time like this, well—that was Atticus.

Boo saw me run instinctively to the bed where Jem was sleeping, for the same shy smile crept across his face. Hot with embarrassment, I tried to cover up by covering Jem up.

"Ah-ah, don't touch him," Atticus said.

Mr. Heck Tate sat looking intently at Boo through his horn-rimmed glasses. He was about to speak when Dr. Reynolds came down the hall.

"Everybody out," he said, as he came in the door. "Evenin', Arthur, didn't notice you the first time I was here."

Dr. Reynolds's voice was as breezy as his step, as though he had said it every evening of his life, an announcement that astounded me even more than being in the same room with Boo Radley. Of course . . . even Boo Radley got sick sometimes, I thought. But on the other hand I wasn't sure.

Dr. Reynolds was carrying a big package wrapped in newspaper. He put it down on Jem's desk and took off his coat. "You're quite satisfied he's alive, now? Tell you how I knew. When I tried to examine him he kicked me. Had to put him out good and proper to touch him. So scat," he said to me.

"Er—" said Atticus, glancing at Boo. "Heck, let's go out on the front porch. There are plenty of chairs out there, and it's still warm enough."

I wondered why Atticus was inviting us to the front porch instead of the livingroom, then I understood. The livingroom lights were awfully strong.

We filed out, first Mr. Tate—Atticus was waiting at the door for him to go ahead of him. Then he changed his mind and followed Mr. Tate.

People have a habit of doing everyday things even under the oddest conditions. I was no exception: "Come along, Mr. Arthur," I heard myself saying, "you don't know the house real well. I'll just take you to the porch, sir."

He looked down at me and nodded.

I led him through the hall and past the livingroom.

"Won't you have a seat, Mr. Arthur? This rocking-chair's nice and comfortable."

My small fantasy about him was alive again: he would be sitting on the porch . . . right pretty spell we're having, isn't it, Mr. Arthur?

Yes, a right pretty spell. Feeling slightly unreal, I led him to the chair farthest from Atticus and Mr. Tate. It was in deep shadow. Boo would feel more comfortable in the dark.

Atticus was sitting in the swing, and Mr. Tate was in a chair next to him. The light from the livingroom windows was strong on them. I sat beside Boo.

"Well, Heck," Atticus was saying, "I guess the thing to do—good Lord, I'm losing my memory . . ." Atticus pushed up his glasses and pressed his fingers to his eyes. "Jem's not quite thirteen . . . no, he's already thirteen—I can't remember. Anyway, it'll come before county court—"

"What will, Mr. Finch?" Mr. Tate uncrossed his legs and leaned forward.

"Of course it was clear-cut self defense, but I'll have to go to the office and hunt up—"

"Mr. Finch, do you think Jem killed Bob Ewell? Do you think that?"

"You heard what Scout said, there's no doubt about it. She said Jem got up and yanked him off her—he probably got hold of Ewell's knife somehow in the dark . . . we'll find out tomorrow."

"Mis-ter Finch, hold on," said Mr. Tate. "Jem never stabbed Bob Ewell."

Atticus was silent for a moment. He looked at Mr. Tate as if he appreciated what he said. But Atticus shook his head.

"Heck, it's mighty kind of you and I know you're doing it from that good heart of yours, but don't start anything like that."

Mr. Tate got up and went to the edge of the porch. He

spat into the shrubbery, then thrust his hands into his hip pockets and faced Atticus. "Like what?" he said.

"I'm sorry if I spoke sharply, Heck," Atticus said simply, "but nobody's hushing this up. I don't live that way."

"Nobody's gonna hush anything up, Mr. Finch."

Mr. Tate's voice was quiet, but his boots were planted so solidly on the porch floorboards it seemed that they grew there. A curious contest, the nature of which eluded me, was developing between my father and the sheriff.

It was Atticus's turn to get up and go to the edge of the porch. He said, "H'rm," and spat dryly into the yard. He put his hands in his pockets and faced Mr. Tate.

"Heck, you haven't said it, but I know what you're thinking. Thank you for it. Jean Louise—" he turned to me. "You said Jem yanked Mr. Ewell off you?"

"Yes sir, that's what I thought . . . I—"

"See there, Heck? Thank you from the bottom of my heart, but I don't want my boy starting out with something like this over his head. Best way to clear the air is to have it all out in the open. Let the county come and bring sandwiches. I don't want him growing up with a whisper about him, I don't want anybody saying, 'Jem Finch . . . his daddy paid a mint to get him out of that.' Sooner we get this over with the better."

"Mr. Finch," Mr. Tate said stolidly, "Bob Ewell fell on his knife. He killed himself."

Atticus walked to the corner of the porch. He looked at the wisteria vine. In his own way, I thought, each was as stubborn as the other. I wondered who would give in first. Atticus's stubbornness was quiet and rarely evident, but in some ways he was as set as the Cunninghams. Mr. Tate's was unschooled and blunt, but it was equal to my father's.

"Heck," Atticus's back was turned. "If this thing's hushed up it'll be a simple denial to Jem of the way I've tried to raise him. Sometimes I think I'm a total failure as a parent, but I'm all they've got. Before Jem looks at anyone else he looks at me, and I've tried to live so I can look squarely back at him . . . if I connived at something like this, frankly I couldn't meet his eye, and the day I can't do that I'll know I've lost him. I don't want to lose him and Scout, because they're all I've got."

"Mr. Finch." Mr. Tate was still planted to the floorboards. "Bob Ewell fell on his knife. I can prove it."

Atticus wheeled around. His hands dug into his pockets. "Heck, can't you even try to see it my way? You've got children of your own, but I'm older than you. When mine are grown I'll be an old man if I'm still around, but right now I'm—if they don't trust me they won't trust anybody. Jem and Scout know what happened. If they hear of me saying downtown something different happened—Heck, I won't have them any more. I can't live one way in town and another way in my home."

Mr. Tate rocked on his heels and said patiently, "He'd flung Jem down, he stumbled over a root under that tree and—look, I can show you."

Mr. Tate reached in his side pocket and withdrew a long switchblade knife. As he did so, Dr. Reynolds came to the door. "The son—deceased's under that tree, doctor, just inside the schoolyard. Got a flashlight? Better have this one."

"I can ease around and turn my car lights on," said Dr. Reynolds, but he took Mr. Tate's flashlight. "Jem's all right. He won't wake up tonight, I hope, so don't worry. That the knife that killed him, Heck?"

"No sir, still in him. Looked like a kitchen knife from the handle. Ken oughta be there with the hearse by now, doctor, 'night."

Mr. Tate flicked open the knife. "It was like this," he said. He held the knife and pretended to stumble; as he leaned forward his left arm went down in front of him. "See there? Stabbed himself through that soft stuff between his ribs. His whole weight drove it in."

Mr. Tate closed the knife and jammed it back in his pocket. "Scout is eight years old," he said. "She was too scared to know exactly what went on."

"You'd be surprised," Atticus said grimly.

"I'm not sayin' she made it up, I'm sayin' she was too scared to know exactly what happened. It was mighty dark out there, black as ink. 'd take somebody mighty used to the dark to make a competent witness . . ."

"I won't have it," Atticus said softly.

"God damn it, I'm not thinking of Jem!"

Mr. Tate's boot hit the floorboards so hard the lights in

Miss Maudie's bedroom went on. Miss Stephanie Crawford's lights went on. Atticus and Mr. Tate looked across the street, then at each other. They waited.

When Mr. Tate spoke again his voice was barely audible. "Mr. Finch, I hate to fight you when you're like this. You've been under a strain tonight no man should ever have to go through. Why you ain't in the bed from it I don't know, but I do know that for once you haven't been able to put two and two together, and we've got to settle this tonight because tomorrow'll be too late. Bob Ewell's got a kitchen knife in his craw."

Mr. Tate added that Atticus wasn't going to stand there and maintain that any boy Jem's size with a busted arm had fight enough left in him to tackle and kill a grown man in the pitch dark.

"Heck," said Atticus abruptly, "that was a switchblade you were waving. Where'd you get it?"

"Took it off a drunk man," Mr. Tate answered coolly.

I was trying to remember. Mr. Ewell was on me . . . then he went down. . . . Jem must have gotten up. At least I thought . . .

"Heck?"

"I said I took it off a drunk man downtown tonight. Ewell probably found that kitchen knife in the dump somewhere. Honed it down and bided his time . . . just bided his time."

Atticus made his way to the swing and sat down. His hands dangled limply between his knees. He was looking at the floor. He had moved with the same slowness that night in front of the jail, when I thought it took him forever to fold his newspaper and toss it in his chair.

Mr. Tate clumped softly around the porch. "It ain't your decision, Mr. Finch, it's all mine. It's my decision and my responsibility. For once, if you don't see it my way, there's not much you can do about it. If you wanta try, I'll call you a liar to your face. Your boy never stabbed Bob Ewell," he said slowly, "didn't come near a mile of it and now you know it. All he wanted to do was get him and his sister safely home."

Mr. Tate stopped pacing. He stopped in front of Atticus, and his back was to us. "I'm not a very good man, sir, but I am sheriff of Maycomb County. Lived in this town all my life an' I'm goin' on forty-three years old. Know everything that's happened here since before I was born. There's a black boy dead for no reason, and the man responsible for it's dead. Let the dead bury the dead this time, Mr. Finch. Let the dead bury the dead.''

Mr. Tate went to the swing and picked up his hat. It was lying beside Atticus. Mr. Tate pushed back his hair and put his hat on.

"I never heard tell that it's against the law for a citizen to do his utmost to prevent a crime from being committed, which is exactly what he did, but maybe you'll say it's my duty to tell the town all about it and not hush it up. Know what'd happen then? All the ladies in Maycomb includin' my wife'd be knocking on his door bringing angel food cakes. To my way of thinkin', Mr. Finch, taking the one man who's done you and this town a great service an' draggin' him with his shy ways into the limelight—to me, that's a sin. It's a sin and I'm not about to have it on my head. If it was any other man it'd be different. But not this man, Mr. Finch."

Mr. Tate was trying to dig a hole in the floor with the toe of his boot. He pulled his nose, then he massaged his left arm. "I may not be much, Mr. Finch, but I'm still sheriff of Maycomb County and Bob Ewell fell on his knife. Good night, sir."

Mr. Tate stamped off the porch and strode across the front yard. His car door slammed and he drove away.

Atticus sat looking at the floor for a long time. Finally he raised his head. "Scout," he said, "Mr. Ewell fell on his knife. Can you possibly understand?"

Atticus looked like he needed cheering up. I ran to him and hugged him and kissed him with all my might. "Yes sir, I understand," I reassured him. "Mr. Tate was right."

Atticus disengaged himself and looked at me. "What do you mean?"

"Well, it'd be sort of like shootin' a mockingbird, wouldn't it?"

Atticus put his face in my hair and rubbed it. When he got up and walked across the porch into the shadows, his youthful step had returned. Before he went inside the house, he stopped in front of Boo Radley. "Thank you for my children, Arthur," he said.

31

When Boo Radley shuffled to his feet, light from the living-room windows glistened on his forehead. Every move he made was uncertain, as if he were not sure his hands and feet could make proper contact with the things he touched. He coughed his dreadful raling cough, and was so shaken he had to sit down again. His hand searched for his hip pocket, and he pulled out a handkerchief. He coughed into it, then wiped his forehead.

Having been so accustomed to his absence, I found it incredible that he had been sitting beside me all this time, present. He had not made a sound.

Once more, he got to his feet. He turned to me and nodded toward the front door.

"You'd like to say good night to Jem, wouldn't you, Mr. Arthur? Come right in."

I led him down the hall. Aunt Alexandra was sitting by Jem's bed. "Come in, Arthur," she said. "He's still asleep. Dr. Reynolds gave him a heavy sedative. Jean Louise, is your father in the livingroom?"

"Yes ma'am, I think so."

"I'll just go speak to him a minute. Dr. Reynolds left some . . ." her voice trailed away.

Boo had drifted to a corner of the room, where he stood with his chin up, peering from a distance at Jem. I took him by the hand, a hand surprisingly warm for its whiteness. I tugged him a little, and he allowed me to lead him to Jem's bed.

Dr. Reynolds had made a tent-like arrangement over Jem's arm, to keep the cover off, I guess, and Boo leaned forward and looked over it. An expression of timid curiosity was on his face, as though he had never seen a boy before. His mouth was slightly open, and he looked at Jem from head to foot. Boo's hand came up, but he let it drop to his side.

"You can pet him, Mr. Arthur, he's asleep. You couldn't if he was awake, though, he wouldn't let you . . ." I found myself explaining. "Go ahead."

Boo's hand hovered over Jem's head.

"Go on, sir, he's asleep."

His hand came down lightly on Jem's hair.

I was beginning to learn his body English. His hand tightened on mine and he indicated that he wanted to leave.

I led him to the front porch, where his uneasy steps halted. He was still holding my hand and he gave no sign of letting me go.

"Will you take me home?"

He almost whispered it, in the voice of a child afraid of the dark.

I put my foot on the top step and stopped. I would lead him through our house, but I would never lead him home.

"Mr. Arthur, bend your arm down here, like that. That's right, sir."

I slipped my hand into the crook of his arm.

He had to stoop a little to accommodate me, but if Miss Stephanie Crawford was watching from her upstairs window, she would see Arthur Radley escorting me down the sidewalk, as any gentleman would do.

We came to the street light on the corner, and I wondered how many times Dill had stood there hugging the fat pole, watching, waiting, hoping. I wondered how many times Jem and I had made this journey, but I entered the Radley front gate for the second time in my life. Boo and I walked up the steps to the porch. His fingers found the front doorknob. He gently released my hand, opened the door, went inside, and shut the door behind him. I never saw him again.

Neighbors bring food with death and flowers with sickness and little things in between. Boo was our neighbor. He gave us two soap dolls, a broken watch and chain, a pair of good-luck pennies, and our lives. But neighbors give in return. We never put back into the tree what we took out of it: we had given him nothing, and it made me sad.

I turned to go home. Street lights winked down the street all the way to town. I had never seen our neighborhood from this angle. There were Miss Maudie's, Miss Stephanie's—there was our house, I could see the porch swing—Miss

Rachel's house was beyond us, plainly visible. I could even see Mrs. Dubose's.

I looked behind me. To the left of the brown door was a long shuttered window. I walked to it, stood in front of it, and turned around. In daylight, I thought, you could see to the postoffice corner.

Daylight . . . in my mind, the night faded. It was daytime and the neighborhood was busy. Miss Stephanie Crawford crossed the street to tell the latest to Miss Rachel. Miss Maudie bent over her azaleas. It was summertime, and two children scampered down the sidewalk toward a man approaching in the distance. The man waved, and the children raced each other to him.

It was still summertime, and the children came closer. A boy trudged down the sidewalk dragging a fishingpole behind him. A man stood waiting with his hands on his hips. Summertime, and his children played in the front yard with their friend, enacting a strange little drama of their own invention.

It was fall, and his children fought on the sidewalk in front of Mrs. Dubose's. The boy helped his sister to her feet, and they made their way home. Fall, and his children trotted to and fro around the corner, the day's woes and triumphs on their faces. They stopped at an oak tree, delighted, puzzled, apprehensive.

Winter, and his children shivered at the front gate, silhouetted against a blazing house. Winter, and a man walked into the street, dropped his glasses, and shot a dog.

Summer, and he watched his children's heart break. Autumn again, and Boo's children needed him.

Atticus was right. One time he said you never really know a man until you stand in his shoes and walk around in them. Just standing on the Radley porch was enough.

The street lights were fuzzy from the fine rain that was falling. As I made my way home, I felt very old, but when I looked at the tip of my nose I could see fine misty beads, but looking cross-eyed made me dizzy so I quit. As I made my way home, I thought what a thing to tell Jem tomorrow. He'd be so mad he missed it he wouldn't speak to me for days. As I made my way home, I thought Jem and I would get grown but there wasn't much else left for us to learn, except possibly algebra.

I ran up the steps and into the house. Aunt Alexandra had gone to bed, and Atticus's room was dark. I would see if Jem might be reviving. Atticus was in Jem's room, sitting by his bed. He was reading a book.

"Is Jem awake yet?"

"Sleeping peacefully. He won't be awake until morning."

"Oh. Are you sittin' up with him?"

"Just for an hour or so. Go to bed, Scout. You've had a long day."

"Well, I think I'll stay with you for a while."

"Suit yourself," said Atticus. It must have been after midnight, and I was puzzled by his amiable acquiescence. He was shrewder than I, however: the moment I sat down I began to feel sleepy.

"Whatcha readin'?" I asked.

Atticus turned the book over. "Something of Jem's. Called *The Gray Ghost*."

I was suddenly awake. "Why'd you get that one?"

"Honey, I don't know. Just picked it up. One of the few things I haven't read," he said pointedly.

"Read it out loud, please, Atticus. It's real scary."

"No," he said. "You've had enough scaring for a while. This is too—"

"Atticus, I wasn't scared."

He raised his eyebrows, and I protested: "Leastways not till I started telling Mr. Tate about it. Jem wasn't scared. Asked him and he said he wasn't. Besides, nothin's real scary except in books."

Atticus opened his mouth to say something, but shut it again. He took his thumb from the middle of the book and turned back to the first page. I moved over and leaned my head against his knee. "H'rm," he said. "*The Gray Ghost*, by Seckatary Hawkins. Chapter One . . ."

I willed myself to stay awake, but the rain was so soft and the room was so warm and his voice was so deep and his knee was so snug that I slept.

Seconds later, it seemed, his shoe was gently nudging my ribs. He lifted me to my feet and walked me to my room. "Heard every word you said," I muttered. ". . . wasn't sleep at all, 's about a ship an' Three-Fingered Fred 'n' Stoner's Boy. . . ."

He unhooked my overalls, leaned me against him, and pulled them off. He held me up with one hand and reached for my pajamas with the other.

"Yeah, an' they all thought it was Stoner's Boy messin' up their clubhouse an' throwin' ink all over it an' . . ."

He guided me to the bed and sat me down. He lifted my legs and put me under the cover.

"An' they chased him 'n' never could catch him 'cause they didn't know what he looked like, an' Atticus, when they finally saw him, why he hadn't done any of those things . . . Atticus, he was real nice. . . ."

His hands were under my chin, pulling up the cover, tucking it around me.

"Most people are, Scout, when you finally see them."

He turned out the light and went into Jem's room. He would be there all night, and he would be there when Jem waked up in the morning.

New York Herald Tribune: "Tender and searing . . . splendid."

Chicago Tribune: "Of rare excellence . . . a novel of strong contemporary national significance."

Time Magazine: "Tactile brilliance . . . has an edge that cuts through cant . . . astonishing."

St. Louis Post Dispatch: "Exciting and surprising climax . . ."

Saturday Review Syndicate: "Stands alone as the best first novel of the year . . . rare, refreshing."

Los Angeles Times: "Memorable . . . vivid . . . a gentle, persuasive humor and a glowing goodness."

Life Magazine: "Remarkable triumph . . . Miss Lee writes with a wry compassion that makes her novel soar."

Minneapolis Tribune: "The reader will find an immense satisfaction . . . and a desire, on finishing it, to start again on page one."

Unequaled praise from everywhere for a unique bestseller—

Harper Lee's

TO KILL A MOCKINGBIRD

★

The New York Times: "Marvelous . . . Miss Lee's original characters are people to cherish in this winning first novel."

Harper's Magazine: "A novel of great sweetness, humor, compassion, and of mystery carefully sustained."

Boston Herald: "Has pace and power . . . overflowing with life."

The New Yorker: "Skilled, unpretentious and totally ingenuous . . . tough, melodramatic, acute, funny."

San Francisco Examiner: "Miss Lee wonderfully builds the tranquil atmosphere of her Southern town, and as adroitly causes it to erupt a shocking lava of emotions."

(continued on next page)